PHARMACOTHERAPY IN CHRONIC OBSTRUCTIVE PULMONARY DISEASE

LUNG BIOLOGY IN HEALTH AND DISEASE

Executive Editor

Claude Lenfant
Director, National Heart, Lung, and Blood Institute
National Institutes of Health
Bethesda, Maryland

1. Immunologic and Infectious Reactions in the Lung, *edited by C. H. Kirkpatrick and H. Y. Reynolds*
2. The Biochemical Basis of Pulmonary Function, *edited by R. G. Crystal*
3. Bioengineering Aspects of the Lung, *edited by J. B. West*
4. Metabolic Functions of the Lung, *edited by Y. S. Bakhle and J. R. Vane*
5. Respiratory Defense Mechanisms (in two parts), *edited by J. D. Brain, D. F. Proctor, and L. M. Reid*
6. Development of the Lung, *edited by W. A. Hodson*
7. Lung Water and Solute Exchange, *edited by N. C. Staub*
8. Extrapulmonary Manifestations of Respiratory Disease, *edited by E. D. Robin*
9. Chronic Obstructive Pulmonary Disease, *edited by T. L. Petty*
10. Pathogenesis and Therapy of Lung Cancer, *edited by C. C. Harris*
11. Genetic Determinants of Pulmonary Disease, *edited by S. D. Litwin*
12. The Lung in the Transition Between Health and Disease, *edited by P. T. Macklem and S. Permutt*
13. Evolution of Respiratory Processes: A Comparative Approach, *edited by S. C. Wood and C. Lenfant*
14. Pulmonary Vascular Diseases, *edited by K. M. Moser*
15. Physiology and Pharmacology of the Airways, *edited by J. A. Nadel*
16. Diagnostic Techniques in Pulmonary Disease (in two parts), *edited by M. A. Sackner*
17. Regulation of Breathing (in two parts), *edited by T. F. Hornbein*
18. Occupational Lung Diseases: Research Approaches and Methods, *edited by H. Weill and M. Turner-Warwick*
19. Immunopharmacology of the Lung, *edited by H. H. Newball*
20. Sarcoidosis and Other Granulomatous Diseases of the Lung, *edited by B. L. Fanburg*
21. Sleep and Breathing, *edited by N. A. Saunders and C. E. Sullivan*
22. *Pneumocystis carinii* Pneumonia: Pathogenesis, Diagnosis, and Treatment, *edited by L. S. Young*
23. Pulmonary Nuclear Medicine: Techniques in Diagnosis of Lung Disease, *edited by H. L. Atkins*
24. Acute Respiratory Failure, *edited by W. M. Zapol and K. J. Falke*
25. Gas Mixing and Distribution in the Lung, *edited by L. A. Engel and M. Paiva*

26. High-Frequency Ventilation in Intensive Care and During Surgery, *edited by G. Carlon and W. S. Howland*
27. Pulmonary Development: Transition from Intrauterine to Extrauterine Life, *edited by G. H. Nelson*
28. Chronic Obstructive Pulmonary Disease: Second Edition, *edited by T. L. Petty*
29. The Thorax (in two parts), *edited by C. Roussos and P. T. Macklem*
30. The Pleura in Health and Disease, *edited by J. Chrétien, J. Bignon, and A. Hirsch*
31. Drug Therapy for Asthma: Research and Clinical Practice, *edited by J. W. Jenne and S. Murphy*
32. Pulmonary Endothelium in Health and Disease, *edited by U. S. Ryan*
33. The Airways: Neural Control in Health and Disease, *edited by M. A. Kaliner and P. J. Barnes*
34. Pathophysiology and Treatment of Inhalation Injuries, *edited by J. Loke*
35. Respiratory Function of the Upper Airway, *edited by O. P. Mathew and G. Sant'Ambrogio*
36. Chronic Obstructive Pulmonary Disease: A Behavioral Perspective, *edited by A. J. McSweeny and I. Grant*
37. Biology of Lung Cancer: Diagnosis and Treatment, *edited by S. T. Rosen, J. L. Mulshine, F. Cuttitta, and P. G. Abrams*
38. Pulmonary Vascular Physiology and Pathophysiology, *edited by E. K. Weir and J. T. Reeves*
39. Comparative Pulmonary Physiology: Current Concepts, *edited by S. C. Wood*
40. Respiratory Physiology: An Analytical Approach, *edited by H. K. Chang and M. Paiva*
41. Lung Cell Biology, *edited by D. Massaro*
42. Heart–Lung Interactions in Health and Disease, *edited by S. M. Scharf and S. S. Cassidy*
43. Clinical Epidemiology of Chronic Obstructive Pulmonary Disease, *edited by M. J. Hensley and N. A. Saunders*
44. Surgical Pathology of Lung Neoplasms, *edited by A. M. Marchevsky*
45. The Lung in Rheumatic Diseases, *edited by G. W. Cannon and G. A. Zimmerman*
46. Diagnostic Imaging of the Lung, *edited by C. E. Putman*
47. Models of Lung Disease: Microscopy and Structural Methods, *edited by J. Gil*
48. Electron Microscopy of the Lung, *edited by D. E. Schraufnagel*
49. Asthma: Its Pathology and Treatment, *edited by M. A. Kaliner, P. J. Barnes, and C. G. A. Persson*
50. Acute Respiratory Failure: Second Edition, *edited by W. M. Zapol and F. Lemaire*
51. Lung Disease in the Tropics, *edited by O. P. Sharma*
52. Exercise: Pulmonary Physiology and Pathophysiology, *edited by B. J. Whipp and K. Wasserman*
53. Developmental Neurobiology of Breathing, *edited by G. G. Haddad and J. P. Farber*
54. Mediators of Pulmonary Inflammation, *edited by M. A. Bray and W. H. Anderson*
55. The Airway Epithelium, *edited by S. G. Farmer and D. Hay*

56. Physiological Adaptations in Vertebrates: Respiration, Circulation, and Metabolism, *edited by S. C. Wood, R. E. Weber, A. R. Hargens, and R. W. Millard*
57. The Bronchial Circulation, *edited by J. Butler*
58. Lung Cancer Differentiation: Implications for Diagnosis and Treatment, *edited by S. D. Bernal and P. J. Hesketh*
59. Pulmonary Complications of Systemic Disease, *edited by J. F. Murray*
60. Lung Vascular Injury: Molecular and Cellular Response, *edited by A. Johnson and T. J. Ferro*
61. Cytokines of the Lung, *edited by J. Kelley*
62. The Mast Cell in Health and Disease, *edited by M. A. Kaliner and D. D. Metcalfe*
63. Pulmonary Disease in the Elderly Patient, *edited by D. A. Mahler*
64. Cystic Fibrosis, *edited by P. B. Davis*
65. Signal Transduction in Lung Cells, *edited by J. S. Brody, D. M. Center, and V. A. Tkachuk*
66. Tuberculosis: A Comprehensive International Approach, *edited by L. B. Reichman and E. S. Hershfield*
67. Pharmacology of the Respiratory Tract: Experimental and Clinical Research, *edited by K. F. Chung and P. J. Barnes*
68. Prevention of Respiratory Diseases, *edited by A. Hirsch, M. Goldberg, J.-P. Martin, and R. Masse*
69. *Pneumocystis carinii* Pneumonia: Second Edition, *edited by P. D. Walzer*
70. Fluid and Solute Transport in the Airspaces of the Lungs, *edited by R. M. Effros and H. K. Chang*
71. Sleep and Breathing: Second Edition, *edited by N. A. Saunders and C. E. Sullivan*
72. Airway Secretion: Physiological Bases for the Control of Mucous Hypersecretion, *edited by T. Takishima and S. Shimura*
73. Sarcoidosis and Other Granulomatous Disorders, *edited by D. G. James*
74. Epidemiology of Lung Cancer, *edited by J. M. Samet*
75. Pulmonary Embolism, *edited by M. Morpurgo*
76. Sports and Exercise Medicine, *edited by S. C. Wood and R. C. Roach*
77. Endotoxin and the Lungs, *edited by K. L. Brigham*
78. The Mesothelial Cell and Mesothelioma, *edited by M.-C. Jaurand and J. Bignon*
79. Regulation of Breathing: Second Edition, *edited by J. A. Dempsey and A. I. Pack*
80. Pulmonary Fibrosis, *edited by S. Hin. Phan and R. S. Thrall*
81. Long-Term Oxygen Therapy: Scientific Basis and Clinical Application, *edited by W. J. O'Donohue, Jr.*
82. Ventral Brainstem Mechanisms and Control of Respiration and Blood Pressure, *edited by C. O. Trouth, R. M. Millis, H. F. Kiwull-Schöne, and M. E. Schläfke*
83. A History of Breathing Physiology, *edited by D. F. Proctor*
84. Surfactant Therapy for Lung Disease, *edited by B. Robertson and H. W. Taeusch*
85. The Thorax: Second Edition, Revised and Expanded (in three parts), *edited by C. Roussos*

86. Severe Asthma: Pathogenesis and Clinical Management, *edited by S. J. Szefler and D. Y. M. Leung*
87. *Mycobacterium avium*–Complex Infection: Progress in Research and Treatment, *edited by J. A. Korvick and C. A. Benson*
88. Alpha 1–Antitrypsin Deficiency: Biology • Pathogenesis • Clinical Manifestations • Therapy, *edited by R. G. Crystal*
89. Adhesion Molecules and the Lung, *edited by P. A. Ward and J. C. Fantone*
90. Respiratory Sensation, *edited by L. Adams and A. Guz*
91. Pulmonary Rehabilitation, *edited by A. P. Fishman*
92. Acute Respiratory Failure in Chronic Obstructive Pulmonary Disease, *edited by J.-P. Derenne, W. A. Whitelaw, and T. Similowski*
93. Environmental Impact on the Airways: From Injury to Repair, *edited by J. Chrétien and D. Dusser*
94. Inhalation Aerosols: Physical and Biological Basis for Therapy, *edited by A. J. Hickey*
95. Tissue Oxygen Deprivation: From Molecular to Integrated Function, *edited by G. G. Haddad and G. Lister*
96. The Genetics of Asthma, *edited by S. B. Liggett and D. A. Meyers*
97. Inhaled Glucocorticoids in Asthma: Mechanisms and Clinical Actions, *edited by R. P. Schleimer, W. W. Busse, and P. M. O'Byrne*
98. Nitric Oxide and the Lung, *edited by W. M. Zapol and K. D. Bloch*
99. Primary Pulmonary Hypertension, *edited by L. J. Rubin and S. Rich*
100. Lung Growth and Development, *edited by J. A. McDonald*
101. Parasitic Lung Diseases, *edited by A. A. F. Mahmoud*
102. Lung Macrophages and Dendritic Cells in Health and Disease, *edited by M. F. Lipscomb and S. W. Russell*
103. Pulmonary and Cardiac Imaging, *edited by C. Chiles and C. E. Putman*
104. Gene Therapy for Diseases of the Lung, *edited by K. L. Brigham*
105. Oxygen, Gene Expression, and Cellular Function, *edited by L. Biadasz Clerch and D. J. Massaro*
106. Beta$_2$-Agonists in Asthma Treatment, *edited by R. Pauwels and P. M. O'Byrne*
107. Inhalation Delivery of Therapeutic Peptides and Proteins, *edited by A. L. Adjei and P. K. Gupta*
108. Asthma in the Elderly, *edited by R. A. Barbee and J. W. Bloom*
109. Treatment of the Hospitalized Cystic Fibrosis Patient, *edited by D. M. Orenstein and R. C. Stern*
110. Asthma and Immunological Diseases in Pregnancy and Early Infancy, *edited by M. Schatz, R. S. Zeiger, and H. N. Claman*
111. Dyspnea, *edited by D. A. Mahler*
112. Proinflammatory and Antiinflammatory Peptides, *edited by S. I. Said*
113. Self-Management of Asthma, *edited by H. Kotses and A. Harver*
114. Eicosanoids, Aspirin, and Asthma, *edited by A. Szczeklik, R. J. Gryglewski, and J. R. Vane*
115. Fatal Asthma, *edited by A. L. Sheffer*
116. Pulmonary Edema, *edited by M. A. Matthay and D. H. Ingbar*
117. Inflammatory Mechanisms in Asthma, *edited by S. T. Holgate and W. W. Busse*
118. Physiological Basis of Ventilatory Support, *edited by J. J. Marini and A. S. Slutsky*

119. Human Immunodeficiency Virus and the Lung, *edited by M. J. Rosen and J. M. Beck*
120. Five-Lipoxygenase Products in Asthma, *edited by J. M. Drazen, S.-E. Dahlén, and T. H. Lee*
121. Complexity in Structure and Function of the Lung, *edited by M. P. Hlastala and H. T. Robertson*
122. Biology of Lung Cancer, *edited by M. A. Kane and P. A. Bunn, Jr.*
123. Rhinitis: Mechanisms and Management, *edited by R. M. Naclerio, S. R. Durham, and N. Mygind*
124. Lung Tumors: Fundamental Biology and Clinical Management, *edited by C. Brambilla and E. Brambilla*
125. Interleukin-5: From Molecule to Drug Target for Asthma, *edited by C. J. Sanderson*
126. Pediatric Asthma, *edited by S. Murphy and H. W. Kelly*
127. Viral Infections of the Respiratory Tract, *edited by R. Dolin and P. F. Wright*
128. Air Pollutants and the Respiratory Tract, *edited by D. L. Swift and W. M. Foster*
129. Gastroesophageal Reflux Disease and Airway Disease, *edited by M. R. Stein*
130. Exercise-Induced Asthma, *edited by E. R. McFadden, Jr.*
131. LAM and Other Diseases Characterized by Smooth Muscle Proliferation, *edited by J. Moss*
132. The Lung at Depth, *edited by C. E. G. Lundgren and J. N. Miller*
133. Regulation of Sleep and Circadian Rhythms, *edited by F. W. Turek and P. C. Zee*
134. Anticholinergic Agents in the Upper and Lower Airways, *edited by S. L. Spector*
135. Control of Breathing in Health and Disease, *edited by M. D. Altose and Y. Kawakami*
136. Immunotherapy in Asthma, *edited by J. Bousquet and H. Yssel*
137. Chronic Lung Disease in Early Infancy, *edited by R. D. Bland and J. J. Coalson*
138. Asthma's Impact on Society: The Social and Economic Burden, *edited by K. B. Weiss, A. S. Buist, and S. D. Sullivan*
139. New and Exploratory Therapeutic Agents for Asthma, *edited by M. Yeadon and Z. Diamant*
140. Multimodality Treatment of Lung Cancer, *edited by A. T. Skarin*
141. Cytokines in Pulmonary Disease: Infection and Inflammation, *edited by S. Nelson and T. R. Martin*
142. Diagnostic Pulmonary Pathology, *edited by P. T. Cagle*
143. Particle–Lung Interactions, *edited by P. Gehr and J. Heyder*
144. Tuberculosis: A Comprehensive International Approach, Second Edition, Revised and Expanded, *edited by L. B. Reichman and E. S. Hershfield*
145. Combination Therapy for Asthma and Chronic Obstructive Pulmonary Disease, *edited by R. J. Martin and M. Kraft*
146. Sleep Apnea: Implications in Cardiovascular and Cerebrovascular Disease, *edited by T. D. Bradley and J. S. Floras*
147. Sleep and Breathing in Children: A Developmental Approach, *edited by G. M. Loughlin, J. L. Carroll, and C. L. Marcus*

148. Pulmonary and Peripheral Gas Exchange in Health and Disease, *edited by J. Roca, R. Rodriguez-Roisen, and P. D. Wagner*
149. Lung Surfactants: Basic Science and Clinical Applications, *R. H. Notter*
150. Nosocomial Pneumonia, *edited by W. R. Jarvis*
151. Fetal Origins of Cardiovascular and Lung Disease, *edited by David J. P. Barker*
152. Long-Term Mechanical Ventilation, *edited by N. S. Hill*
153. Environmental Asthma, *edited by R. K. Bush*
154. Asthma and Respiratory Infections, *edited by D. P. Skoner*
155. Airway Remodeling, *edited by P. H. Howarth, J. W. Wilson, J. Bousquet, S. Rak, and R. A. Pauwels*
156. Genetic Models in Cardiorespiratory Biology, *edited by G. G. Haddad and T. Xu*
157. Respiratory-Circulatory Interactions in Health and Disease, *edited by S. M. Scharf, M. R. Pinsky, and S. Magder*
158. Ventilator Management Strategies for Critical Care, *edited by N. S. Hill and M. M. Levy*
159. Severe Asthma: Pathogenesis and Clinical Management, Second Edition, Revised and Expanded, *edited by S. J. Szefler and D. Y. M. Leung*
160. Gravity and the Lung: Lessons from Microgravity, *edited by G. K. Prisk, M. Paiva, and J. B. West*
161. High Altitude: An Exploration of Human Adaptation, *edited by T. F. Hornbein and R. B. Schoene*
162. Drug Delivery to the Lung, *edited by H. Bisgaard, C. O'Callaghan, and G. C. Smaldone*
163. Inhaled Steroids in Asthma: Optimizing Effects in the Airways, *edited by R. P. Schleimer, P. M. O'Byrne, S. J. Szefler, and R. Brattsand*
164. IgE and Anti-IgE Therapy in Asthma and Allergic Disease, *edited by R. B. Fick, Jr., and P. M. Jardieu*
165. Clinical Management of Chronic Obstructive Pulmonary Disease, *edited by T. Similowski, W. A. Whitelaw, and J.-P. Derenne*
166. Sleep Apnea: Pathogenesis, Diagnosis, and Treatment, *edited by A. I. Pack*
167. Biotherapeutic Approaches to Asthma, *edited by J. Agosti and A. L. Sheffer*
168. Proteoglycans in Lung Disease, *edited by H. G. Garg, P. J. Roughley, and C. A. Hales*
169. Gene Therapy in Lung Disease, *edited by S. M. Albelda*
170. Disease Markers in Exhaled Breath, *edited by N. Marczin, S. A. Kharitonov, M. H. Yacoub, and P. J. Barnes*
171. Sleep-Related Breathing Disorders: Experimental Models and Therapeutic Potential, *edited by D. W. Carley and M. Radulovacki*
172. Chemokines in the Lung, *edited by R. M. Strieter, S. L. Kunkel, and T. J. Standiford*
173. Respiratory Control and Disorders in the Newborn, *edited by O. P. Mathew*
174. The Immunological Basis of Asthma, *edited by B. N. Lambrecht, H. C. Hoogsteden, and Z. Diamant*
175. Oxygen Sensing: Responses and Adaptation to Hypoxia, *edited by S. Lahiri, G. L. Semenza, and N. R. Prabhakar*

176. Non-Neoplastic Advanced Lung Disease, *edited by J. R. Maurer*
177. Therapeutic Targets in Airway Inflammation, *edited by N. T. Eissa and D. P. Huston*
178. Respiratory Infections in Allergy and Asthma, *edited by S. L. Johnston and N. G. Papadopoulos*
179. Acute Respiratory Distress Syndrome, *edited by M. A. Matthay*
180. Venous Thromboembolism, *edited by J. E. Dalen*
181. Upper and Lower Respiratory Disease, *edited by J. Corren, A. Togias, and J. Bousquet*
182. Pharmacotherapy in Chronic Obstructive Pulmonary Disease, *edited by B. R. Celli*
183. Acute Exacerbations of Chronic Obstructive Pulmonary Disease, *edited by N. M. Siafakas, N. R. Anthonisen, and D. Georgopoulos*
184. Lung Volume Reduction Surgery for Emphysema, *edited by H. E. Fessler, J. J. Reilly, Jr., and D. J. Sugarbaker*
185. Idiopathic Pulmonary Fibrosis, *edited by J. P. Lynch III*

ADDITIONAL VOLUMES IN PREPARATION

Therapy for Mucus-Clearance Disorders, *edited by B. K. Rubin and C. P. van der Schans*

Pleural Disease, *edited by D. Bouros*

Interventional Pulmonary Medicine, *edited by J. F. Beamis, P. N. Mathur, and A. C. Mehta*

Oxygen/Nitrogen Radicals: Lung Injury and Disease, *edited by Val Vallyathan*

Lung Development and Regeneration, *edited by D. J. Massaro, G. Massaro, and P. Chambon*

The opinions expressed in these volumes do not necessarily represent the views of the National Institutes of Health.

PHARMACOTHERAPY IN CHRONIC OBSTRUCTIVE PULMONARY DISEASE

Edited by

Bartolome R. Celli

St. Elizabeth's Medical Center
and Tufts University School of Medicine
Boston, Massachusetts, U.S.A.

MARCEL DEKKER, INC. NEW YORK • BASEL

Although great care has been taken to provide accurate and current information, neither the author(s) nor the publisher, nor anyone else associated with this publication, shall be liable for any loss, damage, or liability directly or indirectly caused or alleged to be caused by this book. The material contained herein is not intended to provide specific advice or recommendations for any specific situation.

Trademark notice: Product or corporate names may be trademarks or registered trademarks and are used only for identification and explanation without intent to infringe.

Library of Congress Cataloging-in-Publication Data
A catalog record for this book is available from the Library of Congress.

ISBN: 0-8247-4029-7

This book is printed on acid-free paper.

Headquarters
Marcel Dekker, Inc., 270 Madison Avenue, New York, NY 10016, U.S.A.
tel: 212-696-9000; fax: 212-685-4540

Distribution and Customer Service
Marcel Dekker, Inc., Cimarron Road, Monticello, New York 12701, U.S.A.
tel: 800-228-1160; fax: 845-796-1772

Eastern Hemisphere Distribution
Marcel Dekker AG, Hutgasse 4, Postfach 812, CH-4001 Basel, Switzerland
tel: 41-61-260-6300; fax: 41-61-260-6333

World Wide Web
http://www.dekker.com

The publisher offers discounts on this book when ordered in bulk quantities. For more information, write to Special Sales/Professional Marketing at the headquarters address above.

Current printing (last digit):

10 9 8 7 6 5 4 3 2 1

PRINTED IN THE UNITED STATES OF AMERICA

INTRODUCTION

As we all know, chronic obstructive pulmonary disease (COPD) is not a new phenomenon. However, while it has been recognized for a very long time, it may not have received the public and scientific attention it deserves. Some actually say that COPD has been ignored. This may be an overstatement, but the fact remains that for many decades, progress in the treatment of this chronic lung disease has been stagnant. This has been in great part due to the recognition that one of the main, if not *the* main, risk factors is smoking. Ever since the publication nearly forty years ago of the United States Surgeon General's report on the health effects of smoking, considerable societal and scientific efforts have focused almost exclusively on the elimination of tobacco smoking.

Today these efforts continue at all levels, but in the case of COPD, we are also seeing the beginnings of a surge of behavioral, basic, and clinical research. The goal is to address the disease, as well as its prevention. Examples from other diseases, not the least of which is cardiovascular disease, have successfully demonstrated that a "war" on a disease is more likely to be won by implementing a multifaceted approach, rather than focusing on one aspect—smoking, in the case of COPD. Suffice it to note that, at least in the United States, the death rate from coronary heart disease has decreased more than 50% in thirty years, while the death rate from COPD is increasing at a rate greater than any other chronic disease.

This book is clear evidence of what is happening with COPD in the clinical and research communities. Who would have predicted years ago that a volume on pharmacotherapy of COPD would be published? But, here it is today!

In my view, this volume brings a new—and much needed—focus to approaches to treatment of COPD. Yes, the pharmacotherapy of COPD is now a reality. Clinicians need to know, and to use, the drug armamentarium that is available today. But this book does much more, as it has the capacity to stimulate new approaches to drug development. Ongoing basic research relative to COPD has already opened leads that are being actively pursued. Undoubtedly, it will not be long before we see new classes of drugs going into clinical trials, and then new brands in each class going into the clinic.

The Lung Biology in Health and Disease series of monographs is very fortunate that Dr. Bartolome Celli agreed to edit this volume. His interest in COPD and his passion in caring for the COPD patient are well recognized. He assembled authors who are well known and respected by all. There is no doubt that this volume is the beginning of a new journey from which patients all over the world will benefit.

Claude Lenfant, M.D.
Bethesda, Maryland, U.S.A.

PREFACE

As we enter the first decade of the 21st century, we can be proud of the big achievements in health care that characterized the last one hundred years. The lifespan of a human born in the early 1900s was 48 years; today we believe it is our right to reach our 70s and still contemplate another healthy decade or two. Indeed, vaccinations, water management, antisepsis and antibiotics, and greater understanding of the causes and therapy of many diseases have made longevity the rule rather than the exception. We have witnessed a decrease in the mortality rate from the major causes of death: heart attacks, strokes, and cancer. However, there is a silent killer, which looms menacingly as we begin this new millennium. This disease is chronic obstructive pulmonary disease (COPD), a forgotten chronic illness that has become the fourth major cause of death in the United States, and the world overall, and is projected to be the third most important one in the year 2020.

Unfortunately and undeservingly, COPD has been thought to be progressive and poorly responsive to therapy. This stems primarily from the basic belief that the airflow limitation used to diagnose the disease is largely irreversible. Indeed, if we have defined the disease using a single physiological variable that does not reverse with bronchodilators and we then show that the obstruction does not respond well to therapy, it is no wonder that the general belief is that the disease is progressive and relentless. This has been detrimental in that the general feeling, by patients and their caregivers, has been desperation, frustration, and lack of hope.

The reality is totally different. The last years have seen a dramatic influx of solid studies exploring many forms of therapy that have had great impact on the outcomes of these patients. Indeed, we now know that several forms of therapy improve survival: smoking cessation, oxygen therapy for hypoxemic patients, and lung volume reduction therapy in selected patients with inhomogeneous emphysema do increase survival rates. In addition, pulmonary rehabilitation improves dyspnea, exercise performance, and health status. Within this rich armamentarium, pharmacological therapy is central to the overall management. Indeed, if asked, most of us will think of medication as the first line of therapy for our patients.

This book addresses the major advances that have occurred in the area of pharmacological therapy for COPD over the last decades. It first provides the reader with a review of outcome measurements in order to increase awareness of the fact that airflow limitation, and, for that matter, lung function, as important as they may be, are not the only outcomes that reflect the impact of COPD. Indeed, we have begun to modify the way in which we think of COPD, from one in which the most important effect of any therapy is to modify the obstruction to one in which the therapy is evaluated in terms of its capacity to modify other equally important outcomes. I have often referred to the great advances that have been achieved in the treatment of hypertension, when the focus changed from the treatment of the high value of the blood pressure per se to the effect of the change on other outcomes such as strokes, congestive heart failure, and myocardial infarction. Indeed, the book concentrates not only on the classic physiological outcomes such as the spirometry and static lung volumes but also on the effect of pharmacotherapy on other physiological events, such as dynamic hyperinflation, that have been shown to provide important clues in the pathogenesis of exercise-induced dyspnea. The book also addresses the newer outcomes that have become tools to evaluate the effect of therapy. Indeed, the systematic evaluation of dyspnea and health status in many recent studies has provided a new dimension to our understanding of the management of patients with COPD. Further, the inclusion of exacerbation as an outcome that is crucial to modify has revolutionized how we view the comprehensive therapy of the disease.

The second part of the book centers on the actual effect of the different pharmacological agents on those outcomes. When we look back and see that we have gone from one single agent, theophylline, to several classes of agents, all of which are becoming more selective and potent, we begin to realize our need to better understand their effect and use. Although we all agree that the actual effect of the different medications on the degree of airflow obstruction is relatively modest, its magnitude is not different, percent-wise, from the magnitude of the effect of the antihypertensive agents in high blood pressure. Further, when we appreciate the effect of the different agents on other, more important outcomes, we begin to realize how much we have improved our capacity to help patients suffering from this disease.

In the last chapter I integrate all of the content of the book into one practical synthesis, aimed at the busy practitioner. However, I strongly recommend that the reader progressively enjoy the knowledge that the individual chapters provide. All the contributors are known for their expertise in their field and have made an effort to bring the most recent information to readers.

The evidence presented in this book supports our optimism. It is no longer justified to adopt a negative attitude toward COPD. Fortunately, the great advances we have witnessed pale in comparison with those that will come. The completion of the first two mega-trials—one comparing the effect of tiotropium with placebo on the baseline rate of decline of forced expiratory volume in one second and the other comparing the effect of inhaled fluticasone and salmeterol on survival—will represent a new level of evidence that may become the gold standard. In the meantime, we must make use of what is already a rich body of knowledge to complement the armamentarium currently available to us.

I do not want to close without expressing my gratitude to the contributors who have provided their time and knowledge; to Claude Lenfant, M.D., who had the foresight to begin this now legendary series of books and encouraged me to tackle this project; to the editors at Marcel Dekker, Inc., who know about bringing ideas to print; and to the pharmaceutical industry, which has made possible the testing and production of many agents that are invaluable to our patients. I trust that the future is bright, and that within our lifetime we will begin to see the decline of COPD as a major cause of death and disability.

Bartolome R. Celli

CONTRIBUTORS

Joan Albert Barberà Hospital Clinic, Institut d'Investigacions Biomèdiques August Pi i Sunyer, Universitat de Barcelona, Barcelona, Spain

Peter J. Barnes Imperial College, London, England

Mario Cazzola A. Cardarelli Hospital, Naples, Italy

Bartolome R. Celli St. Elizabeth's Medical Center and Tufts University, Boston, Massachusetts, U.S.A.

Gary T. Ferguson Pulmonary Research Institute of Southeast Michigan, Livonia, and Wayne State University School of Medicine, Detroit, Michigan, U.S.A.

Antoni Ferrer Hospital de Sabadell and Universitat Autònoma de Barcelona, Barcelona, Spain

Mitchell Friedman Tulane University Health Sciences Center, New Orleans, Louisiana, U.S.A.

Jian-Qing He St. Paul's Hospital, Vancouver, British Columbia, Canada

Paul W. Jones St. George's Hospital Medical School, London, England

Ikuma Kasuga St. Paul's Hospital, Vancouver, British Columbia, Canada

Steven Kesten Boehringer Ingelheim Pharmaceuticals, Ridgefield, Connecticut, U.S.A.

Donald A. Mahler Dartmouth Medical School, Lebanon, New Hampshire, U.S.A.

Maria Gabriella Matera Second University of Naples, Naples, Italy

Walter T. McNicholas University College Dublin and St. Vincent's University Hospital, Dublin, Ireland

Denis E. O'Donnell Queen's University, Kingston, Ontario, Canada

Peter D. Paré St. Paul's Hospital, Vancouver, British Columbia, Canada

Romain Pauwels University Hospital, Ghent, Belgium

Stephen I. Rennard University of Nebraska Medical Center, Omaha, Nebraska, U.S.A.

Roberto Rodriguez-Roisin Hospital Clinic, Institut d'Investigacions Biomèdiques August Pi i Sunyer, Universitat de Barcelona, Barcelona, Spain

Katherine A. Webb Queen's University, Kingston, Ontario, Canada

Jadwiga A. Wedzicha St. Bartholomew's Hospital, London, England

Theodore J. Witek Boehringer Ingelheim GmbH, Ingelheim am Rhein, Germany

Noe Zamel University of Toronto, Toronto, Ontario, Canada

Alicia R. ZuWallack Kent County Memorial Hospital, Warwick, and College of Pharmacy, University of Rhode Island, Kingston, Rhode Island, U.S.A.

Richard L. ZuWallack St. Francis Hospital and Medical Center, Hartford, and University of Connecticut School of Medicine, Farmington, Connecticut, U.S.A.

CONTENTS

Part Two MEASURING OUTCOMES

A. Physiology

PHARMACOTHERAPY IN CHRONIC OBSTRUCTIVE PULMONARY DISEASE

1

Providing Evidence of Therapeutic Benefit in Clinical Drug Development

STEVEN KESTEN

Boehringer Ingelheim Pharmaceuticals
Ridgefield, Connecticut, U.S.A.

THEODORE J. WITEK

Boehringer Ingelheim GmbH
Ingelheim am Rhein, Germany

I. Introduction

The primary goal of the clinical development of pharmacological therapeutics is to provide useful agents for clinical practice. As such, sufficient evidence must demonstrate that the efficacy and safety observations characterize a therapeutic window that improves the care of patients. Drug development follows regulations and guidelines in order for authorities to provide an independent review of data on a drug's efficacy and safety and to adequately convey the findings of drug development trials in prescribing information.

Attributes evaluated over the course of clinical development can be useful in determining appropriate therapy for individual patients once a drug is authorized for marketing. In chronic obstructive pulmonary disease (COPD), bronchodilators have been the mainstay of therapy and their development over the last several decades has been based in demonstrating improvements in forced expiratory volume in 1 sec. (FEV_1). In accordance with the Global Initiative for Obstructive Lung Disease (GOLD) [1], clinical development in COPD is now more considerate of additional benefits that respiratory therapeutics may afford, such as dyspnea (and other symptom relief), reduction of exacerbations, and overall health status measures that evaluate a patient's quality of life.

The emergence of these endpoints in appropriate design and execution of clinical trials will assist the practioner in learning more about the potential role that therapeutics may play in a given patient.

II. Regulation in the Development of Drugs

A. Regulation of Prescription Drugs: General Background

In the United States, the federal government's entry into the regulation of drugs began in 1906 with the Federal Pure Food and Drug Act. As its name implies, this law was written to ensure the purity of drugs. The government's regulation of drugs to assure their safety and efficacy, however, followed upon adverse public health events. In 1938 Congress passed the Federal Food, Drug, and Cosmetic Act. The act was to be enforced by the Food and Drug Administration (FDA) and required proof of a drug's safety prior to commercialization. Toxicity studies became a required part of the FDA's approval of a New Drug Application (NDA). The federal law was strengthened by an amendment in 1962 that required proof of a new drug's efficacy for the use intended, in addition to proof of its safety. The amendment also required pharmacological and toxicological studies as a part of the Investigational New Drug (IND) application. The FDA must approve an IND application before a drug is tested in humans in the United States.

B. Drug Development Process

Distinct periods of evaluation for a new drug remain useful in describing the development process. There are generally three phases of clinical research and development. Phase I testing incorporates the preliminary pharmacological evaluation and is usually limited to a small number of volunteers. In these initial tests the safety and tolerance of a drug in humans is evaluated, and the drug's pharmacokinetics and appropriate dosage range are evaluated.

Phase II testing covers controlled, double-blind, clinical trials of the drug in a relatively small number of patients (50–200) over a relatively short period of time (weeks to months). Following a positive assessment of studies, extensive clinical trials are undertaken in Phase III testing. Thousands of patients may participate in Phase III trials, which are often carried out as multicenter trials following the same protocol. If the data from Phase III testing further demonstrate the safety and efficacy of the drug, its sponsor may then submit the documentation of preclinical and clinical trials under a NDA. Following a review by the FDA, the NDA may be approved, or it may need to be amended with additional information before the drug gains approval for marketing.

This traditional phased approach has often been followed as it pertains to respiratory therapeutics. For example, bronchodilator properties of an agent can easily be demonstrated in a relatively small cohort of patients. Establishing dose–response will often involve a greater number of patients in Phase II dose-ranging studies. Thus, one can have a relatively good assurance that a bronchodilator will prove efficacious in bronchodilating in larger Phase III trials. In trials evaluating attributes beyond bronchodilation, however, Phase II "proof of principle" can be more difficult. Endpoints such as the frequency and severity of exacerbations, which may be required for an immune modulator, for example, will require a larger number of patients and a larger evaluation period. Thus, the development of surrogate endpoints of ultimate drug benefit will be beneficial, although the demonstration of clinical efficacy ultimately will be required.

The final period of drug evaluation involves postmarketing surveillance, and is often referred to as Phase IV. Here, a record of adverse reactions to the drug is compiled in order to provide information on its long-term safety in a broad-based population. Additionally, Phase IV studies may be conducted to explore hypothesis on drug attributes that were observed during development or discovered once the drug is marketed. Indications outside the product label require a supplemental application to authorities.

III. Key Considerations in Clinical Program Designs

A. Patient Selection

In clinical practice, the physician sees the entire spectrum of patients with COPD. In clinical development, the goal should be clarified as to whether the development is targeted to a broad population or a specific subset. For example, a bronchodilator would be targeted to a broad population, whereas a ventilatory stimulant would be studied only for those with respiratory failure secondary to COPD. In general, a development program should aim to provide the most applicable and practical information to the prescriber. Nevertheless, certain inclusion and exclusion criteria are necessary to ensure optimal execution and interpretation.

One of the disadvantages of narrowing a study population with exclusion criteria in clinical trials is that the full spectrum of patients is not exposed during development. This, in conjunction with the large exposures following a product introduction, highlights the importance of pharmacovigilance in postmarket safety.

Defining patients for recruitment in COPD clinical trials can rely on general physician diagnosis (along with spirometry, age, and smoking criteria) [3]. Additionally, recruitment may require a historical diagnosis of chronic bronchitis [3], or may characterize patients based on, for example, documenting impaired gas exchange via diffusion capacity measures [4]. In one recent series of bronchodilator trials [4] it was found that 23–24% across treatment groups had chronic bronchitics, 44–49% had pure emphysema, and 27–32% had mixed disease. These distinctions may help particularly if they impact effects of therapy.

B. Endpoints and Sample Size

The endpoints that are selected for evaluation in clinical development are driven by the drug's anticipated attributes and ultimately form the basis for the prescribing information provided to the practioner. In the United States, for example, a drug's stated indication is based on a-priori stated endpoints in, usually, two randomized, well-controlled clinical trials. The sample size of most Phase III trials is driven by the statistical power necessary to demonstrate that an observation is not due to chance. In calculating sample size, however, a key variable is anticipated effect size. For many clinical endpoints, one must make a judgment as to what effect size is likely to have on clinical importance. Thus, studies should consider such clinical implications when establishing sample size.

C. Clinically Important Difference

For many instruments used in COPD research, a threshold for a clinically important difference has been established. This often involves an anchor-based approach in which changes in a specific health outcome are matched to a general scale of well-being [5]. For example, when patients feel overall slightly better based on a graded scale anchored from worse to better, the corresponding score in a health status measure is deemed to be clinically meaningful. With this approach, a score of approximately 4 units is regarded as having a clinically meaningful effect in the St. George's Respiratory Questionnaire (SGRQ), a common health status instrument used to evaluate a COPD patient's quality of life [6,7]. This effect size has been corroborated by a similar approach, but using a clinician's global evaluation [8].

Likewise, instruments to evaluate symptomatic changes also need to have effect size prespecified. In dyspnea evaluations, for example, a change of 1 unit in the validated Transition Dyspnea Index (TDI) focal score was also found to be the minimal clinically important difference [9,10]. The characterization of this change being clinically meaningful is inherent in the instrument's descriptors of scoring. A post-hoc analysis in long-term tiotropium trials dichotomized a cohort as responders based on a 1-unit change and demonstrated that those who improve their breathlessness also use less supplemental albuterol, have improved SGRQ scores, and less frequent exacerbations [9].

D. Validated Instruments

The selection of instruments to evaluate health status and symptoms should be validated to optimize interpretation of results. For example, instruments measuring the same endpoints (e.g., Medical Research Council [MRC] dyspnea versus Baseline Dyspnea Index [BDI]) should correlate to provide concurrent validity. Likewise, one should observe significant associations between independent but related endpoints (i.e., improved lung function and reduced breathlessness) to demonstrate construct validity. Here, correlation coefficients are typically in the low range, indicating that measures are associated but are indeed not measuring the same outcome (Fig. 1). The reader is referred to specific reviews which address this important consideration in instrument selection and data analysis [7,11,12].

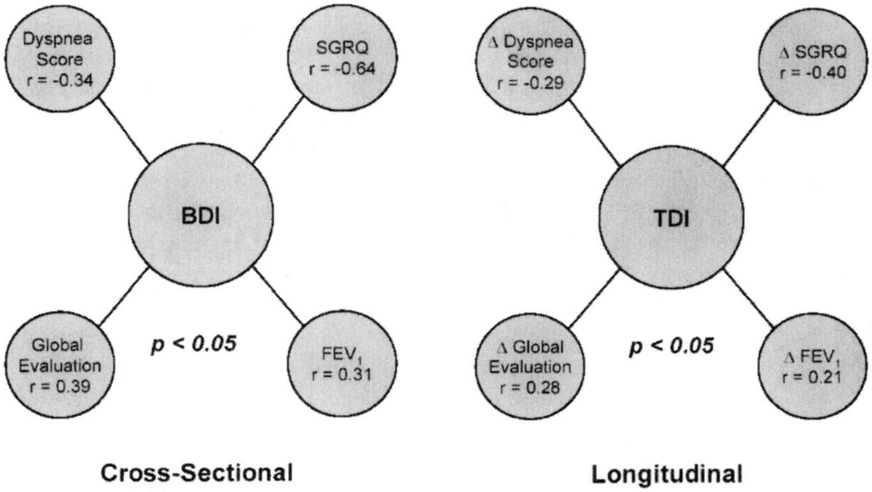

Figure 1 Correlation coefficients for measured outcomes in six month placebo-controlled trials of tiotropium in COPD.

IV. Key Considerations in Endpoints: Application to COPD

COPD serves as a useful example how clinical drug development has assisted in advancing knowledge regarding historic outcomes and in establishing the importance of examining more patient-focused outcomes.

A. FEV_1 as the Historical Gold Standard

Inherent in the development of a pharmaceutical product is proof that benefit exists based on an understanding of its biological mechanism of action and its pharmacokinetic and pharmacodynamic properties. Examples for COPD are that there should be demonstration of smooth muscle relation for bronchodilators and anti-inflammatory properties for corticosteroids. More specifically, for bronchodilators the duration of bronchodilation should be based on in-vitro evidence of prolonged muscle relaxation from agonism or antagonism of associated receptors. Ideally, the pharmacodynamic properties should be based on a biological explanation that is often related to pharmacokinetics. The recent example of tiotropium highlights the point. Tiotropium exhibits kinetic receptor subtype selectivity in which the dissociation from M3 receptors is approximately 35 hr and provides the explanation for prolonged bronchodilation with once-daily dosing [13]. These areas are clearly shown for bronchodilators, whereas the foundation for corticosteroids is somewhat unclear despite evidence of clinical benefit in subpopulations of patients [14].

For COPD, the historic gold standard for pharmacological therapy has been spirometry and, in particular, FEV_1. Most agents approved for use today were based on trials with improvement of FEV_1 as the primary endpoint. The development of bronchodilators will always rely on some clinical demonstration of improvement in FEV_1 in patients with COPD. In fact, the same has been previously true for corticosteroids. Earlier systemic steroid trials simply compared the rapidity of improvement in FEV_1 over relatively short periods in patients presenting with exacerbations of COPD [15]. Such studies led to the widespread acceptance of steroids for exacerbations. Furthermore, long-term trials of inhaled steroids have specified a primary outcome of slowing the accelerated decline in FEV_1; however, this effect has not been demonstrated [14,16].

It is increasingly recognized that FEV_1 is at best a surrogate for many of the goals of COPD management. The previous absence of other means of evaluation has also contributed to reliance in spirometry as the foundation of proof of benefit. Older bronchodilators such as short-acting inhaled β-agonists and anticholinergics gained approval and widespread acceptance with the only evidence being improvements in FEV_1. This approach has benefited patients with COPD, as such drugs are extremely important in management. However, the last decade has been accompanied by the realization that problems exist in how we define spirometric improvements and the limitation of presently accepted concepts on spirometric evaluation. As well, there is increasing acceptance of other clinically important means of evaluating benefit of pharmacological preparations for COPD.

B. Characterization of Reversibility

Accuracy of Diagnosis in COPD Clinical Trials

Acute improvements in lung function following administration of short-acting inhaled bronchodilators have historically been used as a test to distinguish asthma from COPD, based on the misconception that COPD is generally irreversible [17]. The demonstrated therapeutic effectiveness of bronchodilators in the management of COPD from clinical drug development has extended our understanding of the disease process and have shown that a meaningful proportion of COPD patients have a reversible component to their disease and objectively improve following bronchodilator inhalation [18]. The Global Initiative for Chronic Obstructive Pulmonary Disease (GOLD), in their definition of COPD, state: "COPD is a disease state characterized by airflow limitation that is not fully reversible" [1]. Organizations representing the pulmonary community have developed recommended criteria for acute bronchodilator response in adults [19,20]. While these criteria may vary among organizations and have been somewhat controversial, most have recommended that reversibility be based on a predefined percent improvement in FEV_1 relative to the initial predose value. Values of 12–15% improvement from baseline in FEV_1 are typically considered to be significantly greater than what would be expected by chance variation in a nonreversible patient and to represent a meaningful bronchodilator response [19,20].

The American Thoracic Society statement on COPD reports that approximately 30% of patients have an increase of 15% or more in FEV_1 after inhalation of a β-agonist aerosol [18]. However, the reference is based on a study by Anthonisen et al. published in 1986 [21]. There are relevant differences between recently published clinical trials and those reported by Anthonisen et al. with respect to testing agent (isoproterenol versus albuterol or ipratropium) and the duration of washout (6 hr for inhaled bronchodilators in the study by Anthonisen et al.). In addition, it should be pointed out that the 30% value reported referred only to single testing. It is critical to recognize how imprecise it is to permanently label a patient as irreversible or reversible based on a single test.

We reported an analysis based on pulmonary function data obtained during two randomized, multicenter, double-blind, parallel-group, Phase III clinical trials comparing the safety and efficacy of inhaled 40 μg ipratropium and 200 μg salbutamol in combination ($n = 358$) to either agent alone (200 μg salbutamol, $n = 347$; 40 μg ipratropium, $n = 362$) in COPD patients following initial treatment and after 29, 57, and 85 days of therapy [22]. Bronchodilator response rate was analyzed as a 12% and 15% improvement in FEV_1 compared to test-day baseline values. The mean ($\pm$SD) baseline FEV_1 was 0.95 ± 0.41 L (36 ± 14% predicted). Ipratropium and albuterol in combination produced a response in a significantly greater percentage of patients than salbutamol or ipratropium for response defined as either a 12% or 15% increase in FEV_1, evaluated at initial treatment (i.e., day 1) from 15 min to 2 hr postdosing (89%, 81%, and 80% responders for combination, salbutamol, and ipratropium, respectively). Approximately 80% of patients receiving salbutamol alone appeared to be reversible using a 15% criterion. In addition, it was observed that a response on a single test day was not predictive of a similar response on a subsequent test day. For the salbutamol and ipratropium groups, approximately 54% and 63% of patients did not demonstrate a 15% improvement in FEV_1 by the 2-hr time point on all test days. Again, on a given test day, a patient may be considered irreversible.

Several other reported studies have evaluated the reliability and utility of the acute bronchodilator response in patients COPD. In a trial evaluating the reproducibility of the bronchodilator test over 3 years, Anthonisen and colleagues noted that the interindividual and intraindividual acute FEV_1 responses to isoproterenol were considerable and difficult to separate from random variations of FEV_1 [21]. Similarly, Dompeling et al. studied the reproducibility of the bronchodilator response in 183 subjects over 2 years [23]. This publication also noted significant variation not only in the prebronchodilator FEV_1 but also in the peak change from baseline FEV_1. Moreover, Kesten et al. reported that there were no clinically significant differences observed in the acute bronchodilator response between asthma and COPD subjects [24]. In this study, however, they did note significant differences in the baseline FEV_1 between to two diseases. Generally, the results of these studies have shown that the acute bronchodilator response test does not accurately characterize the disease or the response to pharmacotherapy in patients with COPD.

The class of bronchodilator used for response testing has also been examined for reproducibility at different time points and for predicting long-term effects of pharmacotherapy. Rennard et al. published that patients were able to benefit from the long-term use of salmeterol independent of the day 1 responsiveness to the long-acting β_2-agonist, salmeterol [25]. Dorinsky et al. reported that the combination of ipratropium and salbutamol was superior in identifying patients who were bronchodilator-responsive [22].

The aforementioned publications imply that the bronchodilator test is neither predictable for long-term spirometric outcomes with bronchodilator therapy nor clearly differentiating COPD from asthma.

Reversibility in COPD Clinical Trials

A recent publication by Rennard et al. reported the results of a large COPD clinical trial comparing salmeterol, placebo, and ipratropium [25]. Reversibility with standard doses of either salbutamol or ipratropium was assessed. Using the criterion of a minimum increase in FEV_1 of 12% and 200 mL, approximately 59% of patients responded to salbutamol and 44% to ipratropium. A study by Cazzola et al. documented that 200 μg salbutamol resulted in a total of 74% responsive patients within a time frame from 15 min to 2 hr using the criterion of 15% increase in FEV_1 [26]. Braun et al. recorded a response rate of 61% to 200 μg salbutamol and 60% to 40 μg ipratropium within 15 min or 82% and 85%, respectively, at any time during the 6-hr observation period [27]. Measured as FEV_1 $AUC_{0-6\ hr}$, the response to ipratropium was 25% higher, a typical finding in a population with COPD. In the tiotropium 1-year placebo-controlled trials, approximately 72% of patients treated with tiotropium achieved a minimum of 15% improvement in FEV_1 (compared to 24% of the placebo group) [28].

COPD Patients With and Without First-Dose Predefined FEV_1 Increases

Although, the value of reversibility testing is limited, the basic question being asked is whether so-called irreversible patients benefit from treatment with tiotropium. In order to answer the questions, an analysis of efficacy in patients who might be considered "irreversible" was performed. The analysis was based on the 1-year placebo-controlled trial. Patients were retrospectively categorized as having either "reversible" or "irreversible" airflow obstruction upon their initial screening visit based, on the criterion of a minimum improvement in FEV_1 of 12% and 200 mL. Following 1-year of study patients who received tiotropium demonstrated statistically and clinically significant improvement of FEV_1 and FVC compared to placebo regardless of day 1 reversibility measurement. Not unexpectedly, the improvements observed in the irreversible group were less than those seen in the reversible patient population. More important, patients who were deemed either reversible or irreversible on day 1 and treated with tiotropium demonstrated significant improvements in both dyspnea (as measured by the Transition Dyspnea Index), health-related quality of life (as assessed by the St. George's Respiratory Questionnaire), and rescue requirement for short-acting β-agonists compared with placebo [28].

Summary

Baseline bronchodilator responsiveness is neither an appropriate instrument in the diagnosis of COPD nor does it reliably predict responses to long-term treatment. Patients with and without a first-dose acute bronchodilator response benefit from treatment with bronchodilators and may achieve clinically meaningful and highly significant improvements in lung function, dyspnea, and health-related quality of life. Clinical drug development with bronchodilators dispelled the notion of COPD as a "irreversible" disease and led to seeking out other evaluations for the therapeutic effectiveness. Therefore, improvements in spirometry should move beyond acute peak improvements. Options for consideration include improvements seen at the end of the dosing interval and area-under-the-curve calculations incorporating relevant periods of time. As COPD is a chronic disease that affects an individual throughout the day, a single-time-point measurement can be viewed as not adequately profiling benefits. Finally, recent data have highlighted the importance of reductions in hyperinflation and improvements in lung volumes [29]. These changes are also important outcomes to consider beyond FEV_1 in clinical drug development.

C. Differences Between Active Bronchodilators

An argument that can been used to define differences between active drugs is based on available information and existing guidelines. The yearly rate of decline of FEV_1 is between 31 mL (COPD patients, sustained quitters) and 62 mL (continuing smokers) [30]. Therefore, an increase of approximately 50 mL could be considered meaningful, as it corresponds to 1-year loss of lung function status in patients with COPD. Recent regulatory guidelines suggest that the choice of a meaningful difference a "delta of one half or one third of the established superiority of the comparator to placebo, especially if the new agent has safety or compliance advantages" [30]. On average, the response to short-acting bronchodilators such as albuterol and ipratropium over 4 hr posttreatment has been approximately 150 mL in COPD patients. Therefore, in COPD, one-third of the standard bronchodilator response is about 50 mL and can thus be used to differentiate two agents, a value also corresponding to the 1-year average loss of FEV_1.

D. Outcomes Beyond Lung Function

It is well established that a relationship exists between bronchodilation and health outcomes such as dyspnea, exacerbations, and health-related quality of life. However, health outcomes are of such critical importance in COPD that pharmacological treatments that improve dyspnea, exacerbations, and health-related quality of life deserve separate attention noting such benefits. FEV_1 is at best a surrogate marker for what is a key clinical goal of any intervention for COPD, the alleviation of symptoms. Indeed, the Global Initiative for Chronic Obstructive Pulmonary Disease (GOLD) recorded the following goals of effective COPD management [1]:

Prevent disease progression
Relieve symptoms
Improve exercise tolerance
Improve health status
Prevent and treat complications
Prevent and treat exacerbations
Reduce mortality

The importance of spirometry and the relevance of demonstrating as a primary outcome that a bronchodilator does indeed produce improvements in spirometry is critical in the clinical development of such medications. However, development programs for recent bronchodilators have been and are being designed to capture improvements in spirometry, as well as establishing other benefits in COPD, such as improvement in symptoms, exacerbations, and quality of life.

Dyspnea

COPD is characterized by progressive airflow limitation that is only partially reversible. While the disease is diagnosed and often categorized through the objective measurement of airways obstruction (i.e., spirometric values), dyspnea is the most clinically relevant parameter to the patient and the health care provider. As stated by the Global Initiative for Chronic Obstructive Pulmonary Disease (GOLD), "Dyspnea is the reason most patients seek medical attention and is a major cause of disability and anxiety associated with the disease" [1].

Therapies that improve spirometry do not necessarily improve dyspnea. Many instruments evaluating dyspnea exist, and a full description is beyond the scope of this review. The Baseline Dyspnea Index (BDI) and Transition Dyspnea Index (TDI) provide a multidimensional measurement of dyspnea based on the daily living activities of patients, and provide data on the progression of the disease [31]. As previously noted, a change of at least 1 unit in the TDI focal score constitutes the minimal clinically important difference (MCID). Several peer-reviewed publications utilizing the BDI/TDI have highlighted a general lack of improvement in dyspnea with commonly used inhaled bronchodilators despite clinically meaningful improvements in FEV_1

and forced vital capacity (FVC) [25,32]. While mean improvements are useful to examine, they do not quantitate changes in an individual patient. A reasonable approach used to demonstrate benefits is to calculate the proportion of subjects achieving a clinically meaningful change and then the number of patients needed to treat to have one patient achieve the MCID (otherwise referred to as number needed to treat or NNT). In addition, this methodology may also be useful in discriminating differences between active drugs.

Spirometry and dyspnea are not redundant measurements. The measurement of dyspnea is related to but distinct from spirometric evaluations of airflow limitation, and hence inclusion of dyspnea measurements adds additional information to spirometry about this important aspect of the underlying disease. In the 1-year tiotropium placebo-controlled trials the associations of spirometry and BDI/TDI were statistically significant ($p < 0.05$). However, the low correlations observed are consistent with previous reports from other trials and that the endpoints are not measuring the same effect, i.e., they are not redundant [9] (Table 1).

Exacerbations

Exacerbations are an important outcome to patients with COPD and to health care providers. COPD is often associated with periodic worsening of symptoms, commonly referred to as exacerbations. Exacerbations generally manifest as a complex of respiratory symptoms with varying severity and duration. Severe exacerbations require hospitalization and can result in death. Hospitalizations due to exacerbations of COPD, particularly when admission to an intensive care unit is required, are predictive of an earlier mortality from COPD [33,34]. Exacerbation frequency has been associated with worsening quality of life [35], an important clinical outcome that was specified in the report from the Global Initiative for Chronic Obstructive

Table 1 Correlations of BDI and TDI Focal Scores (Pearson Correlation Coefficients) with Spirometry as Observed in 1-Year Double-Blind Clinical Trials of Tiotropium Compared to Placebo

		BDI	TDI
FEV_1	Baseline	0.26	
	Change		0.22
FVC	Baseline	0.21	
	Change		0.22

Pulmonary Disease (GOLD) as follows: "It is well recognized that exacerbations impair patients' quality of life and decrease their health status" [1].

In addition to the clinical consequences, exacerbations represent an enormous economic burden to health care systems. In the United Kingdom in 1996, total costs were estimated at approximated $4 billion, with $0.8 billion being direct costs [36]. In 1993 in the United States, COPD was responsible for approximately $24 billion in direct and indirect costs, with approximately $15 billion attributed to direct costs [36]. The major cost in treatment relates to exacerbations and in particular hospitalization for exacerbations [37].

The number of exacerbation variables that can be evaluated in clinical trial results. They include numbers of exacerbations and hospitalizations due to exacerbations, number of exacerbations and associated hospitalization days, Kaplan-Meier estimates of probability of exacerbation, and log rank tests evaluating the time to COPD exacerbations.

The importance of study design, characterization of the population, appropriate sample sizes, and prespecified definitions should not be underestimated. The ability to discern changes as a result of therapeutic interventions in clinical trials is influenced by the frequency of the event. Infrequent events require large population samples. This can partially be overcome through enrichment of the population. For exacerbations, this might consist of an inclusion criterion of previous history of exacerbations, as exacerbations are predictive of future events [3,5]. There is no universally accepted definition of exacerbations. The sensitivity of the definition can influence the frequency of the event. The frequency of an exacerbation will be higher if it is simply defined by an increase of two doses of a short-acting β-agonist versus a requirement for treatment with systemic steroids (or antibiotics). The definition will influence the interpretation of clinical relevance, as the former definition may be regarded as including two much noise (i.e., high sensitivity, low specificity). Certain trials require a period of prolonged stability, thereby excluding a subpopulation of frequent exacerbators in whom the intervention might be most beneficial. It is not infrequent to find reports noting exacerbations as an outcome without a specific definition of the event. Finally, there may be cultural differences for what is regarded as an exacerbation and, in particular, what is the threshold for hospitalization for exacerbations.

In the GOLD report, it is concluded that "Appropriate treatment and measures to prevent further exacerbations should be implemented as quickly as possible" [1]. Furthermore, the importance of exacerbations is highlighted by the inclusion of "prevent and treat exacerbations" among the goals of effective COPD management. Given the enormous impact of exacerbations from the patient standpoint as outlined and for the health care system, it is important to specify the benefits of new therapies for COPD on exacerbations for the health care provider. The evidence must adhere to rigorous standards in order to appropriately evaluate the outcome of COPD exacerbations.

Health Status

As outlined previously, one of the goals of COPD management is to improve health status (i.e., health-related quality of life). There are widely published and well-validated instruments. Examples of disease-specific instruments include the Chronic Respiratory Questionnaire and the St. George's Respiratory Questionnaire [38,39]. An example of a widely used generic instrument is the Multiple Outcomes Survey Short-Form 36 (SF-36) [40]. The CPMP Points to Consider for COPD recommend the use of quality-of-life assessments and specifically mentions the use of the SGRQ as a quality-of-life instrument. The remarks regarding dyspnea hold true for health status evaluation, particularly as they pertain to clinically meaningful differences.

The instruments have shown responsiveness to pharmacological intervention in COPD, although conflicting outcomes have been noted in the literature with regard to certain pharmacological interventions [14,41,42]. As with dyspnea, it is important to specify what constitutes a meaningful outcome. However, consideration must be give to ceiling effects (i.e., few symptoms or impairments, hence minimal room for improvement) and an adequate duration of study. It is not reasonable to expect immediate changes in health status, as one might see for bronchodilation. The ISOLDE trial indicated that it would be several years before meaningful differences might appear with inhaled steroids. Observations in the tiotropium 1-year clinical trials have shown progressive improvements over time, with suggestion of continued differences against the control over the 1-year period of observation [43,44]. Whereas tiotropium showed improvements over baseline, the ISOLDE trial illustrated that benefits could be quantified as slowing of the rate of deterioration over time. Finally, responder analyses (i.e., proportions of patients achieving clinically meaningful differences) and NNT should be considered in evaluating efficacy.

V. Summary

In order to establish efficacy of a bronchodilator initially, it is critical to specify spirometric outcomes as primary evaluations. While spirometry has indeed become the conventional primary endpoint for bronchodilators, it is nevertheless a surrogate endpoint of patient outcome. A clinical trial program for a new therapeutic intervention can be designed in accordance with the drug's intended attributes and careful selection of instruments and analysis.

In this regard, prespecifying secondary outcomes or conducting additional trials with prespecified unique primary endpoints is an acknowledgment of the importance of moving beyond spirometry in evaluating treatment interventions. The consistency of results in the primary and secondary outcomes across different instruments evaluating different but clinically important aspects of COPD is compelling evidence that a therapy benefits the patient beyond improving standard spirometric indices. Clinical drug development has led to increasing understanding of relevant outcomes and what constitutes clinically meaningful differences in patients with COPD.

References

1. Global Initiative for Chronic Obstructive Lung Disease. Global strategy for the diagnosis, management, and prevention of chronic obstructive pulmonary disease. NHLBI/WHO Workshop Report. National Institutes of Health/National Heart, Lung and Blood Institute, Bethesda, MD, April 2001.
2. Witek TJ, Souhrada JF, Serby CW, Disse B. Tiotropium (Ba679): Pharmacology and early clinical observations. In: Spector SS, ed. Anticholinergic Agents in the Upper and Lower Airways. New York: Marcel Dekker, 1999:137–152.
3. Mahler DA, Wire P, Horstman D, Chang C-N, Yates J, Fischer T, Shah T. Effectiveness of fluticasone propionate and Salmeterol combination delivered via the diskus device in the Treatment of Chronic obstructive pulmonary disease. Am J Respir Crit Care Med 2002; 166:1084–1091.
4. Mahler DA, Donohue JF, Barbee RA, Goldman MD, Gross NJ, Wisniewski ME, Yancey SW, Zakes BA, Rickard KA, Anderson WH. Efficacy of salmeterol xinafoate in the treatment of COPD. Chest 1999; 115:957–965.
5. Samsa G, Edelman D, Rothman ML, Williams GR, Lipscomb J, Matchar D. Determining clinically important differences in health status measures: a general approach with illustration to the health utilities index mark II. Pharmacoeconomics 1999; 15(2):141–155.
6. Jones PW, Quirk FH, Baveystock CM. The St. George Respiratory Questionnaire. Respir Med 1991; 85(suppl B):25–31.
7. Jones PW. Health Status measurement in chronic obstructive pulmonary disease. Thorax 2001; 56:880–887.
8. Jones PW, Witek TJ. Determination of clinically significant effects in health status with St. George's Respiratory Questionnaire (SGRQ). Chest 2001; 120:269S.
9. Witek TJ Jr., Mahler DA. Minimal important difference of the transition dyspnea index in a multinational clinical trial. Eur Respir J 2003; 21:267–272.
10. Witek TJ Jr., Mahler DA. Meaningful effect size and patterns of response of the transition dyspnea index. J Clin Epidemiol 2003; 56:248–255.
11. Jones PW. Interpreting thresholds for a clinically significant change in health status in asthma and COPD. Eur Respir J 2002; 19:398–404.

12. Eakin EG, Sassi-Dambron DE, Ries AC, Kaplan RM. Reliability and validity of dyspnea measures in patients with obstructive lung disease. Int J Behav Med 1995; 2:118–134.
13. Disse B, Speck GA, Rominger KL, Witek TJ, Hammer R. Tiotropium (Spiriva): Mechanistical considerations and clinical profile in obstructive lung disease. Life Sci 1999; 64:457–464.
14. Burge PS, Calverley PMA, Jones PW, et al. Randomised, double-blind, placebo controlled study of fluticasone propionate inpatients with moderate to severe chronic obstructive disease: the ISOLDE trial. Br Med J 2000; 320:1297–1303.
15. Thompson WH, Nielson CP, Carvalho P, et al. Controlled trial of oral prednisone in outpatients with acute COPD exacerbation. Am J Respir Crit Care Med 1996; 154:407–412.
16. The Lung Health Study Research Group. Effect of inhaled triamcinolone on the decline in pulmonary function in chronic obstructive pulmonary disease. N Engl J Med 2000; 343:1902–1909.
17. Weinberger M, Hendeles L, Ahrens. Pharmacologic management of reversible obstructive airways disease. Med Clin N Am 1981; 65:579–613.
18. American Thoracic Society. Standards for the diagnosis and care of patients with chronic obstructive pulmonary disease. Am J Respir Crit Care Med 1995; 152:S77–S120.
19. American Thoracic SocietyLung function testing: selection of reference values and interpretative strategies. Am Rev Respir Dis 1991; 144:1202–1218.
20. Tashkin DP. Measurement and significance of the bronchodilator response: bronchodilation and inhibition of bronchoprovocation. In: Spector SHL, ed. Provocation Testing in Clinical Practice. New York: Marcel Dekker, 1995:512–573.
21. Anthonisen NR, Wright EC. Bronchodilator response in chronic obstructive pulmonary disease. Am Rev Respir Dis 1986; 133:814–819.
22. Dorinsky PM, Reisner C, Ferguson GT, Menjoge SS, Serby CW, Witek TJ. The combination of ipratropium and albuterol optimizes pulmonary function reversibility testing in patients with chronic obstructive pulmonary disease (COPD). Chest 1999; 115:966–971.
23. Dompeling E, van Schayck CP, Molema J, Akkemans R, Folgering H, van Grunsven PM, van Weel C. A comparison of six different ways of expressing the bronchodilating response in asthma and COPD; reproducibility and dependence of prebronchodilator FEV1. Eur Respir J 1992; 5:975–981.
24. Kesten S, Rebuck AS. Is the short-term response to inhaled beta-adrenergic agonist sensitive or specific for distinguishing between asthma and COPD? Chest 1994; 105:1042–1045.
25. Rennard SI, Anderson W, Zu Wallack R, Broughton J, Bailey W, Friedman M, Wisniewski M, Rickard K. Use of a long-acting inhaled beta$_2$-adrenergic agonist, salmeterol xinafoate, in patients with chronic obstructive pulmonary disease. Am J Respir Crit Care Med 2001; 163:1087–1092.
26. Cazzola M, Vinciguerra A, Di Perna F, Matera MG. Early reversibility to salbutamol does not always predict bronchodilation after salmeterol in stable chronic obstructive pulmonary disease. Respir Med 1998; 92:1012–1016.

27. Braun SR, Levy SF, Grossman J. Comparison of ipratropium bromide and albuterol in chronic obstructive pulmonary disease: a three center study. Am J Med 1991; 91:28S–32S.
28. Tashkin D, Kesten S. Long-term treatment benefits with tiotropium COPD patients with and without short-term bronchodilator responses. Chest 2003; 123(5):1441–1449.
29. O'Donnell DE, Lam M, Webb KA. Spirometric correlates of improvement in exercise performance after anticholinergic therapy in chronic obstructive pulmonary disease. Am J Respir Crit Care Med 1999; 160:542–549.
30. Scanlon PD, Connett JE, Waller LA, et al. Smoking cessation and lung function in mild-to-moderate chronic obstructive pulmonary disease. The Lung Health Study. Am J Respir Crit Care Med 2000; 161:381–390.
31. Mahler DA, Harver A. Clinical measurement of dyspnea. In: Mahler DA, ed. Dyspnea. Mt. Kisco, NY: Futura, 1990:75–126.
32. Mahler DA, Donohue JF, Barbee RA, Goldman MD, Gross NJ, Wisniewski ME, et al. Efficacy of salmeterol xinafoate in the treatment of COPD. Chest 1999; 115:957–965.
33. Keistinen T, Tuuponen T, Kivela SL. Survival experience of the population needing hospital treatment for asthma or COPD at age 50–54 years. Respir Med 1998; 92:568–572.
34. Seneff MG, Wagner DP, Wagner RP, Zimmerman JE, Knaus WA. Hospital and 1-year survival of patients admitted to intensive care units with acute exacerbation of chronic obstructive pulmonary disease. JAMA 1995; 274:1852–1857.
35. Seemungal TA, Donaldson GC, Paul EA, Bestall JC, Jeffries DJ, Wedzicha JA. Effect of exacerbation on quality of life in patients with chronic obstructive pulmonary disease. Am J Respir Crit Care Med 1998; 157:1418–1422.
36. Murray CGL, Lopez AD. Evidence-based health policy-lessons from the global burden of disease study. Science 1996; 274:740–743.
37. Friedman M, Witek TJ Jr, Serby CW, et al. Pharmacoeconomic evaluation of a combination of ipratropium plus albuterol compared to ipratropium alone and albuterol alone in chronic obstructive pulmonary disease. Chest 1999; 115: 635–641.
38. Jones PW, Quirk FH, Baveystock CM, Littlejohns P. A self-complete measure of health status for chronic airflow limitation. Am Rev Respir Dis 1992; 145: 1321–1327.
39. Moran LA, Guyatt GH, Norman GR. Establishing the minimal number of items for a responsive, valid, health-related quality of life instrument. J Clin Epidemiol 2001; 54:571–579.
40. Ware JE, Sherbourne CD. The MOS 36-Item Short-Form Health Survey (SF-36). Med Care 1992; 30:473–483.
41. Jones PW, Bosh TK. Quality of life changes in COPD patients treated with salmeterol. Am J Respir Crit Care Med 1997; 155:1283–1289.
42. Rutten-van Molken M, Roos B, Van Noord JA. An empirical comparison of the St George's Respiratory Questionnaire (SGRQ) and the Chronic Respiratory Disease Questionnaire (CRQ) in a clinical trial setting. Thorax 1999; 54: 995–1003.

43. Casaburi R, Mahler DA, Jones PW, Wanner A, San Pedro G, Zu Wallack RL, Menjoge SS, Serby CW, Witek TJ. A long-term evaluation of once-daily inhaled tiotropium in chronic obstructive pulmonary disease. Eur Respir J 2002; 19:217–224.
44. Vincken W, van Noord JA, Greefhorst APM, Bantje ThA, Kesten S, Korducki L, Cornelissen PJG. Improvement in health status in patients with COPD during one year treatment with tiotropium. Eur Respir J 2002; 19:209–216.

2

Use of Expiratory Airflows and Lung Volumes to Assess Outcomes in COPD

GARY T. FERGUSON

Pulmonary Research Institute of Southeast Michigan, Livonia
and Wayne State University School of Medicine
Detroit, Michigan, U.S.A.

I. Introduction

Measures of lung function have been the gold standard against which outcomes in chronic obstructive pulmonary disease (COPD) have been measured [1–3]. Although fault can be found with this concept and rationales provided for using other outcome measures [4], physiology, diagnosis, and many other characteristics of COPD are directly associated with expiratory airflow limitation [5,6]. Thus, the need to measure lung function stands. The purpose of this chapter is to review and evaluate various measures of expiratory airflows and lung volumes and identify their role in evaluating patients with COPD. The relevance of each measure will then be described and used to recommend those measures best suited for evaluating the impact of therapeutic intervention in patients with COPD.

II. Expiratory Airflows

A. Physiology of Expiratory Airflows

Most airflow measurements are performed during maximal forced expiratory efforts in an attempt to identify airflows that are reduced or limited [1,2,7]. In general, airflow through a tube is dependent on pressure driving airflow through a tube and resistance to airflow within a tube. In the lungs, driving pressures and resistances are influenced by multiple confounding variables, which, in turn, are linked to various mechanical properties of the lungs and to the respiratory muscles [1,2].

During quiet breathing, exhalation is normally a passive process. Relaxation of previously active inspiratory muscles results in a less negative pleural pressure (P_{pl}), which at any given elastic recoil pressure of the lung (P_{el}) increases the alveolar pressure ($P_{alv} = P_{pl} + P_{el}$). The pressure gradient between the alveoli and atmosphere (P_{atm}) provides the driving pressure for expiratory airflow. Exhalation continues until P_{alv} falls to that of P_{atm}, either by complete deflation or by the application of an inspiratory effort sufficient to counteract the recoil pressure (P_{el}) at that lung volume. For maximal expiratory airflows to occur, an inspiratory effort sufficient to maximally inflate the lungs is required. Such an inspiratory effort provides maximal driving pressures from the elastic recoil of the lungs and the chest wall. Active expiratory muscle contraction further increases P_{pl}, leading to the greatest driving force ($P_{alv} - P_{atm}$) possible. Thus, when maximal inspiration is followed by a maximal expiratory effort, a maximal airflow is achieved.

As exhalation proceeds, lung volumes fall, elastic recoil lessens, and traction against the airways is reduced. During this time, a gradient of pressure from P_{alv} to P_{atm} occurs along the airway. When forced exhalation occurs, there is a point where the pressure inside the airway is equal to the pleural pressure outside the airway (P_{pl}). This equal pressure point (EPP) shifts along the airway from larger to smaller airways as exhalation progresses. When the EPP reaches more collapsible smaller airways, the airways compress and airway resistance increases. In effect, a Starling resistor is created, such that the difference between P_{alv} and the pressure at the EPP (P_{pl} rather than P_{atm}) becomes the driving pressure. Any additional expiratory effort increases P_{alv} and P_{pl} equally and the difference between the two pressures becomes fixed, equaling the elastic recoil pressure of the lung (P_{el}) at that lung volume. Thus, in the early portions of maximal exhalation at higher lung volumes, expiratory airflows are very "effort-dependent." However, during mid to lower lung volumes, increasing driving pressure no longer changes airflows and they become "effort-independent." If forced expiratory effort is sustained for a sufficient period of time, the most rapid deflation of the lung possible occurs. By measuring airflows and the volumes of air exhaled over specified periods of time, expiratory airflows can be quantified, standardized, and used to analyze the presence and severity of airflow limitation.

B. Measurement Techniques for Expiratory Airflows

Spirometry

Spirometry is a simple test that measures the volume of gas forcefully exhaled from the lungs over time [8]. Sources of error in spirometry have been well described [9], leading to specific recommendations and standards for spirometry [7,10,11]. Essential to this is the use of validated equipment, performance of the test by qualified personnel, and adherence to quality control recommendations [7]. Spirometry is an effort-dependent test that requires a cooperative patient. Specific criteria for start of test, length of test, end of test, and reproducibility of efforts validate test results. Appropriate environmental corrections for local temperature and barometric pressure are also required. Several studies provide reference values based on age, sex, height, and weight for the various airflow values derived from spirometry [10,12,13]. If the above criteria are met, spirometry is an excellent technique for assessing airflow limitation.

Peak Expiratory Flow Meters

Peak expiratory airflow (PEF) measurements can be obtained using simple, inexpensive, individual expiratory airflow monitoring devices that have gained acceptance as a method for monitoring expiratory airflows, especially in asthmatics [14]. These devices do not assess airflow parameters other than PEF. Results from different peak flow meters can be quite variable [15], tend to be alinear, and may overestimate airflows [16]. Although PEF reference values are available, repeated measurements over time commonly define a subject's best value for comparison to future changes.

C. Specific Measures of Expiratory Airflows

FEV_1

Forced expiratory volume in 1 sec (FEV_1) defines the volume of gas exhaled during the first second of a forced exhalation maneuver (Fig. 1). Of all the airflow measures available, FEV_1 has been the most widely utilized measure to diagnosis airway disease, quantify disease severity, track disease progression, and evaluate response to therapy [17–19]. Normal predicted values are available, and when measured using specified spirometry criteria, provide excellent precision, reliability, and reproducibility [10,13].

Vital Capacity

Vital capacity (VC) defines the volume of gas in the lungs between complete inhalation and complete exhalation. VC is determined by measuring the

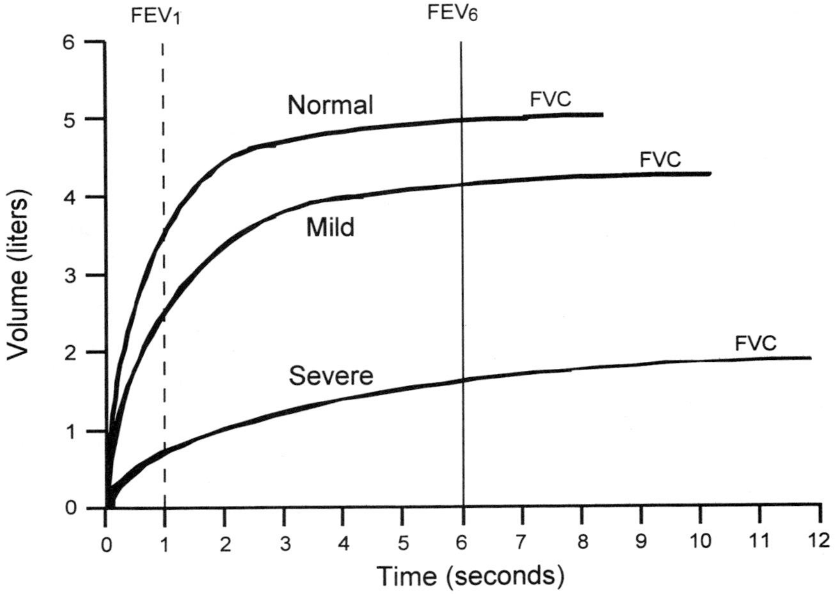

Figure 1 Relationship between volume of air and time during a forced exhalation. Examples of normal, mild, and severe subjects provided. Note the volume of air exhaled in 1 sec (FEV_1), 6 sec (FEV_6), and total volume exhaled (forced vital capacity, FVC).

volume of gas completely "exhaled" after fully inhaling or volume of gas completely "inhaled" after fully exhaling, and can be measured during slow or forced maneuvers. When measuring VC, it is important to define how the result is obtained, as technique and recent lung volume "history" can influence the result [20]. Forced maneuvers can be as much as 5% lower than those obtained during a slow or relaxed effort [21]. Normal predicted values are available, and VC measurements are reliable and reproducible [10].

Forced Versus Slow Vital Capacity

Forced vital capacity (FVC) is the VC measurement obtained during a maximal forced exhalation and is routinely measured as a part of spirometry (Fig. 1). Most studies of normal and disease states report FVC. However, the ability for some subjects to fully exhale during a forced effort can be difficult [3,10,22]. If complete exhalation does not occur, VC measurements are underestimated, negatively impacting on interpretation of airflow limitation [21]. To overcome problems with the FVC maneuver, it has been suggested that

VC should be measured during a slow (SVC) or relaxed effort in addition to the forced maneuver, with the SVC value used instead of the FVC [23]. Alternatively, it has been suggested that the VC maneuver be modified such that the initial portion of exhalation is maximal to obtain FEV_1, but the remainder of the vital capacity maneuver be performed with a more relaxed effort, providing both FEV_1 and SVC within the same effort [22]. Although of interest, this technique has not been well validated.

FEV_1/FVC Ratio

Of all the measurements derived from spirometry, the ratio between FEV_1 and FVC is the most sensitive, specific, and reliable measure of airflow limitation [10]. As with other lung function measurements, normative FEV_1/FVC ratios depend on various subject variables, especially age. Airflow limitation is commonly defined by a single FEV_1/FVC ratio, with a ratio of less than 70% typically used. However, this can lead to false positive and negative diagnoses, especially in the elderly [24]. Comparison of the FEV_1/FVC ratio results to a lower limit of normal criteria adjusted for age and height can eliminate this problem.

FEV_6 and FEV_1/FEV_6 Ratio

The volume of air forcibly exhaled after 6 sec, or FEV_6, has been proposed as a surrogate measurement for FVC [3] (Fig. 1). The FEV_6 is simple to measure, avoids technical problems associated with the FVC maneuver, is reproducible, reduces the time to perform each measurement, and is more comfortable. Predicted normals are now available for FEV_6 and the FEV_1/FEV_6 ratio [25]. Importantly, the FEV_1/FEV_6 ratio is as sensitive and specific as the FEV_1/FVC ratio for defining airflow limitation [26].

FEF_{25-75}

Mid-expiratory airflow measurements, such as FEF_{25-75}, have been proposed as a potentially more sensitive measure of mild airflow obstruction and small-airway disease [27]. However, the variability of this maneuver is greater and the measure has a lower specificity and poorer positive predictive value for airflow obstruction than that associated with the FEV_1/FVC ratio [8].

Peak Expiratory Flow (PEF)

Peak flows occur early during the "effort-dependent" portion of forced exhalation and PEF does not measure airflows during the "effort-independent" portion of forced exhalation, when many important components of COPD, such as alterations in lung compliance, airway tethering, and small-airways disease, come into play [14]. Lung diseases other than COPD can affect PEF measurements, and PEF measurements cannot distinguish between the various disease entities. Thus, PEF measurements are not recommended as diagnostic tests, even with asthma [29]. PEF measurement can be highly variable, even when performed within the stricter guidelines associated with spirometry [7,30].

Flow Volume Loops

Many spirometers include graphic representations that plot airflows relative to lung volumes as they change throughout inspiration and exhalation. These flow volume loops produce characteristic patterns, which are commonly associated with anatomic abnormalities affecting airflows [10]. However, these patterns are not truly diagnostic, are not quantifiable, and are unable to assess changes in expiratory airflows over time or with therapy.

D. COPD and Expiratory Airflows

Pathophysiology

An integral part of the definition of COPD is the presence of airflow limitation [5,6]. Many pathophysiological changes occur in the lungs of patients with COPD, including (1) airway inflammation with mucosal edema and mucus gland hyperplasia, (2) bronchoconstriction associated with increased cholinergic tone, (3) peribronchial inflammation and fibrosis with narrowing of small airways, and (4) destruction of alveolar septae and loss of tissue elasticity. Each of these changes alters airway caliber, airway resistance, and expiratory airflows [31]. Destruction of lung tissue in patients with emphysema produces somewhat unique mechanisms of airflow limitation. Loss of elastic tissue leads to earlier and greater degrees of airway collapse in the smaller airways, increasing airway resistance and reducing expiratory airflows. In addition, a decrease in lung elastance reduces a key force driving expiratory airflows.

Detecting Airflow Limitation in COPD

Expiratory airflows in COPD are best measured using spirometry. The importance of spirometry in identification and diagnosis of COPD patients is emphasized by the fact that COPD cannot be reliably detected by a medical history or physical examination alone [32], while spirometry can detect lung function abnormalities in asymptomatic patients [33]. A key criteria for airflow limitation in COPD is a decrease in the FEV_1/FVC ratio or the FEV_1/FEV_6 ratio. Although other airflow measurements are also altered when airflow limitation is present, they add little to the diagnostic yield. In particular, measures of peak expiratory flows (PEF) and mid-expiratory airflows such as the FEF_{25-75} are no more sensitive and are less reliable when compared to the FEV_1/FVC ratio [28,34].

Quantifying COPD Severity

To date, measurement of the severity of COPD centers on the FEV_1. Currently, staging of COPD disease severity uses FEV_1 alone [5,6]. However, staging of disease severity using FEV_1 alone may not be entirely satisfactory, and the addition of other measures, in conjunction with FEV_1, may ultimately add to a better stratification of disease severity.

COPD Progression

Spirometry has been used extensively in studies of lung health and aging [35,36]. A widely accepted component of COPD is a progressive deterioration in lung function over time, as manifest by an abnormal rate of decline in expiratory airflows. Normal declines in FEV_1 average about 30 mL/year with an upper limit of the normal of 50 mL/year. Rates of decline greater than 50 mL/year identify subjects with a rapid decline in lung function [37]. The presence of expiratory airflow limitation via spirometry (low FEV_1/FVC ratio) is a strong predictor of disease progression toward more severe COPD [38].

III. Lung Volumes

A. Physiology of Lung Volumes

As with expiratory airflows, understanding physiological factors that define lung volumes helps one understand the relationship between lung volumes and disease. The volume of gas within the lungs changes as conditions surrounding the lungs change, and measurements of lung volumes can identify abnormalities associated with specific diseases [39]. In general, elastic properties of the lungs and chest wall and closure of small airways determine specific lung volumes. Functional residual capacity (FRC) is the volume of gas present in the lungs at the end of passive exhalation, when the inward elastic recoil of the lung is equal and opposite to the outward elastic recoil of the chest wall and no muscle effort is required to maintain the lung volume [2,39,40].

At any lung volume other than FRC, respiratory muscle contraction directed either inward (expiratory) or outward (inspiratory) must be applied to counteract the elastic properties of the respiratory system and move the lung and chest wall to the newly specified position. Total lung capacity (TLC) defines the upper boundary of the lung or the volume of gas when the lung is maximally inflated. Assuming adequate respiratory muscle forces are available, TLC is constrained primarily by the elastic recoil of the lung. Any change in the elasticity of the lung will thereby influence TLC and FRC [40].

Residual volume (RV) defines the lower boundary of the lung or the volume of gas when the lung is maximally deflated. Depending on a subject's age, RV is influenced by chest wall compliance and/or by the closure of small airways. In adults, as lung volumes fall, outward traction of elastic tissue tethering airways declines and small airways transiently occlude, trapping gas distal to the occlusion (closing volume). When no further gas is available to exhale, RV is achieved

B. Measurement Techniques for Lung Volume

The measurement of lung volumes requires the determination of the absolute volume of gas for at least one of the key lung volumes, TLC, FRC, or RV. This lung volume can then be combined with other lung volumes measured using spirometry to provide absolute values for the rest of the lung volumes. Several techniques are available to measure lung volumes [40]. These techniques utilize physical laws related to conservation of mass or pressure and volume in a closed, stable system. By perturbing the system with measurable changes, unknown baseline volumes can be derived.

Dilutional Methods

Several methods of gas dilution have been utilized to determine the volume of gas in the lung [40]. A classic method entails breathing a gas mixture containing an inert gas, such as helium, which distributes throughout the respiratory system without being adsorbed or metabolized. The diluted concentration of helium is measured and the volume of gas diluting the helium can be derived, providing the volume of gas in the lung at which the subject began breathing the gas mixture, usually FRC. Alternatively, a single breath of inert gas can be inhaled during an inspiratory VC maneuver. After breath holding and then exhaling, the concentration of inhaled inert gas times the inhaled volume equals the mean concentration of exhaled inert gas times the diluting alveolar volume (V_A), or TLC.

Other dilutional methodologies assess the washout of nitrogen in the lung [41]. The volume of gas exhaled required to virtually eliminate nitrogen from exhaled gas while breathing 100% oxygen, in conjunction with concentrations of nitrogen at the start and end of the test and mean concentrations of inhaled and exhaled nitrogen, allows calculation of the volume of gas at the start of oxygen breathing, or FRC. Finally, nitrogen concentration at the end of an expiratory slow VC maneuver after having previously inhaled 100% oxygen approximates the concentration of nitrogen within the lung at RV and, along with the measurements of mean exhaled nitrogen concentrations and the VC, allows the calculation of RV.

Each of these tests assumes that gas distribution is fairly rapid, homogenous, and complete. If this is not the case, lung volumes can be significantly underestimated [42,43], especially when single breath measurements are used [41,44]. Alternatively, leaks in the system, usually at the mouthpiece, fail to measure dilutional gases, which escape and falsely elevate volume calculations.

Plethysmography

Body plethysmography requires a subject to be enclosed within an airtight box. The subject breaths through a mouthpiece with a shutter which, when occluded, is capable of measuring mouth pressure. The mouthpiece is briefly occluded at the end of exhalation and the subject performs shallow panting efforts against the closed shutter. Changes in mouth pressure during panting approximate changes in intrathoracic pressure. By relating pressure changes in the box to changes in mouth pressure, the volume of gas being compressed and decompressed in the thorax or thoracic gas volume (TGV) can be derived. If the airway is occluded at end exhalation, then TGV equals FRC. If occlusion occurs at a volume other than end exhalation, as long as a seal on the mouthpiece is sustained, then the difference in volume between TGV and FRC can be measured and FRC calculated.

Although it is an excellent method for assessing lung volumes, body plethysmography does have limitations [45]. A subject must tolerate at least short periods of enclosure within the body box and must be able to pant with prescribed panting efforts. A potential area of concern relates to mouth pressures that do not adequately reflect intrathoracic pressure changes during panting. This can be of particular concern if the subject cannot maintain a seal around the mouthpiece or if the subject's cheeks pouch out during panting. Such problems lead to underestimation of thoracic pressures and overestimation of TGV [43,46,47]. Attention to technique can minimize these problems. Alternatively, intrathoracic pressures can be measured directly with an esophageal balloon, although this level of invasion is more than most subjects appreciate.

Chest X-Ray Planimetry

Planimetric measurement of lung areas from chest X-rays, in conjunction with formulas comparing these measurements to lung volumes, can be used to estimate TLC [40]. Equipment for such measurements is generally not available, and the technique is rarely used today.

C. Specific Measures of Lung Volumes

TLC, FRC, RV, V_T, VC, IC, ERV, IRV

TLC, FRC, and RV have been defined above. Using these lung volume measurements plus the tidal volume (V_T) or volume of gas inhaled from FRC during spontaneous breathing, several other lung volume measurements can be defined. As previously noted, the vital capacity (VC) is the volume of gas that can be maximally exhaled (i.e., TLC−RV). Other volume measurements include the inspiratory capacity (IC) or volume of gas that can be maximally inhaled from FRC (TLC−FRC), the inspiratory reserve volume (IRV) or volume of gas that can be maximally inhaled after having already inhaled a normal tidal breath (TLC−FRC + V_T), and the expiratory reserve volume (ERV) or volume of gas that can be maximally exhaled from FRC (FRC−RV) (Fig. 2).

Several lung volume components can be measured with spirometry alone. However, as noted above, determination of the absolute volume of gas associated with each measurement requires linkage to a direct lung volume measurement [48]. The lung volume most commonly measured for this linkage is FRC. Thus, measurement of FRC, in conjunction with measures of IC and VC, provides TLC and RV (e.g., TLC = FRC + IC and RV = TLC−VC). Anything that alters the intensity of maximal inspiratory and expiratory efforts will influence all of these measurements except FRC. Normative values are available for lung volumes, based on demographic information similar to expiratory airflows [49,50].

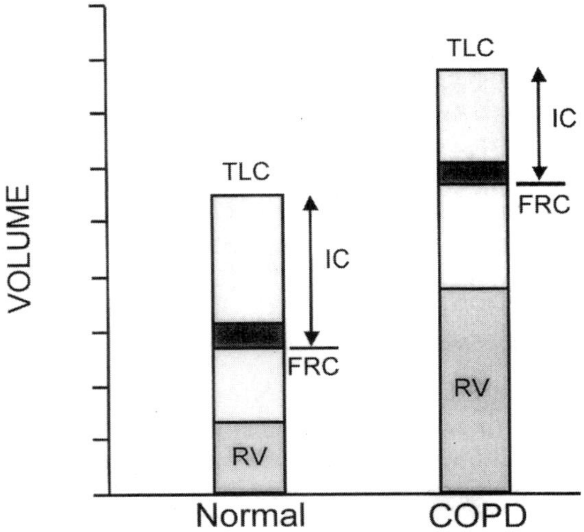

Figure 2 Division of lung volumes in normal subjects and patients with COPD. Note the significant increases in total lung capacity (TLC), functional residual capacity (FRC), and residual volume (RV), as well as the increase in the ratio of FRC to TLC and of RV to TLC. Note also the fall in inspiratory capacity (IC).

End Inspiratory and End Expiratory Lung Volumes (EELV and EILV)

Under normal conditions, subjects passively exhale until the elastic forces of the lung and chest wall equilibrate, so that the end expiratory lung volume (EELV) is the same as FRC. However, circumstances may dictate that exhalation stop at a lung volume other than FRC [51]. This most commonly occurs when subjects actively control ventilation or when the ventilatory pattern is altered by factors such as exercise or disease. End inspiratory lung volume (EILV) is the lung volume that is achieved at the end of a tidal inspiration. As with EELV, any volitional, physiological, or pathological condition that changes EELV or V_T can change EILV.

A key difference when considering EELV and EILV, as compared to other lung volume measurements, is the notion that EELV and EILV are dynamic and can change rapidly, while other lung volumes are more static. This, in turn, changes how these lung volumes are measured. When measuring EELV and EILV, TLC is assumed to be fixed. After obtaining a baseline measurement of TLC (most commonly using plethysmography), TLC becomes the new anchor against which IC and V_T are compared to determine EELV and EILV (EELV = TLC − IC and EILV equals EELV + V_T). The value of this measurement becomes limited if TLC shifts or repeated IC efforts are not reliable [52]. However, several studies suggest that TLC remains fixed, at least during short periods of exercise [53,54], and that repeated measures of IC measures are reproducible [55,56].

D. Impact of COPD on Lung Volumes

Terminology surrounding alterations in lung volumes can be confusing and is less standardized [39]. In particular, the indiscriminate use of the term "hyperinflation" can cause significant problems. When interpreting chest radiographs, "hyperinflation" is used to describe overly large lung volumes at maximum inspiration or TLC. However, during pulmonary function testing, "hyperinflation" commonly refers to a greater than predicted EELV, a volume that is not visualized or appreciated on chest X-ray. Using a single consistent definition will facilitate more precise communication plus a better understanding of specific disease pathophysiology.

Overdistension

When damage to alveoli and elastic tissue occurs as a part of COPD, the lung becomes more compliant. As a consequence, the maximum stretch of the lung during an inspiratory effort increases, yielding a larger TLC. This increase in TLC is referred to as overdistension and is distinct from an increase in FRC, in which TLC may remain normal. Although it is observed in many patients with COPD, overdistension is not always present, likely because of the diverse pathology associated with COPD and a lack of severe changes in lung elastance in many patients. Lung elastance does not change rapidly over time and is independent of expiratory airflows. Thus, factors that acutely alter airflows are not believed to change TLC acutely. Nevertheless, acute changes in TLC or overdistension are seen [52,57]. A potential explanation relates to regional changes in gas distribution in portions of the lung having different compliances, which, when accessed by a given therapy, can change the composite or total compliance of the lung.

Hyperinflation

As noted above, hyperinflation defines an increase in EELV or FRC and is not the size of the lungs at TLC. Although most often defined based on an absolute increase in FRC, comparison of FRC to TLC as a percentage (FRC/TLC ratio) has been standardized and is also used to identify patients with hyperinflation, especially when conditions that can alter TLC may be present. Hyperinflation can occur due to two distinct processes, frequently described as static and dynamic, both of which can be observed in COPD patients.

Static Hyperinflation

When elastance of the lung is altered, as in emphysema, the pressure–volume curve shifts in a manner such that a larger lung volume is required to provide an elastic recoil force sufficient to offset the outward recoil of the chest wall [58,59]. This becomes the new FRC and is considered due to static hyperinflation. Of interest, chronic hyperinflation can produce irreversible changes in the structure and compliance of the chest wall, which may also contribute to static hyperinflation [60].

Dynamic Hyperinflation

Dynamic hyperinflation relates to changes in EELV and is described in greater detail in other chapters. Briefly, when expiratory airflow limitation occurs, patients may not be able to exhale fully prior to initiating a new breath [61]. If this happens on repeated breaths, the volume of gas at end exhalation (EELV) increases and dynamic hyperinflation occurs [58,59]. Although lung elastance plays an indirect role due to its impact on expiratory airflows, the dominant factors contributing to dynamic inflation are expiratory airflow limitation and expiratory times, which determine whether adequate time is available to exhale completely. Thus, dynamic hyperinflation may occur rapidly and vary greatly [62,63].

Gas Trapping Versus Trapped Gas

Loss of elastic recoil in COPD patients is associated with earlier airway collapse and airway closure during exhalation, with an increase in RV and RV/TLC ratio. In addition, when inadequate exhalation occurs during dynamic hyperinflation, RV and the RV/TLC ratio also acutely increase. Indeed, RV and RV/TLC ratio may change earlier and to a greater degree than FRC or EELV. This increase in RV or RV/TLC ratio has been termed "gas trapping" and is considered an early lung volume manifestation of airflow limitation [39]. Unfortunately, inadequate expiratory effort can falsely elevate RV and reduce the specificity of this measurement. Thus, reliance on "gas trapping" as a sole indicator of hyperinflation with airflow limitation is not recommended.

Inhomogeneous gas distribution associated with poorly communicating regions of ventilation or the presence of noncommunicating gas (e.g., bullae) within the lung can cause significant differences in lung volume measurements when determined by dilutional versus plethysmographic methodologies [64]. Comparison of lung volume results from the two different methodologies has been proposed to identify the presence and severity of poorly communicating gas within the lung, with the difference between the two lung volume measurements termed "trapped gas" [43]. Associated with the concept of "trapped gas" is the implication that a reduction in "trapped gas" may occur if airflows within poorly ventilated regions of lung improve [65]. Unfortunately, variability of the individual measurements requires large changes in "trapped gas" to occur in order to be meaningful.

Restriction Secondary to Obstruction

Although VC defines the limits within which a subject breathes and includes both IC and ERV, normal subjects use only a small portion of the ERV when increasing V_T and patients with COPD typically do not recruit ERV at all when increasing V_T [51]. Thus, IC defines the boundaries of V_T recruitment for a patient with COPD, and IRV becomes the volume that is available for recruiting additional volume, if needed [66]. Airflow limitation that causes hyperinflation reduces IC (Fig. 2) and imposes a degree of restriction. Although more pronounced during dynamic hyperinflation associated with exercise, this restriction also plays a significant role during resting breathing [66,67].

IV. Other Measures

A. Airway Resistance and Specific Conductance

An alternative method for assessing airways is airway resistance, which may be considered to represent the physiology associated with airway diseases better than spirometry. However, the measurement of airway resistance has limitations, including the use of a single resistance measure to reflect changes in resistance throughout all of the airways, the tendency for airway resistance to assess larger airways rather than the smaller airways that are more affected in COPD, and the need to adjust for the influence of lung volume on airway resistance.

Airway resistance is measured using body plethysmography techniques. Subjects pant with the mouthpiece shutter open, allowing for measurement of airflows. The shutter is then closed and mouth pressures with panting are measured. Changes in airflows and mouth pressures are used to derive the resistance. Since closed-shutter panting also yields TGV, specific conductance can be calculated (the inverse of resistance divided by lung volume) and used to standardize airway resistance for lung volume. Although they are useful, airway resistance and specific conductance have a fair degree of variability and the sensitivity of these measures in identifying airway abnormalities is less than those obtained by spirometry [34]. On the other hand, measurement of airway resistance does not require maximal respiratory efforts, which can be of benefit when assessing some patients.

B. Upstream Resistance, Closing Volume, and Frequency Dependence of Compliance

Several additional measures have been devised in an attempt to assess small-airway function, including upstream resistance [68], closing volume [69], and frequency dependence of compliance [70]. Each of these has sound physiological rationales for usage. However, in early stages of airway disease, when such measures might be of most value, changes within the lung are not uniform and sensitivity of the tests is reduced [71]. These findings, in conjunction with the more complex and invasive nature of the tests, make them of lesser value.

V. Bronchodilator Reversibility and Airway Hyperreactivity

A. Bronchodilator Reversibility

A key facet of airway diseases relates to changes in expiratory airflows and lung volumes that occur over time or in response to various interventions. Methodologies have been developed to assess the ability of airflows and lung volumes to change, the most common of which is to test for improvement after administering a bronchodilator [10]. Measures of bronchodilator reversibility are typically associated with changes in expiratory airflows. Criteria have been established defining reversibility as an increase in FEV_1 of the greater of 200 mL and 12% of the baseline FEV_1 [10] or an increase in FEV_1 by 10% of the predicted normal FEV_1 [72].

As noted above, bronchodilators have no direct impact on airway elastance, but may cause changes in gas distribution in poorly ventilated portions of the lung, leading to a fall in TLC [57]. More typically, no acute change in TLC occurs following use of bronchodilators [57]. On the other hand, significant changes occur in other lung volumes. Whether described in absolute terms or as a percentage of TLC, FRC and RV often acutely deflate after bronchodilators, primarily as a result improvements in dynamic hyperinflation [57]. Associated with this is an increase in IC [59].

Bronchodilator Reversibility in COPD

Although COPD is described as a progressive, irreversible disease, two-thirds of COPD patients exhibit acute reversibility to bronchodilators, especially when reassessed over time [18,73,74]. Thus, the presence of acute bronchodilator reversibility does not preclude a diagnosis of COPD [75], nor does a lack of acute reversibility imply a lack of benefit for bronchodilator therapy. When evaluating reversibility, little additional insight is gained by analyzing expiratory airflows other than FEV_1 [84]. Unfortunately, bronchodilator reversibility in COPD does not correlate well with other outcomes used to assess response to therapy [76]. As noted above, bronchodilator reversibility can lead to important changes in lung volumes [67,77]. Indeed, in COPD patients, improvement can be manifested solely by reductions in hyperinflation and gas trapping, without measurable improvements in expiratory airflows [78,79] (Fig. 3).

B. Airway Hyperreactivity

An alternative approach in assessing airflows is to induce bronchoconstriction using agents such as methacholine and histamine. Normative ranges for doses required to induce bronchoconstriction are available and can be used to identify the presence and severity of airway hyperreactivity.

Airway Hyperreactivity in COPD

As with bronchodilator reversibility, airway hyperreactivity (AHR) is commonly considered not to be a part of COPD. However, AHR is more common in COPD patients than previously expected [80]. Evidence now suggests that AHR is a predictor of more rapid disease progression in COPD [80,81]. Whether medical interventions reducing AHR in COPD patients alters the course of disease progression is unknown, although trials with inhaled corticosteroids alter AHR, but do not change disease progression [82,83].

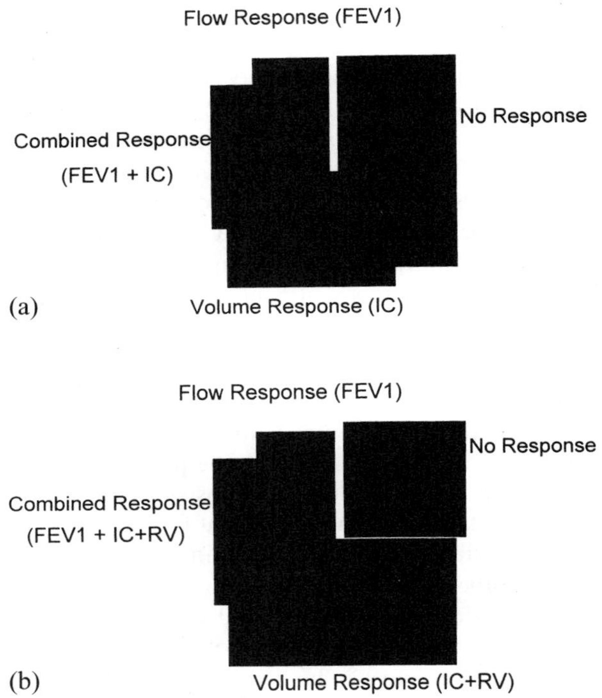

Figure 3 (a) Percentage of hyperinflated COPD patients demonstrating changes in expiratory airflows (FEV_1), lung volumes (IC), both ($FEV_1 + IC$), or neither following bronchodilators. (b) Percentage of COPD patients demonstrating changes in expiratory airflows (FEV_1), lung volumes ($IC + RV$), both ($FEV_1 + IC + RV$), or neither following bronchodilators. Note the percentage of patients exhibiting reductions in dynamic hyperinflation as evidenced by an increase in IC and the percentage of patients exhibiting changes in lung volumes only, without changes in expiratory airflows, following bronchodilators. (Adapted from Newton MF, O'Donnell DE, Forkert L. Response of lung volume to inhaled salbutamol in a large population of patients with hyperinflation. Chest 2002; 121:1042–1050.)

VI. Clinical Relevance

A. Association with Pathology

The traditional standard for comparison of disease in COPD has been pathological changes in lung tissue. FEV_1 correlates closely with pathological changes in the lungs of smokers and patients with COPD [84]. TLC has also been shown to correlate with tissue pathology in COPD, especially when lung destruction secondary to emphysema is assessed.

B. Association with CT Scans

Abnormally low lung densities on high-resolution computerized tomography (HRCT) correlate with pathological severity in emphysema [85]. A modest correlation between FEV_1 and HRCT emphysema severity scores has been suggested [86]. However, emphysema is only one component of COPD contributing to airflow limitation, and other studies suggest that FEV_1 correlates poorly with CT measures of emphysema [87]. Correlation of lung volume measurements to CT scans suggests a modest relationship [88].

C. Association with Outcome Measures

Outcome measures in COPD are discussed in detail in other chapters. However, the relationship of expiratory airflows and lung volumes to these outcomes is important in order to determine the value of these physiological measures in COPD.

Mortality

Severity of disease as assessed by FEV_1 is a strong independent predictor of mortality in patients with COPD [89,90]. In addition, FEV_1 is an excellent measure of global health, predicting all-cause mortality and morbidity [91]. FEV_1 has also been shown to identify patients at high risk for lung cancer [92] and other medical conditions [93].

Exercise Performance

In general, expiratory airflows and bronchodilator reversibility do not correlate well with exercise performance in COPD patients [76] (Fig. 4). On the other hand, lung volume measurements, in particular those associated with hyperinflation, correlate well with exercise performance, with IC correlating best [66,67,94] (Fig. 4).

Work of Breathing and Dyspnea

COPD has a negative impact on respiratory muscles and their ability to perform inspiratory work, in part related to the effects of hyperinflation. Airflow limitation and hyperinflation also increase the work of breathing by increasing threshold, resistive, and elastic work loads [2,31,95]. In spite of

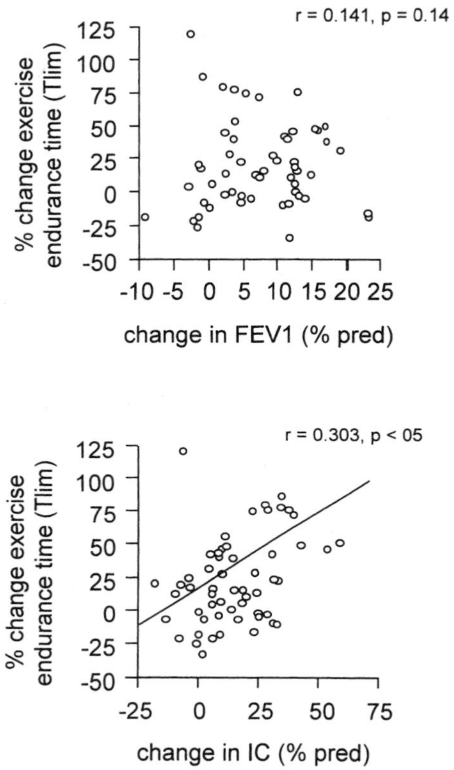

(a)

(b)

Figure 4 (a) Lack of correlation between expiratory airflows (FEV_1) and exercise performance. (b) Correlation between dynamic hyperinflation as assessed by inspiratory capacity (IC) and exercise performance. (Adapted from O'Donnell DE, Lam M, Webb KA. Spirometric correlates of improvement in exercise performance after anticholinergic therapy in chronic obstructive pulmonary disease. Am J Respir Crit Care Med 1999; 160:542–549.)

this, FEV_1 and FVC correlate poorly with measures of dyspnea in COPD. As with exercise performance, measures of hyperinflation, especially IC, correlate well with measures of dyspnea [67,66].

Quality of Life

One would predict that severity of COPD should affect patient quality of life. However, several studies suggest a poor correlation between FEV_1 and quality of life [96]. The correlation does improve when adjusted for other co-morbidities [97]. Measures of hyperinflation, such as IC, correlate better with quality-of-life measures, although still with only modest success.

Exacerbation Rates

Frequency of exacerbations increases with increasing severity of COPD, as determined by FEV_1 [83]. In addition, a more rapid rate of decline in FEV_1 occurs in COPD patients with more frequent exacerbations, especially those with more than three exacerbations per year [98]. Although controversial, it has been suggested that FEV_1 can be used to identify patients likely to benefit from therapies attempting to reduce exacerbation rates, such as inhaled steroids [83], as well as patients needing more potent antibiotics to cover Gram-negative bacteria [99].

Health Care Utilization/Economics

Little information is available on health care utilization relative to lung function. As with quality of life, correlation between lung function and health care utilization is poor, and lung function measurements provide little predictive value [100]. Indeed, other co-morbidities often play a much greater role.

VII. Conclusion and Recommendations

COPD is a disease defined by the presence of expiratory airflow limitation. FEV_1/FVC ratio has been used to identify airflow limitation, while FEV_1 has been the primary endpoint used to assess disease severity, disease progression, and response to therapy. Although other measures of expiratory airflows and lung volumes exist, little information has been available suggesting a value in these measurements when assessing COPD patients.

Recently, the FEV_1/FEV_6 ratio has been shown to provide diagnostic sensitivity and specificity equal to the FEV_1/FVC ratio and can be performed without the difficulties attendant to the FVC maneuver. Use of these ratios continues to be the best measure for diagnosing airflow limitation, even in asymptomatic or at-risk patients. However, use of predicted values for these ratios, rather than the 70% value, may provide even better sensitivity and specificity.

Of all the potential measures available to assess disease severity and rate of disease progression in COPD, none has been shown to be better than the FEV_1. However, use of FEV_1 alone to stage disease severity is limited, and alternative methodologies or composite measures are still needed. This becomes particularly important as recommendations for evaluation and treatment of COPD are linked to disease severity. Traditionally, a change in FEV_1

has been used to assess the value of a therapeutic intervention in COPD. Unfortunately, FEV_1 may not be the best outcome to measure, due to its poor correlation with many clinically meaningful outcomes. Other expiratory airflow measures provide little additional insight when assessing the impact of such therapies.

The value of lung volumes in assessing COPD has recently been highlighted. Subtle, and otherwise nonmeasurable, changes in expiratory airflows that affect lung hyperinflation can be measured. Although FRC and RV identify hyperinflation in COPD, EELV and IC may be of greater importance. Indeed, IC defines the boundaries of lung volume within which ventilation is restricted. Changes in IC are dynamic and can identify meaningful changes which occur in response to acute therapies and may not be detected by measures of expiratory airflows. Changes in IC also correlate well with several clinical outcomes important to patients. IC can be performed as a part of spirometry testing, and equipment needed to measure other lung volumes is not required. Lung volumes, especially IC, should be a part of lung function measurements when assessing outcomes in the treatment of COPD.

References

1. Pride NB. Tests of forced expiration and inspiration. Clin Chest Med 2001; 22:599–622.
2. Corbridge T, Irvin CG. Pathophysiology of chronic obstructive pulmonary disease with emphasis on physiologic and pathologic correlation. In: Casaburi R, Petty TL, eds. Principles and Practice of Pulmonary Rehabilitation. Philadelphia: Saunders, 1993:18–32.
3. Ferguson GT, Enright PL, Buist AS, Higgins MW. Office spirometry for lung health assessment in adults: a consensus statement from the National Lung Health Education Program. Chest 2000; 117:1146–1161.
4. Curtis JR, Martin DP, Martin TR. Patient-assessed health outcomes in chronic lung disease: What are they, how do they help us, and where do we go from here? Am J Respir Crit Care Med 1997; 156:1032–1039.
5. American Thoracic Society. Standards for the diagnosis and care of patients with chronic obstructive pulmonary disease. ATS statement. Am J Respir Crit Care Med 1995; 152:S77–S121.
6. Pauwels RA, Buist AS, Calverley PM, Jenkins CR, Hurd SS. Global strategy for the diagnosis, management, and prevention of chronic obstructive pulmonary disease. NHLBI/WHO Global Initiative for Chronic Obstructive Lung Disease (GOLD) Workshop summary. Am J Respir Crit Care Med 2001; 163: 1256–1276.
7. American Thoracic Society. Standardization of spirometry: 1994 update. Am J Respir Crit Care Med 1995; 152:1107–1136.

8. Crapo RO. Pulmonary function testing. N Engl J Med 1994; 331:25–30.
9. Becklake MR, White N. Sources of variation in spirometric measurements. Identifying the signal and dealing with the noise. Occup Med 1993; 8:241–264.
10. American Thoracic Society. Lung function testing: selection of reference values and interpretive strategies. Am Rev Respir Dis 1991; 144:1202–1218.
11. American Association of Respiratory Care. Clinical practice guidelines: Spirometry, 1996 update. Respir Care 1996; 41:629–636.
12. British Thoracic Society. Guidelines for the measurement of respiratory function. Respir Med 1994; 88:165–194.
13. Crapo RO, Morris AH, Gardner RM. Reference spirometric values using techniques and equipment that meet ATS recommendations. Am Rev Respir Dis 1981; 123:659–664.
14. Guidelines for the diagnosis and management of asthma. Clinical practice guidelines. National Institute of Health Publication 97-4051, 1997:12–18.
15. Jackson AC. Accuracy, reproducibility, and variability of portable peak flowmeters. Chest 1995; 107:648–651.
16. Pederson OF, Miller MR. The peak flow working group: test of portable peak flow meters by explosive decompression. Eur Respir J 1997; 9(suppl 24):23s–25s.
17. Nisar M, Earis JE, Pearson MG, Calverley PM. Acute bronchodilator trials in chronic obstructive pulmonary disease. Am Rev Respir Dis 1992; 146:555–559.
18. Rennard SI, Anderson W, Zu Wallack R, Broughton J, Bailey W, Friedman M, Wisniewski M, Rickard K. Of a long-acting inhaled beta2-adrenergic agonist, salmeterol xinafoate, in patients with chronic obstructive pulmonary disease. Am J Respir Crit Care Med 2001; 163:1087–1092.
19. Van Noord JA, Bantje TA, Eland ME, Korducki L, Cornelissen PJ. A randomised controlled comparison of tiotropium and ipratropium in the treatment of chronic obstructive pulmonary disease. The Dutch Tiotropium Study group. Thorax 2000; 55:289–294.
20. Brusasco V, Pellegrino R, Rodarte JR. Vital capacities in acute and chronic airway obstruction: dependence on flow and volume history. Eur Respir J 1987; 10:1316–1320.
21. Townsend MC, Du Chene AG, Fallat RJ. The effects of underrecorded forced expirations on spirometric lung function indexes. Am Rev Respir Dis 1982; 126:734–737.
22. Stoller JK, Basheda S, Laskowski D, Goormastic M, McCarthy K. Trial of standard versus modified expiration to achieve end-of-test spirometry criteria. Am Rev Respir Dis 1993; 148:275–280.
23. Bubis MJ, Sigurdson M, McCarthy DS, Anthonisen NR. Differences between slow and fast vital capacities in patients with obstructive disease. Chest 1980; 77:626–631.
24. Hardie JA, Buist AS, Vollmer WM, Ellingsen I, Bakke PS, Morkve O. Risk of over-diagnosis of COPD in asymptomatic elderly never-smokers. Eur Respir J 2002; 20:1117–1122.
25. Hankinson JL, Odencrantz JR, Fedan KB. Spirometric reference values from a

sample of the general US population. Am J Respir Crit Care Med 1999; 159:179–187.
26. Enright PL, Connett JE, Bailey WC. FEV_1/FEV_6 predicts lung function decline in adult smokers. Respir Med 2002; 96:444–449.
27. Olsen CR, Hale FC. A method for interpreting acute response to bronchodilators from the spirogram. Am Rev Respir Dis 1968; 98:301–302.
28. Detels R, Tashkin DP, Simmons MS, Carmichael HE Jr, Sayre JW, Rokaw SN, Coulson AH. The UCLA population studies of chronic obstructive respiratory disease. 5. Agreement and disagreement of tests in identifying abnormal lung function. Chest 1982; 82:630–638.
29. Guidelines for the diagnosis and management of asthma. Clinical practice guidelines. National Institute of Health Publication 97-4051, 1997:12–18.
30. Enright PL, Lebowitz MD, Cockroft DW. Physiologic measures: pulmonary function tests. Asthma outcome. Am J Respir Crit Care Med 1994; 149:s9–s18.
31. Hubmayr Rd, Rodarte JR. Cellular effects and physiologic responses: lung mechanics. In: Cherniack NS, ed. Physiologic responses to COPD. Chronic Obstructive Pulmonary Disease, 1991. Philadelphia: Saunders, 1991:79–90.
32. Holleman DR Jr, Simel DL. Does the clinical examination predict airflow limitation? JAMA 1995; 273:131–319.
33. Mannino DM, Gagnon RC, Petty TL, Lydick E. Obstructive lung disease and low lung function in adults in the United States: data from the National Health and Nutrition Examination Survey, 1988–1994. Arch Intern Med 2000; 160: 1683–1689.
34. Berger R, Smith D. Acute postbronchodilator changes in pulmonary function parameters in patients with chronic airways obstruction. Chest 1988; 93:541–546.
35. Fletcher CM, Peto R, Tinker CM, Speizer FE. The natural history of chronic bronchitis and emphysema: an eight year study of early chronic obstructive lung disease in working men in London. New York: Oxford University Press, 1976.
36. Griffith KA, Sherrill DL, Siegel EM, Manolio TA, Bonekat HW, Enright PL. Predictors of loss of lung function in the elderly: the Cardiovascular Health Study. Am J Respir Crit Care Med 2001; 163:61–68.
37. Kerstjens HAM, Rijcken B, Schouten JP, Postma DS. Decline of FEV_1 by age and smoking status: facts, figures, and fallacies. Thorax 1997; 52:820–827.
38. Fletcher C, Peto R. The natural history of chronic airflow obstruction. Br Med J 1977; 1:1645–1648.
39. Leith DE, Brown R. Human lung volumes and the mechanisms that set them. Eur Respir J 1999; 13:468–472.
40. Gibson GJ. Lung volumes and elasticity. Clin Chest Med 2001; 22:623–635.
41. Brugman TM, Morris JF, Temple WP. Comparison of lung volume measurements by single breath helium and multiple breath nitrogen equilibration methods in normal subjects and COPD patients. Respiration 1986; 49:52–60.
42. Boutellier U, Farhi LE. A fundamental problem in determining functional residual capacity or residual volume. J Appl Physiol 1986; 60:1810–1813.
43. Rodenstein DO, Stanescu DC. Reassessment of lung volume measurement by

helium dilution and by body plethysmography in chronic air-flow obstruction. Am Rev Respir Dis 1982; 126:1040–1044.
44. Burns CB, Scheinhorn Dj. Evaluation of single-breath dilution total lung capacity in obstructive lung disease. Am Rev Respir Dis 1984; 130:580–583.
45. Garcia JG, Hunninghake GW, Nugent KM. Thoracic gas volume measurement: increased variability in patients with chronic obstructive ventilatory defects. Chest 1984; 85:272–275.
46. Brown R, Ingram RH Jr, McFadden ER Jr. Problems in the plethysmographic assessment of changes in total lung capacity in asthma. Am Rev Respir Dis 1978; 118:685–692.
47. Pare PD, Wiggs BJR, Coppin CA. Errors in the measurement of total lung capacity in chronic obstructive lung disease. Thorax 1983; 38:468–471.
48. Williams JH Jr, Bencowitz HZ. Differences in plethysmographic lung volumes: effects of linked vs unlinked spirometry. Chest 1989; 95:117–123.
49. Stocks J, Quanjer PhH. Reference values for residual volume, functional residual capacity and total lung capacity. ATS Workshop on Lung Volume Measurements Official statement of the European Respiratory Society. Eur Respir J 1995; 8:492–506.
50. Withers RT, Bourdon PC, Crockett A. Lung volume standards for healthy male lifetime nonsmokers. Chest 1988; 93:91–97.
51. Henke KG, Sharratt M, Pegelow D, Dempsey JA. Regulation of end-expiratory lung volume during exercise. J Appl Physiol 1988; 64:135–146.
52. Freedman S, Tattersfield AE, Pride NB. Changes in lung mechanics during asthma induced by exercise. J Appl Physiol 1975; 38:974–982.
53. Stubbing DG, Pengelly LD, Morse JLC, Jones NL. Pulmonary mechanics during exercise in subjects with chronic airflow obstruction. J Appl Physiol 1980; 49:511–515.
54. Younes M, Kivinen G. Respiratory mechanics and breathing pattern during and following maximal exercise. J Appl Physiol 1984; 57:1773–1782.
55. Yan S, Kaminski D, Sliwinski P. Reliability of inspiratory capacity for estimating end-expiratory lung volume changes during exercise in patients with chronic obstructive pulmonary disease. Am J Respir Crit Care Med 1997; 156:55–59.
56. Dolmage TE, Goldstein RS. Repeatability of inspiratory capacity during incremental exercise in patients with severe COPD. Chest 2002; 121:708–714.
57. Pellegrino R, Bruscaco V. On the causes of lung hyperinflation during bronchoconstriction. Eur Respir J 1997; 10:468–475.
58. Gibson GJ. Pulmonary hyperinflation a clinical overview. Eur Respir J 1996; 9:2640–2649.
59. Brusasco V, Fitting JW. Lung hyperinflation in airway obstruction. Eur Respir J 1996; 9:2440.
60. Pinet C, Estenne M. Effect of preoperative hyperinflation on static lung volumes after lung transplantation. Eur Respir J 2000; 16:482–485.
61. Pellegrino R, Brusasco V. Lung hyperinflation and flow limitation in chronic airway obstruction. Eur Respir J 1997; 10:543–549.

62. O'Donnell DE, Webb KA. Exertional breathlessness in patients with chronic airflow obstruction. The role of lung hyperinflation. Am Rev Respir Dis 1993; 148:1351–1357.
63. Belman MJ, Botnick WC, Shin JW. Inhaled bronchodilators reduce dynamic hyperinflation during exercise in patients with chronic obstructive pulmonary disease. Am J Respir Crit Care Med 1996; 153:967–975.
64. Garcia-Rio F, Pino-Garcia JM, Serrano S, Racionero MA, Terreros-Caro JG, Alvarez-Sala R, Villasante C, Villamor J. Comparison of helium dilution and plethysmographic lung volumes in pregnant women. Eur Respir J 1997; 10: 2371–2375.
65. Waterhouse JC, Pritchard SM, Howard P. Hyperinflation, trapped gas and theophylline in chronic obstructive pulmonary disease. Monaldi Arch Chest Dis 1992; 48:126–129.
66. O'Donnell DE, Revill SM, Webb KA. Dynamic hyperinflation and exercise intolerance in chronic obstructive pulmonary disease. Am J Respir Crit Care Med 2001; 164:770–777.
67. O'Donnell DE, Lam M, Webb KA. Spirometric correlates of improvement in exercise performance after anticholinergic therapy in chronic obstructive pulmonary disease. Am J Respir Crit Care Med 1999; 160:542–549.
68. Michaels R, Sigurdson M, Thurlbeck S, Cherniack R. Elastic recoil of the lung in cigarette smokers: the effect of nebulized bronchodilator and cessation of smoking. Am Rev Respir Dis 1979; 119:707–716.
69. Petty TL, Silvers GW, Stanford RE, Baird MD, Mitchell RS. Small airway pathology is related to increase closing capacity and abnormal slope of phase III in excised human lungs. Am Rev Respir Dis 1980; 121:449–456.
70. Kjeldgaard JM, Hyde RW, Speers DM, Reichert WW. Frequency dependence of total respiratory resistance in early airway disease. Am Rev Respir Dis 1976; 114:501–508.
71. Buist AS, Van Fleet DL, Ross BB. A comparison of conventional spirometric tests and the test of closing volume in an emphysema screening center. Am Rev Respir Dis 1973; 107:735–743.
72. Standardized lung function testing. Official statement of the European Respiratory Society. Eur Respir J 1993; 16(suppl 6):1–100.
73. Anthonisen NR, Wright EC, IPPB trial group. Bronchodilator response in chronic obstructive pulmonary disease. Am Rev Respir Dis 1986; 133:814–819.
74. Dorinsky PM, Reisner C, Ferguson GT, Menjoge SS, Serby CW, Witek TJ Jr, The combination of ipratropium and albuterol optimizes pulmonary function reversibility testing in patients with COPD. Chest 1999; 115:966–971.
75. Kesten S, Rebuck AS. Is the short-term response to inhaled β-adrenergic agonist sensitive or specific for distinguishing between asthma and COPD? Chest 1994; 105:1042–1045.
76. Hay JG, Stone P, Carter J, Church S, Eyre-Brook A, Pearson MG, Woodcock AA, Calverley PM. Bronchodilator reversibility, exercise performance and breathlessness in stable chronic obstructive pulmonary disease. Eur Respir J 1992; 5:659–664.

77. Hadcroft J, Calverley PM. Alternative methods for assessing bronchodilator reversibility in chronic obstructive pulmonary disease. Thorax 2001; 56:713–720.
78. O'Donnell DE, Forkert L, Webb KA. Evaluation of bronchodilator responses in patients with "irreversible" emphysema. Eur Respir J 2001; 18:914–920.
79. Newton MF, O'Donnell DE, Forkert L. Response of lung volume to inhaled salbutamol in a large population of patients with hyperinflation. Chest 2002; 121:1042–1050.
80. Anthonisen NR, Connett JE, Kily JP, Altose MD, Bailey WC, Buist AS, Conway WA, Enright PL, Kanner RE, O'Hara P, Owens GR, Scanlon PD, Tashkin DP, Wise RA, Lung Health Study Research Group. Effects of smoking intervention and the use of an inhaled anticholinergic bronchodilator on the rate of decline of FEV_1, the lung health study. JAMA 1994; 272:1497–1505.
81. Tashkin DP, Altose MD, Connett JE, Kanner RE, Lee WW, Wise RA. Methacholine reactivity predicts changes in lung function over time in smokers with early chronic obstructive pulmonary disease. The Lung Health Study Research Group. Am J Respir Crit Care Med 1996; 153:1802–1811.
82. Effect of inhaled triamcinolone on the decline in pulmonary function in chronic obstructive pulmonary disease. N Engl J Med 2000; 343:1902–1909.
83. Burge PS, Calverley PM, Jones PW, Spencer S, Anderson JA, Maslen TK. Randomised, double blind, placebo controlled study of fluticasone propionate in patients with moderate to severe chronic obstructive pulmonary disease: the ISOLDE trial. Br Med J 2000; 320(7245):1297–1303.
84. Thurlbeck WM. Pathology of chronic obstructive pulmonary disease. Clin Chest Med 1990; 11:389–404.
85. Stern EJ, Frank MS. CT of the lung in patients with pulmonary emphysema: diagnosis, quantification, and correlation with pathologic and physiologic findings. Am J Radiol 1994; 162:791–798.
86. Remy-Jardin M, Edme JL, Boulenguez C, Remy J, Mastora I, Sobaszek A. Longitudinal follow-up study of smoker's lung with thin-section CT in correlation with pulmonary function tests. Radiology 2002; 222:261–270.
87. Gelb AF, Hogg JC, Muller NL, Schein MJ, Kuei J, Tashkin DP, Epstein JD, Kollin J, Green RH, Zamel N, Elliott WM, Hadjiaghai L. Contribution of emphysema and small airways in COPD. Chest 1996; 109:353–359.
88. Turato G, Zuin R, Miniati M, Baraldo S, Rea F, Beghe B, Monti S, Formichi B, Boschetto P, Harari S, Papi A, Maestrelli P, Fabbri LM, Saetta M. Airway inflammation in severe chronic obstructive pulmonary disease: relationship with lung function and radiologic emphysema. Am J Respir Crit Care Med 2002; 166:105–110.
89. Thomason MJ, Strachan DP. Which spirometric indices best predict subsequent death from chronic obstructive pulmonary disease? Thorax 2000; 55: 785–788.
90. Traver GA, Cline MG, Burrows B. Predictions of mortality in COPD: a 15 year follow-up study. Am Rev Respir Dis 1979; 119:895–902.
91. Weiss ST, Segal MR, Sparrow D, Wager C. Relation of FEV_1 and peripheral

blood leukocyte count to mortality. The normative aging study. Am J Epidemiol 1995; 142:493–498.
92. Tockman MS, Anthonisen NR, Wright EC, Donithan MG. Airways obstruction and the risk for lung cancer. Ann Intern Med 1987; 106:512–518.
93. Tockman MS, Pearson JD, Fleg JL, Metter EJ, Kao SY, Rampal KG, Cruise LJ, Fozard JL. Rapid decline in FEV_1. A new risk factor for coronary heart disease mortality. Am J Respir Crit Care Med 1995; 151:390–398.
94. Marariu C, Ghezzo H, Milic-Emili J, Gautier H. Exercise limitation in obstructive lung disease. Chest 1998; 114:965–968.
95. O'Donnell DE, Bertley JC, Chau KL, Webb KA. Qualitative aspects of exertional breathlessness in chronic airflow limitation: pathophysiologic mechanisms. Am J Respir Crit Care Med 1997; 155:109–115.
96. Prigatano GP, Wright EC, Levin D. Quality of life and its predictors in patients with mild hypoxemia and chronic obstructive pulmonary disease. Arch Intern Med 1984; 144:1613–1619.
97. van Manen JG, Bindels PJ, Dekker EW, Ijzermans CJ, Bottema BJ, van der Zee JS, Schade E. Added value of co-morbidity in predicting health-related quality of life in COPD patients. Respir Med 2001; 95:496–504.
98. Seemungal T, Harper-Owen R, Bhowmik A, Moric I, Sanderson G, Message S, Maccallum P, Meade TW, Jeffries DJ, Johnston SL, Wedzicha JA. Respiratory viruses, symptoms, and inflammatory markers in acute exacerbations and stable chronic obstructive pulmonary disease. Am J Respir Crit Care Med 2001; 164:1618–1623.
99. Eller J, Ede A, Schaberg T, Niederman MS, Mauch H, Lode H. Infective exacerbations of chronic bronchitis: relation between bacteriologic etiology and lung function. Chest 1998; 113:1542–1548.
100. Reisner C, Gondek K, Ferguson GT, Menjoge S, Musheno M, Mandel M. Depression severity and smoking history, but not age and FEV_1, highly correlate with total charges and medical resource utilization in chronic obstructive pulmonary disease. Chest 1998; 114:341S.

3

Exercise Testing

DENIS E. O'DONNELL and KATHERINE A. WEBB

Queen's University
Kingston, Ontario, Canada

I. Introduction

Chronic obstructive pulmonary disease (COPD) is progressively disabling and is a leading cause of death throughout the world. The inability to engage in the usual activities of daily living is one of the most distressing experiences of people afflicted with COPD. Exercise intolerance progresses relentlessly as the disease advances, and can lead to virtual immobility and social isolation. Effective symptom control and improvement of exercise capacity are among the major goals for the management of COPD, and are the primary focus of this review.

Bronchodilators have the potential to improve exercise performance by favorably altering ventilatory mechanics and alleviating respiratory discomfort. In clinical practice, the caregiver detemines whether a bronchodilator has helped by asking the patient a few simple questions: "Did the new treatment help your breathing?" More specifically, if the answer is affirmative: "In what way has it helped you?" If the patient responds that he or she can undertake a particular daily task with less breathlessness or for a longer duration since taking the drug, then the caregiver is usually convinced of the drug's benefit. In clinical trials, the same general approach is taken, except that in this instance, a possible placebo effect is measured, the physical task is standardized, and the effect on dyspnea (for a given stimulus) is carefully quantified. Thus, we can determine whether a new medication consistently improves dyspnea and exercise performance in a population.

Exercise testing is being used increasingly for the evaluation of bronchodilator efficacy. In this review, we will examine the mechanisms of exercise intolerance in COPD. We will discuss the interface between physiological impairment and disability, and how abnormal ventilatory mechanics can be pharmacologically manipulated to achieve clinical benefit. Finally, we will describe and compare the various exercise testing protocols currently used to assess the clinical impact of bronchodilator therapy.

II. Exercise Limitation in COPD

Exercise limitation is multifactorial in COPD. Recognized contributing factors include: (1) intolerable exertional symptoms; (2) ventilatory limitation due to impaired respiratory system mechanics and ventilatory muscle dysfunction; (3) metabolic and gas exchange abnormalities; (4) peripheral muscle dysfunction; (5) cardiac impairment; and (6) any combination of these interdependent factors [1]. The predominant contributing factors to exercise limitation vary among patients with COPD or, indeed, within a given patient over time. The more advanced the disease, the more of these factors come into play in complex integrative manner. In patients with severe COPD, ventilatory limitation and severe dyspnea are often the predominant contributors to exercise intolerance and will, therefore, be discussed in some detail.

A. Ventilatory Constraints on Exercise Performance in COPD

COPD is a heterogeneous disorder characterized by dysfunction of the small and large airways and by parenchymal and vascular destruction, in highly variable combinations. Although the most obvious physiological defect in COPD is expiratory flow limitation, due to reduced lung recoil (and airway tethering effects) as well as intrinsic airway narrowing, the most important mechanical consequence of this is a "restrictive" ventilatory deficit due to dynamic lung hyperinflation (DH) [2–4] (Figs. 1 and 2). When expiratory flow limitation reaches a critical level, lung emptying becomes incomplete during resting tidal breathing and lung volume fails to decline to its natural equilibrium point, i.e., the relaxation volume of the respiratory system. End-expiratory lung volume (EELV), therefore, becomes dynamically and not statically determined, and represents a higher resting lung volume than in health [3]. In flow-limited patients, EELV is therefore a continuous variable, which fluctuates widely with rest and activity. When ventilation (i.e., tidal

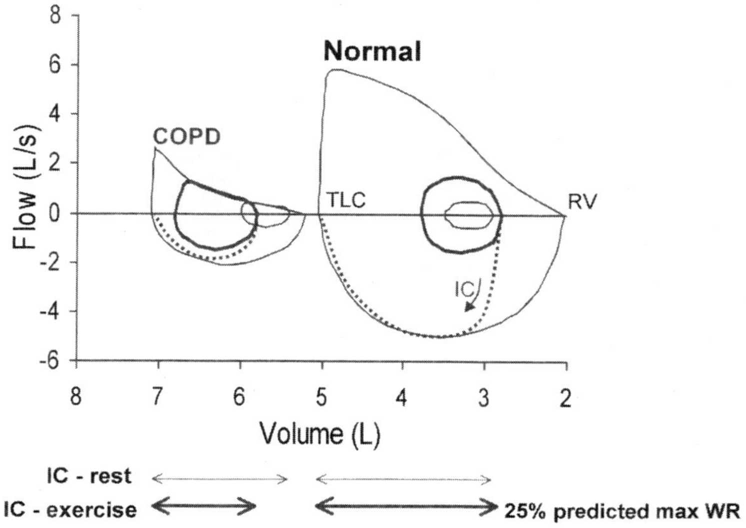

Figure 1 Flow-volume loops showing the effects of exercise on tidal volume in COPD and in health. The outer loops represent the maximal limits of flow and volume. The smallest loops represent the resting tidal volumes. The thicker loops represent the increased tidal volumes and flows seen with exercise. The dotted lines represent the IC maneuver to TLC which is used to anchor tidal flow-volume loops within the respective maximal loops. Healthy subjects are able to increase both their tidal volumes and inspiratory and expiratory flows. In COPD, expiratory flow is already maximal during resting ventilation. Dynamic hyperinflation optimizes expriatory flow rates but causes restrictive mechanics.

volume and/or breathing frequency) increases in flow-limited patients, as for example during exercise, an increase in EELV (or DH) is inevitable (Figs. 1 and 2). DH (and its negative mechanical consequences) can occur in the healthy elderly, but at much higher levels of ventilation and oxygen consumption (VO_2) than in COPD [5–7]. For practical purposes, the extent of DH during exercise depends on the extent of expiratory flow limitation, the level of baseline lung hyperinflation, the prevailing ventilatory demand, and the breathing pattern [2].

The pattern of DH development during exercise in COPD patients is highly variable. Clearly, some patients do not increase EELV during exercise, whereas others show dramatic increases (i.e., >1 L) [2,8,9]. We recently studied the pattern and magnitude of DH during incremental cycle exercise in 105 patients with COPD ($FEV_{1.0} = 37 \pm 13\%$ predicted; mean $\pm$SD) [4]. In contrast to age-matched healthy control subjects, the majority (80%) of this

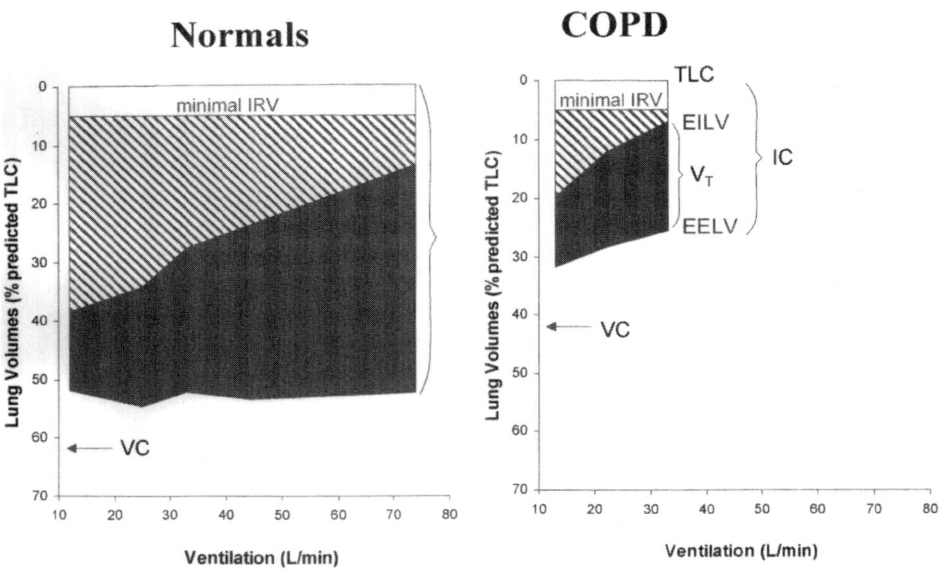

Figure 2 Changes in operational lung volumes are shown as ventilation increases with exercise in 105 COPD patients and in 25 age-matched healthy subjects. End-expiratory lung volume (EELV) increases above the relaxation volume of the respiratory system in COPD, as reflected by a decrease in inspiratory capacity (IC), while EELV in health either remains unchanged or decreases. "Restrictive" constraints on tidal volume (V_T, *solid area*) expansion during exercise are significantly greater in the COPD group from both below (increased EELV) and above (reduced IRV as EILV approaches TLC). (Reproduced with permission from Ref. 2.)

sample demonstrated significant increases in EELV above resting values: on average, dynamic inspiratory capacity (IC) decreased significantly, by 0.37 ± 0.39 L (or $14 \pm 15\%$ predicted; means $\pm$SD) from rest [2]. Similar levels of DH have recently been reported in COPD patients after completing a 6-min walking test while breathing without an imposed mouthpiece [10]. The extent of DH during exercise is inversely correlated with the level of resting lung hyperinflation: patients who were severely hyperinflated at rest showed minimal further DH during exercise [2].

B. Tidal Volume Restriction and Exercise Intolerance

An important mechanical consequence of DH is severe mechanical constraints on tidal volume (V_T) expansion during exercise: V_T is truncated from below by the increasing EELV and constrained from above by the TLC envelope and the relatively reduced inspiratory reserve volume (IRV) (Figs. 1 and 2). Thus, compared with age-matched healthy individuals at a comparable low work rate and ventilation, COPD patients showed substantially greater increases in dynamic end-inspiratory lung volume (EILV), a greater ratio of V_T to IC, and marked reduction in the IRV (Fig. 2). In 105 COPD patients, the EILV was found to be $94 \pm 5\%$ of TLC at a peak symptom-limited VO_2 of only 12.6 ± 5.0 ml/kg/min. At this volume, the diaphragm is maximally shortened and greatly compromised in its ability to generate larger inspiratory pressures [2].

The resting IC [not the resting vital capacity (VC)] and, in particular, the dynamic IC during exercise represent the true operating limits for V_T expansion in any given patient. Therefore, when V_T approximates the peak dynamic IC during exercise or the dynamic EILV encroaches on the TLC envelope, further volume expansion is impossible, even in the face of increased central drive and electrical activation of the diaphragm [11].

In our study, we performed a multiple regression analysis with symptom-limited peak VO_2 as the dependent variable and several relevant physiological measurements as independent variables (including the $FEV_{1.0}$/FVC ratio and the ratio of ventilation to maximal ventilatory capacity). The peak V_T (standardized as percent predicted VC) emerged as the strongest contributory variable, explaining 47% of the variance in peak VO_2 [2]. In turn, the peak V_T correlated strongly with both the resting and peak dynamic IC [2]. This latter correlation was particularly strong ($r = 0.9$) in approximately 80% of the sample who had a diminished resting and peak dynamic IC (i.e., <70% predicted). Tantucci et al. [12] have provided evidence that such patients with a diminished resting IC have demonstrable resting expiratory flow limitation by the negative expiratory pressure (NEP) technique. Recent studies have confirmed that patients with COPD who have a reduced resting IC and evidence of resting expiratory flow limitation have poorer exercise performance when compared with those who have a better-preserved resting IC and no evidence of expiratory flow limitation at rest [2,13,14].

C. Dynamic Hyperinflation and Inspiratory Muscle Dysfunction

While DH serves to maximize tidal expiratory flow rates during exercise, it has serious consequences with respect to dynamic ventilatory mechanics, inspiratory muscle function, perceived respiratory discomfort, and, probably, cardiac function (Table 1). DH results in "high-end," alinear pressure–volume mechanics in contrast to health, in which the relationship between pressure and volume is relatively constant throughout exercise. This results in increased elastic and inspiratory threshold loading [i.e., intrinsic positive end-

Table 1 Negative Effects of Dynamic Lung Hyperinflation During Exercise

↑ Elastic/threshold loads Inspiratory muscle weakness	} ↑ Pes/PI_{max} "effort"
Reduced tidal volume expansion → tachypnea	} ↓ CLdyn ↑ VD/VT ↑ $PaCO_2$
Early ventilatory limitation to exercise	
↑ Exertional dyspnea	
↓ Cardiovascular function	

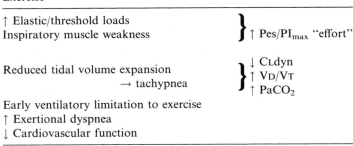

Abbreviations: Pes/PI_{max} = tidal esophageal pressure swing as a fraction of the maximal inspiratory pressure; CLdyn = dynamic lung compliance; VD/VT = physiological dead space; $PaCO_2$ = partial pressure of arterial carbon dioxide.

expiratory pressure (autoPEEP) effect] of muscles already burdened with increased resistive work [3,4,15]. The elastic and resistive loads on the ventilatory muscles substantially increase the mechanical work and the oxygen cost of breathing at a given ventilation in COPD, compared with health.

The tachypnea associated with an increased elastic load causes increased velocity of muscle shortening during exercise, which results in further functional inspiratory muscle weakness [3]. Exercise tachypnea also results in reduced dynamic lung compliance, which has an exaggerated frequency dependence in COPD [3]. DH alters the length tension relationship of the inspiratory muscles, particularly the diaphragm, and compromises its ability to generate pressure. Due to weakened inspiratory muscles and the intrinsic mechanical loads already described, tidal inspiratory pressures represent a high fraction of their maximal force-generating capacity [15–18]. Moreover, DH results in a disproportionate increase in the end-expiratory ribcage volume, which likely decreases the effectiveness of sternocleidomastoid and scalene muscle activity [19]. Therefore, DH may alter the pattern of ventilatory muscle recruitment to a more inefficient pattern, with negative implications for muscle energetics [19].

The net effect of DH during exercise in COPD is that the V_T response to increasing exercise is progressively constrained, despite near-maximal inspiratory efforts [15]. The ratio of respiratory effort [(i.e., the tidal esophageal pressure swings relative to the maximum inspiratory pressure (P_{es}/PI_{max})] to the tidal volume response (i.e., V_T/VC or V_T/predicted VC) is significantly higher at any given work rate or ventilation in COPD compared with health [15].

D. Dynamic Hyperinflation and Dyspnea

Dyspnea intensity during exercise has been shown to correlate well with concomitant measures of dynamic lung hyperinflation [15,20]. In a multiple regression analysis with Borg ratings of exertional dyspnea intensity as the dependent variable, versus a number of independent physiological variables, the change in EILV (expressed as percent of TLC) during exercise emerged as the strongest independent correlate ($r = 0.63$, $p = 0.001$) in 23 patients with advanced COPD (average $FEV_{1.0} = 36\%$ predicted) [20]. The change in EELV and change in V_T (components of EILV) emerged as significant contributors to exertional breathlessness and, together with increased breathing frequency, accounted for 61% of the variance in exercise Borg ratings [20]. A second study showed equally strong correlations between the intensity of perceived inspiratory difficulty during exercise and EILV/TLC ($r = 0.67$, $p < 0.01$) or EELV/TLC ($r = 0.69$, $p < 0.001$) [15] (Fig. 3). Dyspnea intensity also correlated well with the ratio of effort (P_{es}/PI_{max}) to tidal volume response (V_T/VC) [15]. This increased effort–displacement ratio in COPD ultimately reflects neuromechanical dissociation, or uncoupling, of the ventilatory pump.

Further indirect evidence of the importance of DH in contributing to exertional dyspnea in COPD has come from a number of studies. These

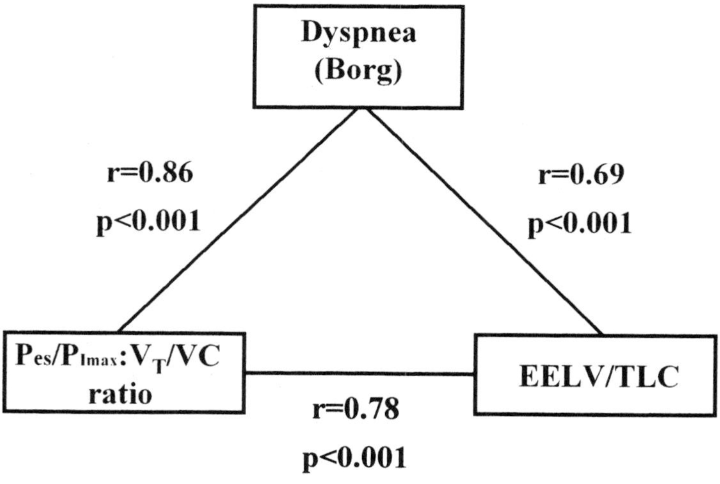

Figure 3 Statistical correlations between Borg dyspnea ratings, end-expiratory lung volume (EELV), and the ratio of inspiratory effort (tidal esophageal pressure relative to the maximum inspiratory pressure, P_{es}/PI_{max}) to the tidal volume response (V_T standardized for vital capacity) at a standardized level of exercise in COPD. (Data from Ref. 15.)

studies showed that dyspnea was effectively ameliorated by interventions that reduced operating lung volumes (either pharmacologically or surgically) or counterbalanced the negative effects of DH on the inspiratory muscles (continuous positive airway pressure) [22–28]. Consistently strong correlations have been reported between reduced Borg ratings of dyspnea and reduced DH during exercise in a number of studies following various bronchodilators and lung volume reduction surgery [21–28] (see below).

E. The Neurophysiological Basis of Exertional Dyspnea in COPD

Current evidence suggests that dyspnea is not only a function of the amplitude of central motor output, but is also importantly modulated by peripheral feedback from a host of respiratory mechanoreceptors (for comprehensive reviews see references [29–32]. Lung and chest wall over-distention may activate vagal receptors in the lung and airways; altering afferent inputs from multiple receptors in the rib cage and associated musculature, as well as from the shortened diaphragm and accessory muscles of breathing [33–35]. A dominant qualitative descriptor of exertional dyspnea selected by COPD patients is the sense of unsatisfied inspiration, i.e., "I can't get enough air in" [15]. We have postulated that this distressing respiratory sensation arises from the inability to expand tidal volume appropriately in the face of an increased inspiratory effort (or increased central drive) during exercise [15]. This disparity between inspiratory effort and the mechanical (volume) response of the respiratory system has been termed neuromechanical dissociation or uncoupling [15]. The psychophysical basis of neuromechanical dissociation likely resides in the complex central processing and integration of signals that mediate (1) central motor command output [36–38], and (2) sensory feedback from various mechanoreceptors that provide precise instantaneous proprioceptive information about muscle displacement (muscle spindles and joint receptors), tension development (Golgi tendon organs), and change in respired volume or flow (lung and airway mechanoreceptors) [39,40]. Awareness of the disparity between effort and ventilatory output may elicit patterned psychological and neurohumoral responses that culminate in respiratory distress, which is an important affective dimension of perceived inspiratory difficulty.

F. How do Bronchodilators Improve Exercise Performance in COPD?

Fundamentally, bronchodilators cause smooth muscle relaxation of the central and peripheral airways. Thus, specific airway resistance diminishes and mean tidal inspiratory and expiratory flow rates increase. When tidal expiratory flow rates increase, lung emptying is enhanced with each breath, thereby reducing air trapping and lung hyperinflation at rest. In more advanced disease, bronchodilators do not actually abolish expiratory flow limitation at rest or during exercise, but permit increased tidal expiratory flow rates over lower operating lung volumes [29,41]. Therefore, as a result of bronchodilators, it is now possible to achieve the required alveolar ventilation at a lower oxygen cost of breathing. It has become clear that improvements in peripheral airway function are not necessarily reflected by a postbronchodilator increase in $FEV_{1.0}$, particularly in more severe COPD. However, reduced lung hyperinflation following bronchodilators provides indirect assessment of improved small-airway function. Substantial decreases in residual volume (RV) and functional residual volume (FRC), with reciprocal increases in VC and IC, often occur when changes in $FEV_{1.0}$ are either minor or absent [42,43]. In fact, in severe disease, there is a poor correlation between changes in lung volumes (VC and RV) and changes in $FEV_{1.0}$ after bronchodilator therapy, indicating that these are largely independent physiological variables [42,43]. Recent studies have shown that greater lung volume responses to single-dose bronchodilator therapy occur in patients with the most severe disease [42].

As previously discussed, the resting IC has been shown to correlate well with symptom-limited peak VO_2 in severe COPD [14]. Therefore, increases in IC (reflecting decreases in hyperinflation) during rest and exercise should delay the onset of critical mechanical limitation to ventilation and should improve dyspnea and exercise performance (see above). β_2-agonists and anticholinergic agents have been shown to reduce absolute lung volumes at rest and during exercise in COPD [22,24]. Moreover, these bronchodilators reduced mechanical restriction, as indicated by an increase in inspiratory reserve volume, during submaximal exercise and at the peak symptom-limited breakpoint of exercise [22,24]. A reduction in restriction allows greater tidal volume expansion, with greater levels of ventilation and a delay in the onset of intolerable dyspnea. Bronchodilators decrease both the elastic and resistive loads on the inspiratory muscles and, therefore, less inspiratory muscle effort is needed for greater tidal volume expansion. It is postulated that relief of exertional dyspnea following pharmacological lung volume reduction is linked to improvements in neuromechanical coupling of the respiratory system.

Based on a number of studies which have examined the effects of pharmacological and surgical volume reduction, improvements in resting IC of approximately 10% predicted (0.3–0.4 L) generally translate into clinically important improvements in dyspnea and exercise capacity [22–27]. Postbronchodilator improvements in resting IC are generally seen in patients who are flow-limited at rest and who have a low baseline IC of <70% predicted [12]. Even though the change in resting RV appears to be the most sensitive index of bronchodilator action (in terms of magnitude of effect), changes in resting and dynamic IC are more closely associated with improvements in both symptom intensity and exercise performance [44].

III. Exercise Testing: Field Tests

A. Timed Walking Distances

Since resting physiological measurements, such as the $FEV_{1.0}$, are poorly predictive of maximal exercise capacity (i.e., peak oxygen consumption) or exercise endurance [2], and since changes in postbronchodilator $FEV_{1.0}$ do not reliably predict improved exercise endurance [9], direct assessment of exercise performance is required to assess functional disability and the impact of therapy [2,9]. Exercise tests vary considerably in their level of sophistication. The simple observation of a patient as he or she walks along the corridor, or climbs a flight of stairs, provides useful qualitative information. Supervised timed walking distances, such as the 12-min walk distance (12-MWD) and the more convenient 6-minute walk distance (6-MWD) tests, have been used extensively as a measure of functional disability [45–48]. Concurrent measurements of dyspnea intensity (using validated scales) and arterial oxygen saturation enhance the value of this test.

Although the 6-MWD is a useful clinical indicator of functional disability and correlates with both morbidity and mortality, it has limitations. Such tests are highly motivation-dependent and it is impossible to control the pace of walking (or power output) during the test. This becomes important particularly when comparisons of two tests are being made in the same individual over time. Since there is also a learning effect during serial testing, particularly in previously inactive patients, it is recommended that two familiarization tests be conducted, and that the final (or best) test should be accepted as the baseline test prior to drug randomization [49,50]. If tests are to be compared over time, great care must be taken by the supervisor to standardize the instruction and encouragement of the patient—something that is often difficult to accomplish [49]. Adequate facilities to conduct the test (i.e., long unimpeded corridors) are also likely to influence test performance and reproducibility. The inability to carry out pertinent physiological measurements during the 6-MWD is a potential disadvantage. Due to these limitations, modifications in timed walking distance tests have been made. For example, 6-min testing using a treadmill, where the power output can be controlled and where physiological measurements can be more easily undertaken, may have advantages over the traditional hallway testing [51,52]. However, the responsiveness of this latter test to bronchodilator therapy remains to be established.

B. Bronchodilators and Walking Distance

The 6-MWD has been shown to be adequately responsive to interventions such as exercise training and volume reduction surgery [53]. However, the sensitivity of the tests for interventions other than exercise training, has been questioned. Modest improvements in walking distance, compared with placebo, have been measured following all bronchodilator classes (Fig. 4). Four studies have examined the effects of ipratropium bromide on walking distance [54–57], only two of which have shown a positive effect [55,56]. This effect on exercise performance tended to be greater with higher dosages of this drug. It is noteworthy that the demonstration of a dose–response curve for exercise endurance, in the setting of a relatively flat $FEV_{1.0}$ response, has previously been demonstrated following oral theophylline therapy [23]. Further studies are clearly required to determine if similar dose-response relationships for symptom relief and improved exercise performance apply to other bronchodilator classes. Two studies showed a significant increase in the 6-MWD (by approximately 20 m) following single-dose oxitropium (200 μg) [58,59]. Six out of seven studies have shown that short-acting β_2-agonists (salbutamol) improved 6 or 12-MWD significantly (reported range 39–100 m), despite only modest changes in $FEV_{1.0}$ [54–56,60–63]. Three studies have

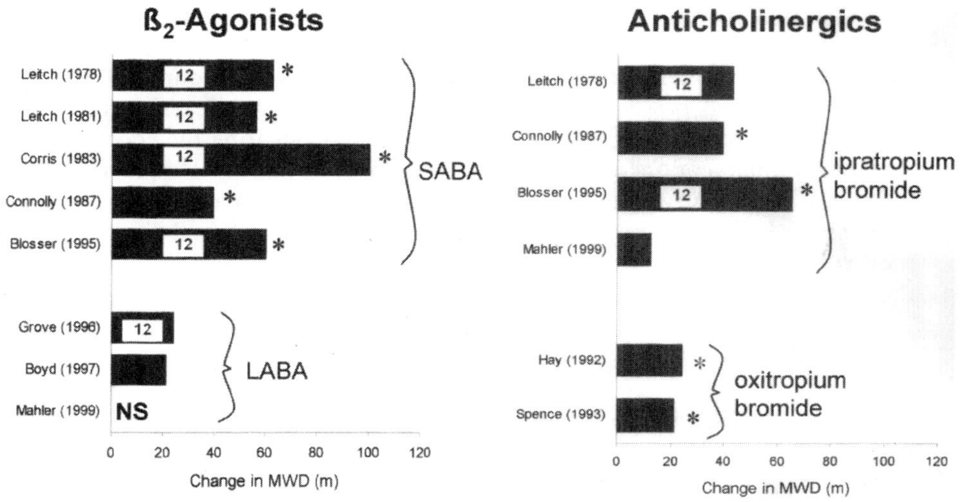

Figure 4 Changes in timed walking distance found in various studies in response to different bronchodilator agents. Tests were 6-MWD unless noted with a "12" as 12-MWD. SABA = short-acting β_2-agonists; LABA = long-acting β_2-agonists. *Significant difference in favor of active drug.

been conducted on the effects on the long-acting β_2-agonist, salmeterol, on walking distance, none of which showed a significant increase compared with placebo [57,64,65].

There is no consensus as to what represents a clinically minimally important improvement in walking distance following a therapeutic intervention. Redelmeier et al. [66] have suggested that a change of 54 m in the 6-MWD is required in order for it to be noticeable to the patient. However, improvements of this magnitude are often not seen with bronchodilator therapy and it can be argued that, on an individual basis, much smaller improvements are clinically meaningful and are readily detectable by patients and their caregivers.

C. The Shuttle Test

The incremental shuttle test was designed to overcome some of the limitations of the 6-MWD, and there is evidence of its reliability and responsiveness, at least to exercise training [67]. With this test, the pace (or work rate) is progressively increased using an auditory cue, which allows observation of the patient over a range of activity levels. The patient walks fixed distances of 10 m between two cones [67,68]. The time available to complete each 10-m distance is progressively decreased, and the distance walked when the patient stops becomes the outcome measure of interest. The test is terminated when patients develop intolerable symptoms and heart rate reaches 85% of maximum.

The endurance shuttle test, performed at a fixed fraction of the preestablished peak power output during the incremental shuttle test, is likely to be more responsive than the incremental test in evaluating the effects of therapeutic interventions such as ambulatory oxygen [69,70]. However, its sensitivity in the evaluation of bronchodilator efficacy remains unknown. There is anecdotal evidence that, in patients with severe functional disability, the 6-MWD is more sensitive in assessing bronchodilator efficacy. However, the shuttle test may prove superior for less disabled patients.

IV. Exercise Testing: Laboratory Tests

A. Cardiopulmonary Exercise Testing (CPET)

Incremental cardiopulmonary exercise testing, performed in a laboratory setting, represents a more rigorous approach to the measurement of physiological and perceptual responses to exercise. It has been argued that incremental testing by cycle ergometry poorly mimics the activities of daily living and therefore may not be relevant in assessing bronchodilator efficacy in symptomatic patients. In general, reported changes in peak symptom-limited

VO_2 and work rates with bronchodilator therapy have been modest, and their clinical relevance remains unknown. Two studies showed small, but statistically significant, increases in peak VO_2 following ipratropium therapy by approximately 40 mL/min [71,72]. As previously indicated with respect to walking tests, higher doses of ipratropium tended to show larger effects on maximal exercise performance. It was unclear whether these modest increases in VO_2 reflected an increase in ventilation following bronchodilation, since peak work rate is often not reported in some studies. Four out of five studies showed a positive effect of oxitropium (200 μg) on peak symptom-limited VO_2 (range 32–182 mL/min) [59,73–76]. The relatively poor responsiveness (ability to detect change) of incremental testing in bronchodilator evaluation was confirmed in a recent study by Oga et al. [77]. In a placebo-controlled study, these authors compared the effects of oxitropium on: (1) peak symptom-limited VO_2 by incremental testing, (2) 6-MWD, and (3) constant-load cycle exercise endurance at 80% of the preestablished peak work rate. In this study, the constant-load cycle test was clearly superior in terms of magnitude of response, suggesting greater sensitivity of this testing protocol for the purposes of bronchodilator evaluation.

B. Constant-Load Exercise Testing

The constant-load cycle exercise test is being used increasingly as a responsive test for evaluating bronchodilator efficacy. When this test is combined with relevant physiological and symptom measurements, it can provide additional valuable insights into the mechanisms of improvement following pharmacological therapy [9]. Constant-load cycle ergometry, at 50–60% of the patients predetermined maximal work rate, has been shown to have excellent reproducibility [9], and to be responsive to interventions such as bronchodilators [9], oxygen therapy [78], and exercise training [79]. Measurements of dyspnea intensity during exercise, using the Borg scale or visual analog scaling methods, have been shown to be reliable and responsive in COPD [9]. The primary symptom that limits exercise should also be recorded following both the active drug and placebo. With effective bronchodilator therapy, dyspnea may be displaced by leg discomfort as the proximate locus of sensory limitation.

V. Failure to Improve Exercise Performance After Bronchodilators

It must be remembered that, regardless of the testing protocol, a lack of improvement in exercise performance does not necessarily mean that the drug is not clinically beneficial. Improvements in exercise endurance would not be anticipated in patients who have good exercise capacity to start with or in patients in whom exercise is limited by factors other than ventilatory constraints and dyspnea. For example, bronchodilators may not improve exercise performance if the proximate limitation of exercise is leg discomfort or is due to musculoskeletal, cardiac, or other comorbidities. Responses to bronchodilator agents may also vary over time in a given individual, and the lack of an acute response in the laboratory does not preclude sustained effects on activity levels in the home.

Gosselink et al. [80], have shown that in COPD, the 6-MWD correlates most closely with measurements of peripheral muscle function. If this is the case, bronchodilators would be expected to have only modest acute effects on the 6-MWD. Finally, lack of improvement may reflect the methodological limitations of studies, i.e., inadequate study sample size, insufficient preliminary training sessions, lack of standardization of instruction and encouragement of patients, differences in pretest bronchodilator therapy, and inadequate facilities to conduct the walking test.

VI. Evaluating Mechanisms of Functional Improvement

A. Quantitative Flow-Volume Loop Analysis

Traditionally, exercise testing has focused on measuring cardiopulmonary responses to exercise. This approach gives little information on dynamic ventilatory mechanics during exercise, which is arguably important to assess in COPD. More recently, quantitative flow-volume loop analysis and the measurement of dynamic operating lung volumes have been employed to evaluate prevailing mechanical abnormalities. In COPD, there is evidence that the change in IC with exercise (which tracks the change in EELV) correlates well with direct mechanical measurements, i.e., the ratio of inspiratory effort (P_{es}/PI_{max}) to the tidal volume response during exercise [15,22]. Therefore, operating dynamic lung volumes can be used as an indirect "noninvasive" assessment of ventilatory mechanics.

As we have seen, operating lung volumes during exercise dictate the length–tension and force–velocity characteristics of the ventilatory muscles, and influence breathing pattern as well as the quality and intensity of dyspnea. Moreover, dynamic volume measurements give clear information about the extent of mechanical restriction during exercise in COPD: the inspiratory reserve volume during exercise provides an indication of the existing constraints on tidal volume expansion [2]. Similarly, the reserves of inspiratory flow can be evaluated by measuring the difference between exercise tidal inspiratory flow rates and those generated at the same volume during a simultaneous maximal IC maneouvre. Changes in dynamic lung volume components during exercise can be evaluated with a combination of serial IC and tidal volume measurements (Figs. 1 and 2).

To evaluate the effects of bronchodilators on exertional dyspnea, comparisons of slopes of Borg dyspnea ratings over time and of Borg dyspnea ratings standardized at isotime (e.g., the highest equivalent time attained during exercise with placebo and active drug) during constant load exercise are likely to be most responsive [9] (Fig. 5). Similarly, to evaluate the effect of bronchodilators on lung hyperinflation during exercise, IC during placebo and active drug should be compared at rest, at a standardized exercise time, and at peak exercise. Comparisons of the rest-to-peak change in IC are likely to be less sensitive than comparisons of standardized IC measurements, since the former may not be different despite a significant reduction in absolute lung volumes (i.e., a parallel shift of the IC/time slope) [9]. Finally, the IC/time slopes may be similar during placebo and the active drug despite increases in ventilation with the latter. The absence of an expected increase in dynamic hyperinflation with an increase in ventilation also indicates improved airway function.

As already mentioned, the crucial abnormality in COPD is expiratory flow limitation. Its presence during exercise is often estimated by measuring

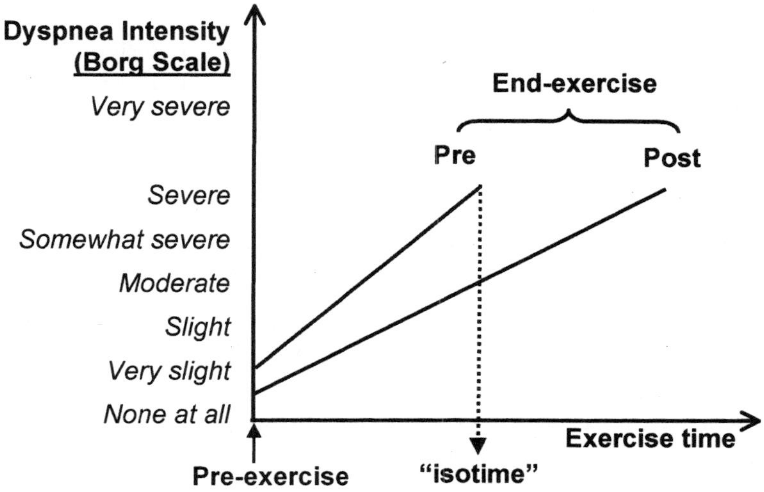

Figure 5 A schematic diagram showing points of analysis for plots of dyspnea intensity (using the modified Borg scale) over time for constant-load exercise tests. Pre- and postintervention comparisons are made pre-exercise (rest), at isotime during exercise, and at symptom-limited end-exercise (peak). Serial tests for each patient are conducted as similarly as possible, using identical work rates at the same time of day.

the extent of overlap of tidal expiratory flow-volume loops with the maximal expiratory flow-volume curve. This assessment provides, at best, imprecise quantitative information about expiratory flow limitation. This "overlap" method may become inaccurate because of errors in placement of the V_T curve on the absolute volume axis due to erroneous IC measurements. In many instances, tidal expiratory flow rates exceed those generated during the VC maneuver at rest. This occurs because of gas and airway compression effects, differences in volume history, and differences in the uniformity of lung emptying during the maximal breath initiated from TLC compared with tidal breathing. Despite these reservations, it is clear that patients with more advanced COPD often have markedly reduced maximal expiratory flow rates at lower lung volumes and, therefore, show complete overlap of the tidal and maximal curves. Expiratory flow limitation can reasonably be assumed to exist in this setting, particularly when there is attendant dynamic hyperinflation. Therefore, in patients who demonstrate dynamic hyperinflation during exercise, tidal expiratory flow rates represent the maximal possible flows that can be generated at that volume. Bronchodilators improve tidal expiratory flow rates and enhance lung emptying, thus increasing IC (Fig. 6).

B. Study Designs Using Constant-Load Protocols

Ideally, a double-blind, placebo-controlled, crossover design should be employed. Thus, patients serve as their own control and the sample size requirement for the study is reduced [9,44]. When the agent being tested has a prolonged half-life and washout period (i.e., tiotropium, inhaled steroids), then a parallel-group design is usually required. Here, a larger study population is needed and matching of the groups in the two arms of the study becomes more challenging. Power and sample size calculations vary with the primary outcome measure of interest for the study. Examples of relevant differences in outcome measures include an improvement in exercise endurance time by 20% of the baseline value, or a reduction in standardized (i.e., isotime exercise) dyspnea ratings by one Borg scale unit.

In general, cycle exercise is the preferred mode of exercise for studies in older patients with COPD. Cycle ergometry is weight supported and does not rely on balance as the treadmill does, it is easy for most patients to perform, and it provides a more consistently stable body position for the measurement of operating lung volumes. Patients should complete an initial incremental CPET to establish the individually targeted constant-load work rate for subsequent testing. Due to a learning effect with repeated exercise testing, study patients should undertake at least two consecutive cycle endurance tests prior to randomization of the intervention. This allows patients to

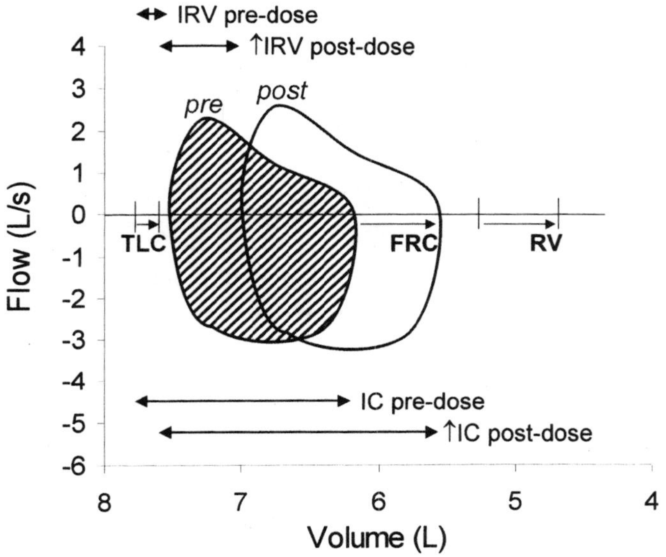

Figure 6 Tidal flow-volume loops are shown at a standardized work rate and time during exercise pre- and postbronchodilator. By reducing airway resistance, bronchodilators improve inspiratory and expiratory flow rates, thus reducing lung hyperinflation and allowing greater tidal volume expansion during exercise. IRV = inspiratory reserve volume; IC = inspiratory capacity; TLC = total lung capacity; FRC = functional residual capacity; RV = residual volume.

become familiar with every aspect of testing, and particularly with subjective measurements. Patients should also be carefully instructed in IC measurement procedures to ensure reproducibility of this test prior to study entry. Detailed methods for these testing procedures are provided elsewhere [2,9].

VII. Utility of Constant-Load Exercise Testing: Examples

A. Short-Acting Anticholinergic Therapy

The effects of nebulized ipratropium bromide (500 μg) were examined in a randomized, double-blind, placebo-controlled, crossover study in 29 patients with advanced COPD ($FEV_{1.0}$ = 40% predicted) [9]. Cycle exercise endurance time at 50–60% of peak work rate improved significantly by 32% of baseline (1.9 min) after ipratropium, with no change after placebo (Fig. 7). IC increased by an average of 14% predicted (0.39 L) at rest, and this difference was

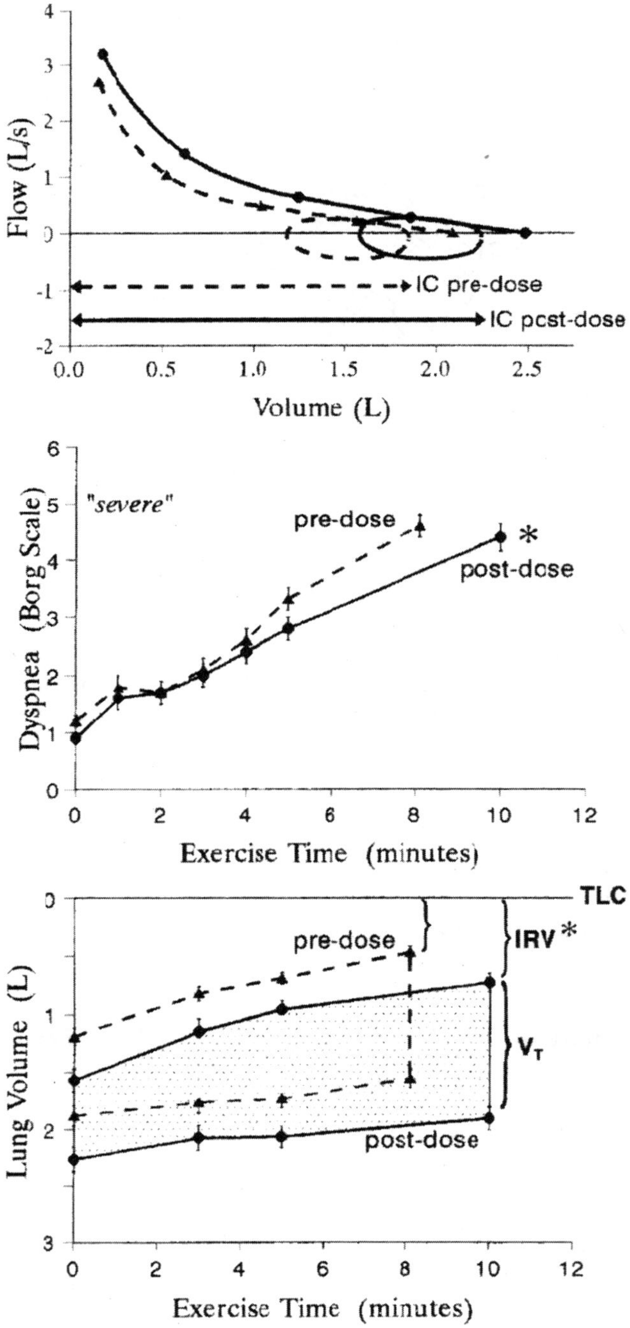
Flow (L/s)
Volume (L)
IC pre-dose
IC post-dose
Dyspnea (Borg Scale)
"severe"
pre-dose
post-dose
*
Exercise Time (minutes)
Lung Volume (L)
TLC
IRV *
V_T
pre-dose
post-dose
Exercise Time (minutes)

maintained throughout exercise. In responses to ipratropium, improvements in dyspnea ratings and exercise endurance times correlated best with the increases in IC, both at rest and at isotime during exercise.

B. Long-Acting β_2-Agonists

The effect of salmeterol on cycle exercise endurance was recently tested in a randomized, double-blind, placebo-controlled, crossover study in 23 patients with COPD ($FEV_{1.0} = 42\%$ predicted) [44]. Measurements were taken after 2 weeks of each intervention: salmeterol (50 mg b.i.d.) or placebo. Exercise endurance time measured at 75% of the peak symptom-limited work rate improved by 39% (1.6 min) after salmeterol, compared with placebo. Salmeterol increased resting IC by 13% predicted (0.33 L), with a continued increase during exercise. This increase in IC allowed greater tidal volume expansion during exercise (Fig. 6), and greater levels of submaximal and peak ventilation (by approximately 3 L/min). As in the previous ipratropium study, improvements in exercise endurance and exertional dyspnea correlated best with increases in resting and dynamic IC after salmeterol. Poor correlations were seen between functional improvement and other volume measurements such as the VC, FVC, and the RV.

C. Long-Acting Anticholinergics

The tiotropium study was the first multinational, multicenter study to employ detailed exercise testing in the evaluation of bronchodilator efficacy, and has shown that such an approach is feasible [81]. Tiotropium bromide is a new selective muscarinic-3 antagonist, which is inhaled once daily using a dry powder dose of 18 μg. A randomized, double-blind, placebo-controlled, parallel-group study, was conducted in 187 patients with advanced COPD ($FEV_{1.0} = 43\%$ predicted, FRC = 160% predicted). Intergroup comparisons of exercise endurance times using a constant-load cycle exercise protocol at 75% of peak symptom-limited work rate were made on days 0, 21, and 42 of the study. Compared with placebo, tiotropium resulted in a progressive increase in endurance time to a mean difference of 105 sec (1.8 min) at day 42. The increase in exercise endurance was associated with a decrease in

---

Figure 7 Responses to nebulized ipratropium bromide (500 μg) are shown. As post-dose maximal expiratory flow-volume relationships improved, tidal flow-volume curves at rest shifted to the right, i.e., an increase in inspiratory capacity (IC) reflected a decrease in lung hyperinflation (*top panel*). Exertional dyspnea decreased significantly ($*p < 0.05$) (*middle panel*). Operating lung volumes improved, i.e., mechanical constraints on tidal volume (V_T) expansion were reduced as IC and inspiratory reserve volume (IRV) increased significantly ($*p < 0.05$) (*lower panel*). (Adapted from Ref. 9.)

exertional dyspnea ratings throughout the course of the study (Fig. 8). As was the case with salmeterol, submaximal and peak V_E increased by 2–3 L/min compared with placebo, reflecting the increased tidal volume expansion capabilities as a result of reduced air trapping. The increases in IC (resting and dynamic), decreases in exertional dyspnea ratings, and the improvements in exercise endurance were closely interrelated in the group receiving tiotropium.

D. Are Acute Increases in Cycle Endurance Times Clinically Important?

The question arises whether acute improvements in exercise endurance measured in the laboratory translate into increases in the activities of daily living in the home. The improvement in endurance time that constitutes a clinically minimally important difference using the constant-load protocol has not been established. It is noteworthy that the peak ventilation, EILV, and VO_2 achieved during constant-load exercise in a number of studies were

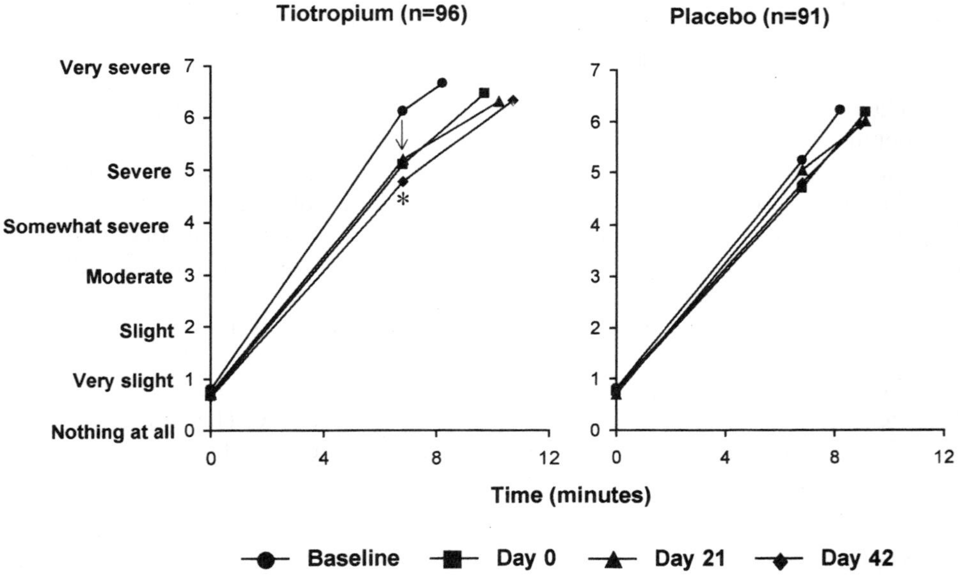

Figure 8 Dyspnea–time plots are shown in response to tiotropium and placebo. *Compared with baseline, exertional dyspnea was significantly reduced at isotime during exercise at days 0, 21, and 42 with tiotropium. Note the progressive improvement in dyspnea and endurance time over the course of the study.

almost identical to the peak measurements achieved during symptom-limited incremental exercise [9,44]. This means that the constant-load protocol is actually a test of maximal exercise performance. Therefore, an improvement in the order of 20% in maximal performance in these severely disabled patients is arguably a clinically relevant improvement, and is comparable in magnitude with the effects seen with other interventions such as ambulatory oxygen [78], exercise training [79], and assisted mechanical ventilation [21] during exercise.

The results of these studies indicate that patients have a greater ventilatory capacity following bronchodilators, and are capable of undertaking a demanding physical task for a longer duration with less respiratory discomfort. In patients with advanced COPD, it has become increasingly clear that small increases in the resting and exercise IC translate into important reductions in elastic work and oxygen cost of breathing.

In the original ipratropium study, prebronchodilator constant-load cycle endurance time was significantly improved from baseline after 3 weeks of regular dosing with the active drug, whereas no such improvement in prebronchodilator endurance time was seen with placebo [9]. The improvements in prebronchodilator endurance time occurred without any increase in the prebronchodilator $FEV_{1.0}$. This suggests that a positive exercise response in the laboratory may predict sustained improvements in exercise performance. Progressive improvement in exercise endurance times during the 42 days of the tiotropium study also suggest additional global skeletal muscle conditioning [81]. In this regard, training effects may arise as a result of spontaneously increased activity levels in the home.

Improvements in exercise performance and dyspnea ratings during the cycle test usually closely correlate with improvements in multidimensional dyspnea questionnaires, such as the Transition Dyspnea Index (TDI), again suggesting that acute improvements in the laboratory herald sustained functional benefits [9]. Clearly, bronchodilators can acutely increase a patient's ability to undertake a given activity. However, to maximally reduce chronic disability, patients should concurrently be encouraged to increase their daily activities, or preferably, to enroll in a structured exercise training program.

VIII. Summary

Exercise testing is being used increasingly as part of the clinical evaluation of bronchodilator efficacy. Bronchodilators improve exercise performance by improving dynamic ventilatory mechanics and by delaying the onset of intolerable exertional dyspnea. Improved exercise performance in response to bronchodilators often occurs in the absence of acute changes in the $FEV_{1.0}$.

New evidence is emerging that all classes of bronchodilating agents can improve dynamic small-airway function and enhance lung emptying, both at rest and during exercise. This pharmacological lung volume reduction explains, in part, the decrease in exertional dyspnea and the increase in ventilatory capacity and exercise endurance in COPD. A variety of field and laboratory tests are available that provide different, but complementary, information about the magnitude of bronchodilator effects. Constant-load endurance exercise protocols, when combined with quantitative flow-volume loop analysis and accurate measurement of dyspnea (using validated questionnaires), can provide valuable insight into the mechanisms of both symptom and functional improvements.

References

1. O'Donnell DE. Exercise limitation and clinical exercise testing in chronic obstructive pulmonary disease. In: Weisman I, Zeballos J, eds. Clinical Exercise Testing. Progress in Respiration Research Karger 2002; 32:138–158.
2. O'Donnell DE, Revill S, Webb KA. Dynamic hyperinflation and exercise intolerance in COPD. Am J Respir Crit Care Med 2001; 164:770–777.
3. Pride NB, Macklem PT. Lung mechanics in disease. In: Fishman AP, ed. Handbook of Physiology, Section 3, Vol. III, Part 2. The Respiratory System. Bethesda, MD: American Physiological Society, 1986:659–692.
4. Younes M. Determinants of thoracic excursions during exercise. In: Whipp BJ, Wasserman K, eds. Lung Biology in Health and Disease, Vol. 42. Exercise, Pulmonary Physiology and Pathophysiology. New York: Marcel Dekker, 1991: 1–65.
5. Johnson BD, Weisman IM, Zeballos RJ, Beck KC. Emerging concepts in the evaluation of ventilatory limitation during exercise: the exercise tidal flow-volume loop. Chest 1999; 116:488–503.
6. Johnson BD, Dempsey JA. Demand vs capacity in the aging pulmonary system. In: Holloszy JO, ed. Exercise and Sports Science Reviews. Baltimore: Williams & Wilkins, 1991:171–210.
7. Johnson BD, Reddan DF, Pegelow KC, Seow KC, Dempsey JA. Flow limitation and regulation of functional residual capacity during exercise in a physically active aging population. Am Rev Respir Dis 1991; 143:960–967.
8. Stubbing DG, Pengelly LD, Morse JLC, Jones NL. Pulmonary mechanics during exercise in subjects with chronic airflow obstruction. J Appl Physiol 1980; 49:511–515.
9. O'Donnell DE, Lam M, Webb KA. Measurement of symptoms, lung hyperinflation and endurance during exercise in chronic obstructive pulmonary disease. Am J Respir Crit Care Med 1998; 158:1557–1565.
10. Marin JM, Carrizo SJ, Gascon M, Sanchez A, Gallego BA, Celli BR. Inspiratory capacity, dynamic hyperinflation, breathlessness and exercise performance dur-

ing the 6-minute-walk test in chronic obstructive pulmonary disease. Am J Respir Crit Care Med 2001; 163:1395–1399.
11. Sinderby C, Spahija J, Beck J, Kaminski D, Yan S, Comtois N, Sliwinski B. Diaphragm activation during exercise in chronic obstructive pulmonary disease. Am J Respir Crit Care Med 2001; 163:1637–1641.
12. Tantucci C, Duguet A, Similowski T, Zelter M, Derenne JP, Milic-Emili J. Effect of salbutamol on dynamic hyperinflation in chronic obstructive pulmonary disease patients. Eur Respir J 1998; 12:799–804.
13. Eltayara L, Becklake MR, Volta CA, Milic-Emili J. Relationship between chronic dyspnea and expiratory flow limitation in patients with chronic obstructive pulmonary disease. Am J Respir Crit Care Med 1996; 154:1726–1734.
14. Diaz O, Villafranco C, Ghezzo H, Borzone G, Leiva A, Milic-Emili J, Lisboa C. Exercise tolerance in COPD patients with and without tidal expiratory flow limitation at rest. Eur Respir J 2000; 16:269–275.
15. O'Donnell DE, Chau LKL, Bertley JC, Webb KA. Qualitative aspects of exertional breathlessness in chronic airflow limitation: pathophysiologic mechanisms. Am J Respir Crit Care Med 1997; 155:109–115.
16. Leblanc P, Summers E, Inman MD, Jones NL, Campbell EJ, Kilian KJ. Inspiratory muscles during exercise: a problem of supply and demand. J Appl Physiol 1988; 64:2482–2489.
17. Rochester DF, Braun NMT. Determinants of maximal inspiratory pressure in chronic obstructive pulmonary disease. Am Rev Respir Dis 1970; 132:42–47.
18. Killian KJ, Jones NI. Respiratory muscles and dyspnea. Clin Chest Med 1988; 9:237–248.
19. Grimby G, Bunn J, Mean J. Relative contribution of rib cage and abdomen to ventilation during exercise. J Appl Physiol 1968; 24:159–166.
20. O'Donnell DE, Webb KA. Exertional breathlessness in patients with chronic airflow limitation: the role of hyperinflation. Am Rev Respir Dis 1993; 148:1351–1357.
21. O'Donnell DE, Sanii R, Younes M. Improvements in exercise endurance in patients with chronic airflow limitation using CPAP. Am Rev Respir Dis 1988; 138:1510–1514.
22. Belman MJ, Botnick WC, Shin JW. Inhaled bronchodilators reduce dynamic hyperinflation during exercise in patients with chronic obstructive pulmonary disease. Am J Respir Crit Care Med 1996; 153:967–975.
23. Chrystyn H, Mulley BA, Peake MD. Dose response relation to oral theophylline in severe chronic obstructive airways disease. Br Med J 1988; 297:1506–1510.
24. O'Donnell DE, Lam M, Webb KA. Spirometric correlates of improvement in exercise performance after anticholinergic therapy in COPD. Am J Respir Crit Care Med 1999; 160:542–549.
25. Martinez FJ, Montes de Oca M, Whyte RI, Stetz J, Gay SE, Celli BR. Lung-volume reduction improves dyspnea, dynamic hyperinflation and respiratory muscle function. Am J Respir Crit Care Med 1997; 155:1984–1990.
26. Laghi F, Jurban A, Topeli A, Fahey PH, Garrity F Jr, Archids JM, DePinto DJ, Edwards LC, Tobin MJ. Effect of lung volume reduction surgery on neuro-

mechanical coupling of the diaphgram. Am J Respir Crit Care Med 1998; 157:475–483.
27. O'Donnell DE, Bertley J, Webb KA, Conlan AA. Mechanisms of relief of exertional breathlessness following unilateral bullectomy and lung volume reduction surgery in advanced chronic airflow limitation. Chest 1996; 110:18–27.
28. Petrof BJ, Calderini E, Gottfried SB. Effect of CPAP on respiratory effort and dyspnea during exercise in severe COPD. J Apply Physiol 1990; 69:178–188.
29. Meek PM, Schwartzstein RMS, Adams L, Altose MD, Breslin EH, Carrieri-Kohlman V, Gift A, Hanley MV, Harver A, Jones PW, Killian K, Knobel A, Lareau S, Mahler DA, O'Donnell DE, Steele B, Stuhlbarg M, Title M. Dyspnea mechanism, assessment and management: a consensus statement (American Thoracic Society). Am J Respir Crit Care Med 1999; 159:321–340.
30. O'Donnell DE. Exertional breathlessness in chronic respiratory disease. In: Mahler DA, ed. Lung Biology in Health and Disease, Vol III: Dyspnea. New York: Marcel Dekker, Inc., 1998:97–147.
31. Killian KJ, Campbell EJM. Dyspnea. In: Roussos C, Macklem PT, eds. Lung Biology in Health and Disease, Vol 29 (Part B). The Thorax. New York: Marcel Dekker, Inc., 1985:787–828.
32. Altose M, Cherniack N, Fishman AP. Respiratory sensations and dyspnea: perspectives. J Appl Physiol 1985; 58:1051–1054.
33. Noble MIM, Eisele JH, Trenchard D, Guz A. Effect of selective peripheral nerve blocks on respiratory sensations. In: Porter R, ed. Breathing: Hering-Breyer Symposium. London: Churchill, 1970:233–246.
34. Zechman FR Jr, Wiley RL. Afferent inputs to breathing: respiratory sensation. In: Fishman AP ed. Handbook of Physiology, Section 3, Vol II, Part 2. The Respiratory System. Bethesda, MD: American Physiology Society, 1986:449–474.
35. Roland PE, Ladegaard-Pederson HA. A quantitative analysis of sensation of tension and kinaesthesia in man: evidence for peripherally originating muscular sense and a sense of effort. Brain 1977; 100:671–692.
36. Chen Z, Eldridge FL, Wagner PG. Respiratory associated rhythmic firing of midbrain neurones in cats: relation to level of respiratory drive. J Appl Physiol 1991; 437:305–325.
37. Chen Z, Eldridge FL, Wagner PG. Respiratory-associated thalamic activity is related to level of respiratory drive. Respir Physiol 1992; 90:99–113.
38. Davenport PW, Friedman WA, Thompson FJ, Franzen O. Respiratory-related cortical potentials evoked by inspiratory occlusion in humans. J Appl Physiol 1986; 60:1843–1948.
39. Gandevia SC, Macefield G. Projection of low threshold afferents from human intercostal muscles to the cerebral cortex. Respir Physiol 1989; 77:203–214.
40. Homma I, Kanamara A, Sibuya M. Proprioceptive chest wall afferents and the effect on respiratory sensation. In: Von Euler C, Katz-Salamon M, eds. Respiratory Psychophysiology. New York: Stockton Press, 1988:161–166.
41. Pellegrino R, Rodarte JR, Brusasco V. Assessing the reversibility of airway obstruction. Chest 1998; 114:1607–1612.

42. Newton MF, O'Donnell DE, Forkert L. Response of lung volume to inhaled salbutamol in a large population of patients with severe hyperinflation. Chest 2002; 121:1042–1050.
43. O'Donnell DE, Forkert L, Webb KA. Evaluation of bronchodilator responses in patients with "irreversible" emphysema. Eur Respir J 2001; 18:914–920.
44. O'Donnell DE, Webb KA. Mechanisms of improved exercise performance in response to salmeterol therapy in COPD. Am J Respir Crit Care Med 2002; 165:A506.
45. McGavin CR, Gupta SP, McHardy G. Twelve-minute walking test for assessing disability in chronic bronchitis. Br Med J 1976; 1:822–823.
46. Butland RJA, Pang J, Gross ER, Woodcock AA, Geddes DM. Two-, 6-, and 12-minute walking tests in respiratory disease. Br Med J 1982; 284:1607–1608.
47. Guyatt GH, Sullivan MJ, Thompson PJ, Fallen EL, Pugsley SO, Taylor DW, Berman L. The 6-minute walk: a new measure of exercise capacity in patients with chronic heart failure. Can Med Assoc J 1985; 132:919–923.
48. Solway S, Brooks D, Lacasse Y, Thomas S. A qualitative systemic overview of the measurement properties of functional walk tests used in the cardiorespiratory domain. Chest 2001; 119:256–270.
49. Guyatt GH, Pugsley SO, Sullivan MJ, Thompson PJ, Berman L, Jones NL, Fallen EL, Taylor DW. Effect of encouragement on walking test performance. Thorax 1984; 39:818–822.
50. Knox AJ, Morrison JF, Muers MF. Reproducibility of walking test results in chronic obstructive airways disease. Thorax 1988; 43:388–392.
51. Stevens D, Elpern E, Sharma K, Szidon P, Ankin M, Kesten S. Comparison of hallway and treadmill six-minute walk tests. Am J Respir Crit Care Med 1999; 160:1540–1543.
52. Swerts PM, Mostert R, Wouters EF. Comparison of corridor and treadmill walking in patients with severe chronic obstructive pulmonary disease. Phys Ther 1990; 70:439–442.
53. Enright PL, Sherrill DL. Reference equations for the six-minute walk in healthy adults. Am J Respir Crit Care Med 1998; 158:1384–1387.
54. Leitch AG, Hopkin JM, Ellis DA, et al. The effect of aerosol ipratropium bromide and salbutamol on exercise tolerance in chronic bronchitis. Thorax 1978; 33:711–713.
55. Connolly CK, Chan NS. Salbutamol and ipratropium in partially reversible airway obstruction. Br J Dis Chest 1987; 81:55–61.
56. Blosser SA, Maxwell SL, Reeves HM, et al. Is an anticholinergic agent superior to a β_2-agonist in improving dyspnea and exercise limitation in COPD? Chest 1995; 108:730–735.
57. Mahler DA, Donohue JF, Barbee RA, et al. Efficacy of salmeterol xinafoate in the treatment of COPD. Chest 1999; 115:957–965.
58. Hay JG, Stone P, Carter J, et al. Bronchodilator reversibility, exercise performance and breathlessness in stable chronic obstructive pulmonary disease. Eur Respir J 1992; 2:659–664.
59. Spence DP, Hay JG, Carter J, et al. Oxygen desaturation and breathlessness

during corridor walking in chronic obstructive pulmonary disease: effect of oxitropium bromide. Thorax 1993; 48:1145–1150.
60. Leitch AG, Morgan A, Ellis DA, et al. Effect of oral salbutamol and slow-release aminophylline on exercise tolerance in chronic bronchitis. Thorax 1981; 36:787–789.
61. Shah SS, Johnston D, Woodcock AA, et al. Breathlessness and exercise tolerance in chronic airflow obstruction: 2-hourly versus 4-hourly salbutamol by inhalation. Curr Med Res Opin 1983; 8:345–349.
62. Corris PA, Neville E, Nariman S, et al. Dose-response study of inhaled salbutamol powder in chronic airflow obstruction. Thorax 1983; 38:292–296.
63. Mohammed AF, Anderson K, Matusiewicz SP, et al. Effect of controlled-release salbutamol in predominantly non-reversible chronic airflow obstruction. Respir Med 1991; 85:495–500.
64. Grove A, Lipworth BJ, Reid P, et al. Effects of regular salmeterol on lung function and exercise capacity in patients with chronic obstructive airways disease. Thorax 1996; 51:689–693.
65. Boyd G, Morice AH, Poundsford JC, et al. An evaluation of salmeterol in the treatment of chronic obstructive pulmonary disease (COPD). Eur Respir J 1997; 10:815–821.
66. Redelmeier DA, Bayoumi AM, Goldstein RS, et al. Interpreting small differences in functional status: the six minute walk test in chronic lung disease patients. Am J Respir Crit Care Med 1997; 155:1278–1282.
67. Singh SJ, Morgan MD, Scott S, Walters D, Harman AB. Development of a shuttle walking test of disability in patients with chronic airways obstruction. Thorax 1992; 47:1019–1024.
68. Singh SJ, Morgan MD, Hardman AE, Rowe C, Bardsley PA. Comparison of oxygen uptake during a conventional treadmill test and the shuttle walking test in chronic airflow limitation. Eur Respir J 1994; 7:2016–2020.
69. Revill SM, Morgan MD, Singh SJ, Williams J, Hardman AB. The endurance shuttle test: a new field test for the assessment of endurance capacity in chronic obstructive pulmonary disease. Thorax 1999; 54:213–222.
70. Revill SM, Singh SJ, Morgan MD. Randomized controlled trial of ambulatory oxygen and an ambulatory ventilator on endurance exercise in COPD. Respir Med 2000; 94:778–783.
71. Ikeda A, Nishimura K, Koyama H, et al. Dose response study of ipratropium bromide aerosol on maximum exercise performance in stable patients with chronic obstructive pulmonary disease. Thorax 1996; 53:48–53.
72. Tsukino M, Nishimura K, Ikeda A, et al. Effects of theophylline and ipratropium bromide on exercise performance in patients with stable chronic obstructive pulmonary disease. Thorax 1998; 53:269–273.
73. Ikeda A, Nishimura K, Koyama H, et al. Oxitropium bromide improves exercise performance in patients with COPD. Chest 1994; 106:1740–1745.
74. Teramoto S, Fukuchi Y, Orimo H. Effects of inhaled anticholinergic drug on dyspnea and gas exchange during exercise in patients with chronic obstructive pulmonary disease. Chest 1993; 103:1774–1782.

75. Teramoto S, Fukuchi Y. Improvements in exercise capacity and dyspnea by inhaled anticholinergic drug in elderly patients with chronic obstructive pulmonary disease. Age Ageing 1995; 24:278–282.
76. Teramoto S, Matsuse T, Sudo E, et al. Long-term effects of inhaled anticholinergic drug on lung function, dyspnea, and exercise capacity in patients with chronic obstructive pulmonary disease. Intern Med 1996; 35:772–778.
77. Oga T, Nishimura K, Tsukino M, Hajiro T, Ikeda A, Izumi T. The effects of oxitropium bromide on exercise performance in patients with stable chronic obstructive pulmonary disease. A comparison of three different exercise tests. Am J Respir Crit Care Med 2000; 161:1897–1901.
78. O'Donnell, D'Arsigny Webb KA. Effects of hyperoxia on ventilatory limitation during exercise in advanced chronic obstructive pulmonary disease. Am J Respir Crit Care Med 2001; 163:892–898.
79. O'Donnell DE, McGuire M, Samis L, Webb KA. The impact of exercise reconditioning on breathlessness in severe chronic airflow limitation. Am J Respir Crit Care Med 1995; 152:2005–2013.
80. Gosselink R, Troosters T, Decramer M. Peripheral muscle weakness contributes to exercise limitation in COPD. Am J Respir Crit Care Med 1996; 153:976–980.
81. O'Donnell DE, Magnussen H, Aguilaniu B, Gerken F, Hamilton A, Fluge T. Spiriva® (tiotropium) improves exercise tolerance in COPD. Am J Respir Crit Care Med 2002; 165:A227.

4

Sleep-Related Breathing Disturbances in COPD

WALTER T. McNICHOLAS

University College Dublin and St. Vincent's University Hospital
Dublin, Ireland

I. Introduction

Sleep is a complex process involving recurring cycles of non-rapid-eye-movement and rapid-eye-movement (REM) sleep, each cycle lasting 90–120 min. Electroencephalographic (EEG) signals differ from those of wakefulness, particularly during non-REM sleep. The exact function of sleep is unclear, but there is no doubt that it is an essential restorative process as evidenced by experiments that have examined the physical and behavioral consequences of sleep deprivation.

Sleep has well-recognized effects on breathing, which in normal individuals have no adverse impact. These effects include a mild degree of hypoventilation with consequent hypercapnia, and a diminished responsiveness to respiratory stimuli. However, in patients with chronic lung disease such as chronic obstructive pulmonary disease (COPD), these physiological changes during sleep may have a profound effect on gas exchange, and episodes of profound hypoxemia may develop, particularly during REM sleep [1], which may predispose to death at night, particularly during acute exacerbations [2]. Furthermore, COPD has an adverse impact on sleep quality itself [3], which may contribute to the complaints of fatigue and lethargy that are well-recognized features of the condition [4].

Impact of Sleep in COPD

1. **Impaired gas exchange**

    Hypoxaemia—particularly during REM sleep
    Hypercapnia—usually mild

2. **Disturbed sleep quality**

    Diminished slow-wave and REM sleep
    Frequent arousals

II. Effects of Sleep on Respiration

The effects of sleep on respiration include changes in central respiratory control, airway resistance, and muscular contractility. A schematic outline of the effects of sleep on respiration is given in Fig. 1.

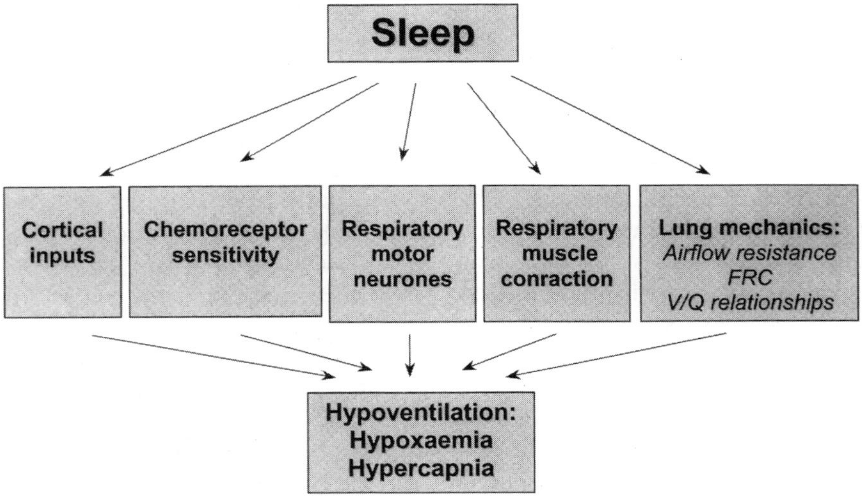

Figure 1 Schematic diagram of the effects of sleep on respiration. In each case, sleep has a negative influence, which has the overall impact of producing hypoventilation and/or hypoxemia and hypercapnia. (FRC = functional residual capacity; V/Q = ventilation-perfusion.)

A. Central Respiratory Effects

Sleep is associated with a diminished responsiveness of the respiratory center to chemical, mechanical, and cortical inputs, particularly during REM sleep [5,6]. Furthermore the respiratory muscles' responsiveness to respiratory center outputs are also diminished during sleep, again particularly during REM, although the diaphragm is less affected than the accessory muscles in this regard. Minute ventilation falls during non-REM and more so during REM sleep, predominantly because of a reduction in tidal volume [7]. During REM sleep, both tidal volume and respiratory frequency are much more variable than in non-REM sleep, particularly during phasic REM. These physiological changes are not associated with any clinically significant deterioration in gas exchange among normal subjects, but may produce profound hypoxemia in patients with respiratory insufficiency [1].

B. Airway Resistance

Normal subjects demonstrate circadian changes in airway caliber, with mild nocturnal bronchoconstriction. Although there have been no published studies on circadian changes in airway caliber among patients with COPD, an exaggerated nocturnal bronchoconstriction among asthmatic patients has been described [8]. An increased cholinergic tone at night is thought to be an important contributor to these changes.

C. Ribcage and Abdominal Contribution to Breathing

The ribcage contribution to breathing is reduced during REM sleep compared with wakefulness and non-REM sleep because of a marked reduction in intercostal muscle activity, whereas diaphragmatic contraction is little affected [9,10]. This fall in intercostal musle activity assumes particular clinical significance in patients who are particularly dependent on accessory muscle activity to maintain ventilation, such as those with COPD, in whom lung hyperinflation reduces the efficiency of diaphragmatic contraction [11].

D. Functional Residual Capacity

A modest reduction in functional residual capacity (FRC) occurs during both non-REM and REM sleep [12], which does not cause significant ventilation to perfusion mismatching in healthy subjects, but can do so, with resulting hypoxemia, in patients with chronic lung disease [13]. Possible mechanisms responsible for this reduction include respiratory muscle hypotonia, cephalad displacement of the diaphragm, and a decrease in lung compliance.

III. Sleep in Chronic Obstructive Pulmonary Disease

Sleep is associated with adverse effects in patients with COPD, principally disordered gas exchange and disturbances in sleep quality. Sleep-related hypoxemia and hypercapnia are well recognized in COPD, particularly during REM sleep, and may contribute to the development of cor pulmonale. Furthermore, COPD patients are particularly likely to die at night, especially if hypoxemic [2]. Nocturnal hypoxemia is most common in "blue-bloater" type patients, who also have a greater degree of awake hypoxemia and hypercapnia than "pink-puffer" type patients [13]. In addition, Fletcher and colleagues have reported that many patients with awake arterial PO_2 (PaO_2) levels in the mildly hypoxemic range can also develop clinically significant nocturnal oxygen desaturation, which appears to predispose to the development of pulmonary hypertension [14].

IV. Mechanisms of Nocturnal Oxygen Desaturation in COPD

Current concepts indicate that nocturnal oxygen desaturation in COPD is largely a consequence of physiological hypoventilation during sleep, with an additional contribution from the impact on gas exchange of altered ventilation to perfusion matching within the lung. Coexisting sleep apnea contributes to nocturnal oxygen desaturation only in a minority of patients with COPD.

A. Hypoventilation

Studies using noninvasive methods of quantifying respiration have shown evidence of sleep-related hypoventilation, particularly during REM sleep, which is associated with periods of hypoxemia in patients with COPD [15–17]. There is a close relationship between the awake PaO_2 and nocturnal oxygen saturation (SaO_2) levels. It is likely that nocturnal oxygen desaturation in patients with COPD is largely the consequence of the combined effects of physiologic hypoventilation during sleep and the fact that hypoxemic patients show a proportionately greater fall in SaO_2 with hypoventilation than normoxemic patients, because of the fact that hypoxemic patients are on, or close to, the steep portion of the oxyhemoglobin dissociation curve.

B. Altered Ventilation-to-Perfusion Relationships

The reduction in accessory muscle contribution to breathing, particularly during REM sleep, results in a decreased FRC, and contributes to worsening ventilation to perfusion relationships during sleep, which also aggravates hypoxemia in COPD. We have demonstrated that transcutaneous PCO_2 ($PtcCO_2$) levels rise to a similar extent in those COPD patients who develop major nocturnal oxygen desaturation as in those who developed only a minor degree of desaturation [16],which suggests a similar degree of hypoventilation in both groups, despite the different degrees of nocturnal oxygen desaturation. The much larger fall in PaO_2 among the major desaturators as compared with the minor desaturators, in conjunction with the similar rise in $PtcCO_2$ in both patient groups, suggests that in addition to a degree of hypoventilation operating in all patients, other factors such as ventilation to perfusion mismatching must also play a part in the excess desaturation of some COPD patients.

C. Coexisting Sleep Apnea Syndrome

The incidence of sleep apnea syndrome in patients with COPD is about 10–15%, which is somewhat higher than would be expected in a normal population of similar age [18]. Factors that may predispose to sleep apnea in patients with COPD include impaired respiratory drive, particularly in "blue-bloater" type COPD patients. Patients with co-existing COPD and sleep apnea typically develop more severe hypoxemia during sleep because such patients may be hypoxemic at the commencement of each apnea, whereas patients with pure sleep apnea tend to resaturate to normal SaO_2 levels in between apneas. Therefore, they are particularly prone to the complications of chronic hypoxemia, such as cor pulmonale and polycythemia.

Mechanisms of Nocturnal Oxygen Desaturation:

1. **Hypoventilation—most important factor**
2. **Impact of oxyhemoglobin dissociation curve**
3. **Ventilation to perfusion mismatching**
4. **Coexisting sleep apnea—only slightly more common in COPD patients than in the general population**

V. Consequences of Nocturnal Hypoxaemia in COPD

Patients with COPD, particularly during exacerbations, have clearly been shown to be at particular risk while asleep, especially from cardiac arrhythmias and death. Ventricular arrhythmias are particularly common in exacerbations during sleep and can be prevented by the correction of hypoxemia

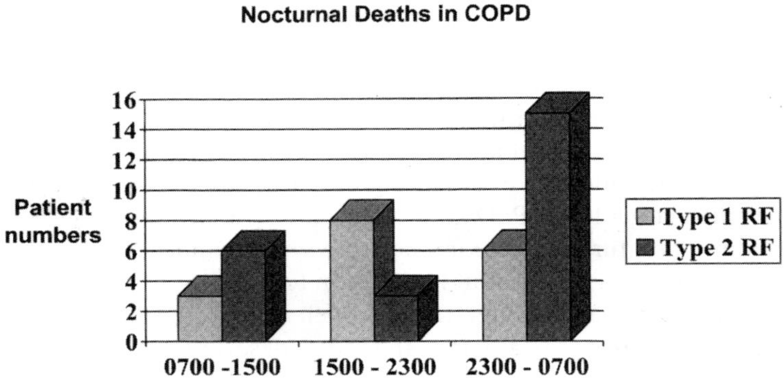

Figure 2 Time of death among patients with COPD comparing those with Type 1 and Type 2 respiratory failure (RF) and demonstrating a significant excess of death at night among those with Type 2 failure. (Adapted from McNicholas WT, FitzGerald MX. Nocturnal death among patients with chronic bronchitis and emphysema. Br Med J 1984; 289: 878.)

[19,20]. Furthermore, a previous report from this department has demonstrated that patients who die in hospital with an exacerbation of COPD are significantly more likely to die at night, in contrast to patients who die from stroke or neoplasm [2]. The excess nocturnal mortality was seen only in patients with severe hypoxemia and hypercapnia (Type 2 respiratory failure), whereas nonhypercapnic patients (Type 1 patients) showed no excess in nocturnal mortality (Fig. 2). These considerations emphasise the importance of adequate monitoring of patients with exacerbations of COPD while asleep.

Consequences of Nocturnal Hypoxemia

1. **Cor pulmonale**
2. **Nocturnal dysrhythmias**
3. **Nocturnal death**

VI. Sleep Quality in COPD

Sleep quality is impaired in patients with COPD, which is likely an important factor in the chronic fatigue, lethargy, and overall impairment in quality of life described by these patients [3,4]. Sleep tends to be fragmented, with frequent arousals and diminished amounts of slow-wave and REM sleep. Unfortunately, sleep impairment is an aspect of COPD that is frequently ignored by many physicians, even in research protocols designed to assess the impact of COPD on quality of life. This aspect assumes particular importance in the context of assessing the impact of pharmacological therapy on quality of life in patients with COPD, since pharmacological agents that improve sleep quality in COPD are likely to have a beneficial clinical impact over and above that associated simply with improvements in lung mechanics and gas exchange, particularly in terms of fatigue and overall energy levels.

VII. Contrasts with Exercise

The mechanisms of hypoxemia during sleep contrast with those during exercise, in which, in the latter, the normal physiological increase in ventilation and in lung volumes during exercise are limited in COPD because of the effects of increased airflow resistance, inadequate ventilatory response, and lack of reduction in dead space. These factors combine to cause relative hypoventilation and V/Q disturbances, leading to hypoxemia in some patients [21].

We have reported that patients with COPD desaturate more than twice as much during sleep than during maximal exercise [17], which contrasts with the findings in patients with interstitial lung disease, who develop greater desaturation during exercise than sleep [22]. This greater O_2 desaturation during sleep supports the finding that in patients with COPD, the demand for coronary blood flow during episodes of nocturnal hypoxemia can be transiently as great as during maximal exercise [23]. This increased myocardial oxygen demand may be a factor in the nocturnal arrhythmias and the higher nocturnal death rate among patients with COPD, particularly since the level of exercise achieved during these studies was much greater than patients would normally reach during daily activities. Nocturnal oxygen desaturation also appears to be important in the development of pulmonary hypertension, even in the absence of significant awake hypoxemia [14].

VIII. Investigation of Sleep-Related Breathing Disturbances in COPD

The serious and potentially life-threatening disturbances in ventilation and gas exchange that may develop during sleep in patients with COPD raise the question of appropriate investigation of these patients. However, it is widely accepted that sleep studies are not routinely indicated in patients with COPD associated with respiratory insufficiency, particularly since the awake PaO_2 level provides a good indicator of the likelihood of nocturnal oxygen desaturation [16,17]. Sleep studies are indicated only when there is a clinical suspicion of an associated sleep apnea syndrome or manifestations of hypoxemia not explained by the awake PaO_2 level, such as cor pulmonale or polycythemia. In most situations in which sleep studies are indicated, a limited study focusing on respiration and gas exchange should be sufficient.

IX. Management of Respiratory Abnormalities During Sleep in COPD

A. General Principles

The first management principle of sleep-related breathing disturbance in COPD should be to optimize the underlying condition, which will almost invariably benefit breathing while asleep. The specific pharmacological therapy of COPD is extensively covered elsewhere in this book, but there are a number of aspects to management particularly relevant to sleep that merit specific consideration. Correction of hypoxemia is particularly important, and considerable interest has focused in recent years on the potential benefits of noninvasive ventilation in COPD, particularly during acute exacerbations. However, this subject is outside the scope of the present chapter.

B. Oxygen Therapy

The most serious consequence of hypoventilation, particularly during sleep, is hypoxemia, and appropriate oxygen therapy plays an important part in the management of any disorder associated with respiratory insufficiency during sleep. Care must be taken that correction of hypoxemia is not complicated by hypercapnia in patients with COPD, since respiratory drive in such patients may be partly dependent on the stimulant effect of hypoxemia. Therefore, the concentration of added oxygen should be carefully titrated to bring the PaO_2 up into the mildly hypoxemic range in order to minimize the tendency to carbon dioxide retention, particularly during sleep. However, the risk of CO_2 retention with supplemental oxygen therapy in such patients may have been overstated in the past, and there is evidence that CO_2 retention with oxygen supplementation during sleep is often modest, and usually nonprogressive [24]. In particular, a recent report from this department has shown little risk of serious carbon dioxide retention with carefully controlled oxygen therapy during exacerbations of COPD, even when relatively high flow oxygen supplementation is required to bring the SaO_2 into the region of 90–92% [25], a finding supported by the report of Agusti and co-authors [26].

The most common methods of low-flow oxygen therapy are nasal cannulae and Venturi facemasks. Patients requiring long-term oxygen therapy are usually given oxygen via nasal cannulae, but in patients with acute exacerbations, face masks are often preferred [26] because of the ability to deliver higher concentrations of oxygen and to give better control of the inspired oxygen concentration (FiO_2). However, facemasks are less comfortable and are much more likely to become dislodged during sleep than nasal cannulae [27].These factors should be considered when choosing the method of oxygen delivery and the relative importance of accurate control of FiO_2, and compliance must be determined when selecting the route of oxygen delivery for each patient. Patients with hypercapnic respiratory failure benefit from the more accurate control of FiO_2 provided by facemasks, but care must be taken to ensure adequate compliance, since the abrupt withdrawal of oxygen supplementation may result in more severe hypoxemia than prior to supplementation. Therefore, patients in this category who tolerate facemasks poorly may be better managed by nasal cannulae.

Management Options for COPD Patients with Sleep-Related Respiratory Disturbance

Supplemental oxygen

- **Controlled flow rates to minimize risk of CO_2 retention**

Pharmacological therapy

- **Anticholinergics**
- **Theophyllines**
- **Almitrine**
- **Protriptyline**

Assisted ventilation

- **Noninvasive by nasal mask**

X. Pharmacological Therapy

A. Anticholinergic Agents

Cholinergic tone is increased at night, and it has been proposed that this contributes to airflow obstruction and deterioration in gas exchange during sleep in patients with obstructive airways disease. A recent report has demonstrated significant improvements in both sleep quality and gas exchange in patients with COPD treated with ipratropium [28]. Objective improvements in sleep quality were particularly seen during REM sleep (Fig. 3), and subjective sleep quality also improved. Mean nocturnal SaO_2 increased by about 1.5% and lowest SaO_2 by about 5%. A preliminary report from this department demonstrated significant improvements in nocturnal SaO_2 with a newer once-daily anticholinergic agent, tiotropium, without significant changes in sleep quality [29]. Improvements in SaO_2 were particularly significant during REM sleep, which is clinically significant since REM sleep is associated with the most severe oxygen desaturation. Mean nocturnal SaO_2 throughout the night was about 2.5% higher with tiotropium than with placebo, regardless of whether the drug was given in the morning or evening.

B. Theophylline

In addition to being a bronchodilator, theophylline has important effects on respiration that may be particularly beneficial in patients with sleep-related respiratory disturbance, including central respiratory stimulation and improved diaphragmatic contractility [30,31]. We have shown this agent to have beneficial effects on oxygen saturation and arterial carbon dioxide levels in COPD during sleep (Fig. 4), which are also seen during resting wakefulness and during exercise [32]. Awake PaO_2 levels were about 8 mmHg higher on theophylline therapy compared with placebo, and mean SaO_2 during sleep was about 2% higher. The mechanism of this effect in COPD appears to be due mainly to a reduction in trapped gas volume rather than bronchodilation [32,33]. However, the principal limiting effect of theophyllines in this context is an adverse effect on sleep quality [32], in contrast to anticholinergic agents, which appears to differ from the effects of theophylline on sleep quality of

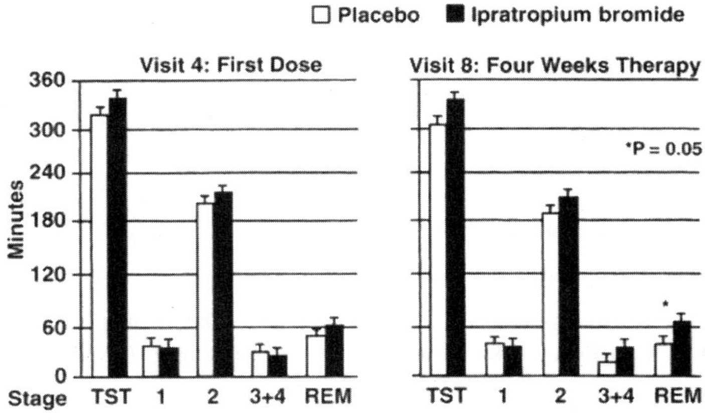

Figure 3 Effects of Ipratropium on sleep quality in COPD. (From Martin RJ, Bucher BL, Smith P, et al. Chest 1999; 115: 1338–1345.)

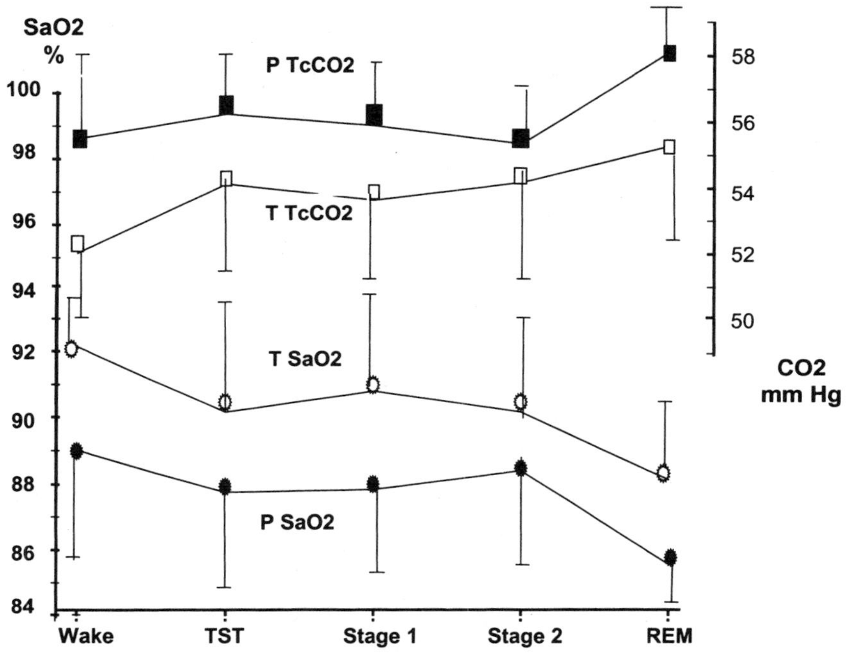

Figure 4 Effects of theophylline on SaO_2 and transcutaneous PCO_2 during sleep in COPD. (From Mulloy E, McNicholas WT. Am Rev Respir Dis 1993; 148: 1030–1036.)

normal subjects [34]. The relatively high incidence of side effects with theophylline therapy, particularly gastrointestinal intolerance, is also a disadvantage.

C. β-Agonists

There are only limited data on the efficacy of β-agonists on the management of sleep-related breathing abnormalities in COPD. One report found a long-acting theophylline superior to salbutamol in terms of nocturnal gas exchange and overnight fall in spirometry, with no difference in effects on sleep quality [35]. However, there are no studies of the impact of long-acting β-agonists on sleep and breathing in COPD.

D. Almitrine

Almitrine is a powerful carotid body agonist, which stimulates ventilation [36]. Almitrine also improves ventilation perfusion relationships within the lung [37], probably by an enhancement of hypoxic pulmonary vasoconstriction [38]. The overall effect is to lessen hypoxemia, and the agent is a useful addition in the management of conditions associated with nocturnal hypoxemia, particularly COPD. Significant improvements in nocturnal SaO_2 have been reported compared with placebo, and these improvements are most pronounced during REM sleep [39]. However, important side effects include pulmonary hypertension, dyspnea (presumably due to the respiratory stimulant effect in patients with chronic airflow limitation), and peripheral neuropathy [40]. The latter complication can be minimized by giving the drug on an intermittent basis with a 1-month holiday after each 2 months of active therapy.

E. Protriptyline and Related Agents

This drug is a tricyclic antidepressant which has a number of other effects that may be beneficial in some patients with sleep-related respiratory insufficiency, including COPD. The most important of these effects is a fragmentation of REM sleep [41], since sleep-related breathing abnormalities tend to be most severe in this sleep stage. Short-term studies have shown a benefit in both awake and sleep blood gas levels in patients with COPD [42], although this benefit may not persist with long-term use of the drug [43]. Furthermore, long-term use is significantly limited by side effects, particularly anticholinergic ones. Therefore, despite its theoretical role, this agent is rarely used in the management of sleep-related breathing disturbances in COPD. In recent years, attention has focused on selective serotonin reuptake inhibitors, which have been shown to benefit patients with sleep apnea syndrome and to have a lower incidence of side effects than the tricyclic agents [44].

XI. Conclusion

Sleep may be associated with serious and potentially life-threatening respiratory disturbances in COPD, yet many physicians pay little attention to this aspect of the disorder. However, it is now recognized that appropriate therapy with oxygen and selected medication(s) can substantially benefit nocturnal gas exchange and may also improve sleep quality, with consequent benefit to daytime performance.

References

1. Douglas NJ, Calverley PMA, Leggett RJE, Brash HM, Flenley DC, Brezinova V. Transient hypoxaemia during sleep in chronic bronchitis and emphysema. Lancet 1979; 1:1–4.

2. McNicholas WT, FitzGerald MX. Nocturnal death among patients with chronic bronchitis and emphysema. Br Med J 1984; 289:878.
3. Cormick W, Olson LG, Hensley MJ, Saunders NA. Nocturnal hypoxaemia and quality of sleep in patients with chronic obstructive lung disease. Thorax 1986; 41:846–854.
4. Breslin E, Van der Schans C, Breubink S, et al. Perception of fatigue and quality of life in patients with COPD. Chest 1998; 114:958–964.
5. Phillipson EA. Control of breathing during sleep. Am Rev Respir Dis 1978; 118:909–939.
6. Phillipson EA, Duffin J, Cooper JD. Critical dependence of respiratory rhythmicity on metabolic CO_2 load. J Appl Physiol 1981; 50:45–54.
7. Stradling JR, Chadwick GA, Frew AJ. Changes in ventilation and its components in normal subjects during sleep. Thorax 1985; 40:364–370.
8. Hetzel MR, Clark TJH. Comparison of normal and asthmatic circadian rhythms in peak expiratory flow rate. Thorax 1980; 35:732–738.
9. Sharp JT, Goldberg NB, Druz WS, Danon J. Relative contributions of rib cage and abdomen to breathing in normal subjects. J Appl Physiol 1975; 39:608–618.
10. Tabachnik E, Muller NL, Bryan AC, Levison H. Changes in ventilation and chest wall mechanics during sleep in normal adolescents. J Appl Physiol 1981; 51:557–564.
11. Johnson MW, Remmers JE. Accessory muscle activity during sleep in chronic obstructive pulmonary disease. J Appl Physiol 1984; 57:1011–1017.
12. Hudgel DW, Devadetta P. Decrease in functional residual capacity during sleep in normal humans. J Appl Physiol 1984; 57:1319–1322.
13. DeMarco FJ Jr, Wynne JW, Block AJ, Boysen PG, Taasan VC. Oxygen desaturation during sleep as a determinant of the "blue and bloated" syndrome. Chest 1981; 79:621–625.
14. Fletcher EC, Luckett RA, Miller T, et al. Pulmonary vascular hemodynamics in chronic lung disease patients with and without oxyhemoglobin desaturation during sleep. Chest 1989; 95:757–766.
15. Caterall JR, Calverley PMA, McNee W, et al. Mechanism of transient nocturnal hypoxemia in hypoxic chronic bronchitis and emphysema. J Appl Physiol 1985; 59:1698–1703.
16. Mulloy E, McNicholas WT. Ventilation and gas exchange during sleep and exercise in patients with severe COPD. Chest 1996; 109:387–394.
17. Stradling JR, Lane DJ. Nocturnal hypoxaemia in chronic obstructive pulmonary disease. Clin Sci 1983; 64:213–322.
18. Chaouat A, Weitzenbum E, Krieger J, Ifoundza I, Oswald M, Kessler R. Association of chronic obstructive pulmonary disease and sleep apnea syndrome. Am J Respir Crit Care Med 1995; 151:82–86.
19. Tirlapur VG, Mir MA. Nocturnal hypoxemia and associated electrocardiographic changes in patients with chronic obstructive airways disease. N Engl J Med 1982; 306(3):125–130.
20. Flick MR, Block AJ. Nocturnal vs. diurnal arrhythmias in patients with chronic obstructive pulmonary disease. Chest 1979; 75:8–11.

21. Gallagher CG. Exercise and chronic obstructive pulmonary disease. Med Clin N Am 1990; 74:619–641.
22. Midgren B, Hansson L, Erikkson L, Airikkala P, Elmqvist D. Oxygen desaturation during sleep and exercise in patients with interstitial lung disease. Thorax 1987; 42:353–356.
23. Shepard JW, Schweitzer PK, Kellar CA, Chun DS, Dolan GF. Myocardial stress. Exercise versus sleep in patients with COPD. Chest 1984; 86:366–374.
24. Goldstein RS, Ramcharan V, Bowes G, McNicholas WT, Bradley D, Phillipson EA. Effects of supplemental oxygen on gas exchange during sleep in patients with severe obstructive lung disease. N Engl J Med 1984; 310:425–429.
25. Moloney ED, Kiely JL, McNicholas W.T. Controlled oxygen therapy and carbon dioxide retention during exacerbations of chronic obstructive pulmonary disease. Lancet 2001; 357:526–528.
26. Agusti AG, Carrera M, Barbe F, Munoz A, Togores B. Oxygen therapy during exacerbations of chronic obstructive pulmonary disease. Eur Respir J 1999; 14:934–936.
27. Costello R, Liston R, McNicholas WT. Compliance at night with low-flow oxygen therapy: a comparison of nasal cannulae and Venturi face masks. Thorax 1995; 50:405–406.
28. Martin RJ, Bucher BL, Smith P, et al. Effect of ipratropium bromide treatment on oxygen saturation and sleep quality in COPD. Chest 1999; 115:1338–1345.
29. McNicholas WT, Calverley PMA, Edwards C, Lee A. Effects of anticholinergic therapy (Tiotropium) on REM-related desaturation and sleep quality in patients with COPD. Am J Respir Crit Care Med 2001; 163(suppl):A281.
30. Eldridge FL, Millhorn DE, Waldrop TG, et al. Mechanism of respiratory effects of methylxanthines. Respir Physiol 1983; 53:239–261.
31. Murciano D, Aubier M, Lecocguic Y, et al. Effects of theophylline on diaphragmatic strength and fatigue in patients with chronic obstructive pulmonary disease. N Engl J Med 1984; 311:349–353.
32. Mulloy E, McNicholas WT. Theophylline improves gas exchange during rest, exercise and sleep in severe chronic obstructive pulmonary disease. Am Rev Respir Dis 1993; 148:1030–1036.
33. Chrystyn H, Mulley BA, Peake MD. Dose response relation to oral theophylline in severe chronic obstructive airways disease. Br Med J 1988; 297:1506–1510.
34. Fitzpatrick MF, Engleman HM, Boellert F. Effect of therapeutic theophylline levels on the sleep quality and daytime cognitive performance of normal subjects. Am Rev Respir Dis 1992; 145:1355–1358.
35. Man GC, Chapman KR, Ali SH, et al. Sleep quality and nocturnal respiratory function with once-daily theophylline (Uniphil) and inhaled salbutamol in patients with COPD. Chest 1996; 110:648–653.
36. Laubie M, Schmitt H. Long-lasting hyperventilation induced by almitrine: evidence for a specific effect on carotid and thoracic chemoreceptors. Eur J Pharmacol 1980; 61:125–136.
37. Reyes A, Roca J, Rodriguez-Roisin R, Torres A, Ussetti P, Wagner PD. Effect of almitrine on ventilation-perfusion distribution in adult respiratory distress syndrome. Am Rev Respir Dis 1988; 137:1062–1067.

38. Romaldini H, Rodriguez-Roisin R, Wagner PD, West JB. Enhancement of hypoxic pulmonary vasoconstriction by almitrine in the dog. Am Rev Respir Dis 1983; 128:288–293.
39. Bell RC, Mullins RC, West LG, Bachand RT, Johanspn WG Jr, The effect of almitrine bismesylate on hypoxaemia in chronic obstructive pulmonary disease. Ann Intern Med 1986; 105:342–346.
40. Howard P. Hypoxia, almitrine, and peripheral neuropathy. Thorax 1989; 44: 247–250.
41. Smith PL, Haponik EF, Allen RP, Bleecker ER. The effects of protriptyline in sleep-disordered breathing. Am Rev Respir Dis 1982; 127:8–13.
42. Carroll N, Parker RA, Branthwaite MA. The use of protriptylline for respiratory failure in patients with chronic airflow limitation. Eur Respir J 1990; 3:746–751.
43. Series F, Cormier M, LaForge J. Long-term effects of protriptyline in patients with chronic obstructive pulmonary disease. Am Rev Respir Dis 1993; 147:1487–1490.
44. Kraiczi H, Hedner J, Dahlof P, Ejnell H, Carlson J. Effect of serotonin uptake inhibition on breathing during sleep and daytime symptoms in obstructive sleep apnea. Sleep 1999; 22(1):61–67.

5

Airway and Alveolar Determinants of Airflow Limitation in COPD

NOE ZAMEL

University of Toronto
Toronto, Ontario, Canada

I. Introduction

The essential feature of chronic obstructive pulmonary diseases (COPD) is airflow limitation. The location of the causes of airflow limitation is in three major areas: large airways, small airways, and alveoli. To proper apply pharmacotherapy in COPD, it is vital to understand the pathophysiology and mechanics of the different sites that cause airflow limitation. This chapter is a concise review of the mechanics of airflow limitation at the level of the large airways, small airways, and alveoli, and how to evaluate the airflow limitation according to the site that it is causing it.

II. Large-Airways Airflow Limitation

The major components of total airway resistance are the nose, oropharynx, and larynx. The resistance at the level of the nose is about half of the total airways resistance. While breathing through the mouth, so that the nose is bypassed, the major components of the airway resistance are the oropharynx, larynx, and the large central airways. During measurements of airways resistance, the larynx resistance can be minimized by breathing in a shallow rapid pattern, like panting, which opens maximally the lumen of the larynx. In contrast to the large central airways, the small peripheral airways, smaller than 2 mm in internal diameter, have very little resistance in healthy subjects, accounting for less than 20% of the total airways resistance when the subject is breathing through the mouth [1,2]. Therefore, significant obstruction at the level of these airways can cause insignificant increase of the total airways resistance. On the other hand, obstruction of the large central airways results in significantly increased total airways resistance.

Table 1 shows how changes of the resistance of the central airways (Rc) and of the peripheral airways (Rp) affect the total airway resistance (Raw). A 100% increase in Rp will result in a 20% elevation of Raw, while a 100% increase of Rc will result in an 80% increase in Raw. A similar elevation in Raw will be required by a 400% increase in Rp. Therefore, an abnormally high Raw cannot distinguish central from peripheral airway obstruction, but a normal Raw in the presence of other tests of airflow limitation is suggestive of peripheral location of the obstruction.

The Raw is usually measured using the whole-body plethysmograph [3], more commonly called the "body box." The Raw varies with the lung volumes, so that its value is lowest at total lung capacity and highest at residual volume in the same person. When Raw is measured in different individuals at equivalent lung volumes, such as functional residual capacity (FRC), there is also a negative relationship with the size of the FRC. For these reasons, the Raw is usually referred to the lung volume at which the measurement is made. The conventional way of reducing the data is to express Raw as its reciprocal, 1/Raw, called airways conductance (Gaw), and to divide it by the lung volume at which the measurement is done. The resultant ratio, Gaw/FRC, is called specific airways conductance (sGaw).

Evaluation of changes of Raw as pharmacotherapeutic endpoint is useful more in asthma than COPD. In asthma, especially in young patients, a

Table 1 Contribution of Central and Peripheral Components of Total Airway Resistance

	Raw	Rc	Rp
Normal	2.0	1.6	0.4
100% increase in Rp	2.4	1.6	0.8
100% increase in Rc	3.6	3.2	0.4
400% increase in Rp	3.6	1.6	2.0

All values are in $cmH_2O/L/sec$. Raw = total airways resistance; Rc = central airway resistance; Rp = peripheral airway resistance.

significant component of airflow limitation can be due to increased Rc, while in COPD the predominant component of airflow limitation is due to elevated Rp [1].

When Raw is measured in the body box, the lung volume at which the measurement is done, usually the FRC, is measured as part of the set of maneuvers. Measurements of lung volumes to evaluate the degree of hyperinflation and gas trapping can be useful endpoints of the efficacy of pharmatherapy in COPD. The assessment of gas trapping is usually done by comparing the lung volumes measured in the body box with gas dilution methods. As Raw is available as part of the procedure, it can be used as a secondary endpoint.

III. Small-Airways Airflow Limitation

There are many ways to determine the presence, severity, and changes of airflow limitation due to obstruction of the small peripheral airways, less than 2 mm in internal diameter. The most traditional way is the spirogram, in which the data are reduced to forced vital capacity, FEV_1, and maximum midexpiratory flow rate. The spirogram is a plot of changes of expiratory volume versus time. The same information contained in the spirogram can be expressed as a plot of the slope of the spirogram (expiratory flow) versus changes of expiratory volume, which is the maximum expiratory flow volume curve (MEFVC). The advantage of the MEFVC format is that it is easier to visualize the pattern of airflow limitation and also offers a more convenient way of reducing the data.

There are three standard models of describing the maximum expiratory flow as related to the mechanical properties of the lungs:

1. Equal pressure point [4]
2. Ptm [5]
3. Chock point [6]

The equal pressure point model is the simplest and the mostly referred in the literature. It is based on dividing the length of the airways into two components, according to the location of the equal pressure point (EPP). The EPP is defined as the point in the airways where the transmural pressure during a forced expiration is zero, that is, the intraluminal pressure is the same as the extraluminal pressure, the later being also the same as pleural pressure. The airway segments from the alveoli to the EPP are called upstream segments and the segments from the EPP to the mouth are called downstream segments. In the downstream segments, as the intraluminal pressure is lower than the extraluminal, there is a passive collapse of these segments, resulting in limiting the expiratory flow to a maximum, which is not dependent on effort. In the upstream segments, as the intraluminal pressure is greater than the extraluminal, these segments are kept open and distended by their positive transmural pressure, in contrast with the negative transmural pressure in the downstream segments.

The driving pressure across the upstream segment is the alveolar pressure at the start of the segment and the intraluminal pressure at the EPP, which is the same as pleural pressure. Therefore, the pressure gradient is alveolar pressure minus pleural pressure, which is the equivalent of lung elastic recoil pressure (Pel). Opposing the maximum expiratory flow (Vmax) is the resistance of the upstream segment (Rus). The Vmax can be expressed as the ratio of Pel/Rus:

$$\text{Vmax} = \text{Pel}/\text{Rus}$$

The length of the upstream segment depends on the location of the EPP. In healthy individuals, during the forced-expiratory vital capacity maneuver, the EPP is located in the large central airways, somehow close to the carina, for over the first two-thirds of the vital capacity. During this period, the length of the upstream segment includes most of the central and all of the peripheral airways. Toward the last third of the forced vital capacity maneuver, the EPP moves progressively toward the alveoli, reaching the small peripheral airways, smaller than 2 mm in internal diameter, over the last fourth of the maneuver. Only during the later part of the maneuver does the length of the upstream segment contains exclusively the peripheral small airways, so that the central large airways are not part of this upstream segment and become part of the downstream segment. Consequently, in healthy subjects, Rus includes Rc and Rp in the first part of the forced vital capacity, but only Rp in the last portion of the maneuver, excluding Rc.

If Rp is only mildly increased, Vmax will be normal in the first part of the forced vital capacity, along with a normal FEV_1, and only it will be reduced in the terminal part of the forced vital capacity. With increasing severity of peripheral airways airflow limitation, as Rp increases more significantly, Vmax will also be reduced in the first part of the forced vital capacity, along with a reduced FEV_1. As Rp increases and/or Pel decreases, the EPP moves toward the alveoli early during the forced vital capacity maneuver, compared with normal conditions, so that Rus expresses the Rp over a longer period of the forced vital capacity, and not only during the terminal part of the maneuver. In the example of Table 1, this occurs when Rp is increased by 400% of normal. Combining measurements of Raw and MEFVC, it is possible to distinguish the predominant site of airflow limitations as located in the central large or in the peripheral small airways.

Another way of estimating the contribution of Rc and Rp to Rus is to determine the density dependence of Vmax. This is done by obtaining MEFVCs breathing air and breathing a mixture of 80% helium with 20% oxygen (HeO_2), which has only one-third of the air density. MEFVCs on air and HeO_2 are superimposed one on top of the other and the increment of Vmax at 50% of the forced vital capacity (ΔVmax) is calculated [7], along with the volume of isoflow [8], which corresponds to the part of the vital capacity where the two MEFVCs become identical. A reduction of ΔVmax or an increase of the volume of isoflow indicates that Rp is the predominant component of Rus, so that the reduction of Vmax reflects airflow limitation at the level of the peripheral small airways. This is usually the case in patients with COPD, and these tests can be used to evaluate the effects of pharmacotherapy at the level of such airways.

IV. Alveolar Airflow Limitation

It has been found recently [9] that in asthmatic patients with moderate to severe airflow limitation and who have a chronic persistent irreversible component of the airflow limitation, approximately 60% of the airflow limitation is due to the airway obstruction and the other 40% is due to loss of lung parenchymal elastic recoil, i.e., loss of Pel. The loss of elastic recoil caused the lungs to hyperinflate, with an abnormal increase of total lung capacity. Although these findings are unexpected in asthma, the loss of lung elastic recoil is expected to be a significant component of airflow limitation in COPD, particularly in emphysema. The contribution of the two components of airflow limitation, airways and alveoli, has not been systematically measured in patients with COPD as it has been in asthmatics. FEV_1 shows a fair to weak negative correlation with computerized tomographic emphysema scores, suggesting that emphysema does not appear to be primarily responsible for severe airflow limitation in most patients with severe COPD, based on measurements of FEV_1 [10]. However, the proper evaluation should be done measuring the MEFVC and the pressure–volume curve of the lungs to measure Pel.

In order to estimate the airway and alveoli components which limit the airflow, Pel and Rus, or its reciprocal Gus (upstream conductance), are measured for a particular lung volume. The observed Vmax can be expressed as

$$\text{Vmax} = \text{Pel}/\text{Rus} \qquad \text{or} \qquad \text{Vmax} = \text{Pel} \times \text{Gus}$$

The reduction of Vmax as percentage of normal predicted can be expressed as

$$\text{Vmax\%pred} = \text{Pel\%pred} \times \text{Gus\%pred}$$

The individual contributions of airways (Gus) and of loss of lung elastic recoil (Pel) in limiting airflow can be estimated in the following way:

For the Gus component:

$$(1 - \text{Vmax\%pred}) \times \{(1 - \text{Gus\%pred})/[(1 - \text{Pel\%pred}) + (1 - \text{Gus\%pred})]\}$$

For the Pel component:

$$(1 - \text{Vmax\%pred}) \times \{(1 - \text{Pel\%pred})/[(1 - \text{Pel\%pred}) + (1 - \text{Gus\%pred})]\}$$

Once the airways and alveoli contributions to airflow limitation have been established, these components can be used as endpoints in the evaluation of the efficacy of pharmacotherapy of COPD in a more specific way than the general approach presently in use. The alveoli component of airflow limitation has been virtually disregarded and the entire emphasis has been placed on the airflow limitation due to airways obstruction. Extensive studies will be required to establish the magnitude of alveolar airflow limitation in COPD and possible ways to treat it accordingly.

References

1. Hogg JC, Macklem PT, Thurlbeck WM. Site and nature of airway obstruction in chronic obstructive lung disease. N Engl J Med 1968; 278:1355.
2. Macklem PT, Mead J. Resistance of central and peripheral airways measured by retrograde catheter. J Appl Physiol 1967; 22:395.
3. Dubois Ab, Botelho SY, Comroe JH Jr. A new method for measuring airways resistance in man using a body plethysmograph. Values in normal subjects and in patients with respiratory disease. J Clin Invest 1956; 35:327.
4. Mead J, et al. Significance of the relationship between lung recoil and maximum expiratory flow. J Appl Physiol 1967; 22:95.
5. Pride NB, et al. Determinants of maximal expiratory flow from the lungs. J Appl Physiol 1967; 23:646.
6. Dawson SV, Elliott EA. Wave-speed limitation on expiratory flow—a unifying concept. J Appl Physiol 1977; 43:498.
7. Despas PJ, Leroux M, Mackelm PT. Site of airway obstruction in asthma as determined by measuring maximal expiratory flow breathing air and a helium-oxygen mixture. J Clin Invests 1972; 51:3255.
8. Hutcheon M, et al. Volume of isoflow: a new test in detection of mild abnormalities of lung mechanics. Am Rev Respir Dis 1974; 11:458.
9. Gelb AF, Zamel N. Unsuspected pseudophysiologic emphysema in chronic persistent asthma. Am J Respir Crit Care Med 2000; 162:1778.
10. Gelb AF, et al. Contribution of emphysema and small airways in COPD. Chest 1996; 109:353.

6

Gas Exchange

ANTONI FERRER

Hospital de Sabadell
and Universitat Autònoma de Barcelona
Barcelona, Spain

JOAN ALBERT BARBERÀ and ROBERTO RODRIGUEZ-ROISIN

Hospital Clinic, Institut d'Investigacions Biomèdiques August Pi i Sunyer, Universitat de Barcelona
Barcelona, Spain

I. Introduction

Imbalance of alveolar ventilation to pulmonary blood flow ($\dot{V}_A/\dot{Q}$) relationships is the vital determinant of gas-exchange abnormalities in chronic obstructive pulmonary disease (COPD) [1]. By contrast, increased intrapulmonary shunting and alveolar to end-capillary diffusion impairment play a negligible role. A major breakthrough in understanding the role of $\dot{V}_A/\dot{Q}$ inequality on gas-exchange abnormalities in COPD has been provided by the development of the multiple inert gas elimination technique (MIGET) [2]. Using this technique it has been possible to assess quantitatively and qualitatively the $\dot{V}_A/\dot{Q}$ distributions in COPD and to unravel the relevance of the different factors that determine the partial pressures of O_2 and CO_2 in arterial blood (PaO_2 and $PaCO_2$, respectively) under different clinical settings. Although the more severe levels of gas exchange impairment are seen in advanced COPD patients, the severity of hypoxemia and hypercapnia relates modestly to the degree of airflow obstruction. Moreover, PaO_2 and $PaCO_2$ values are determined not only by changes occurring in the lung (i.e., $\dot{V}A/\dot{Q}$ imbalance), but also by extrapulmonary factors (i.e., minute ventilation, cardiac output, and oxygen consumption) that are unrelated to the degree of airflow obstruction. Therefore the separate assessment of these intrapulmonary and extrapulmonary determinants of hypoxemia and hypercapnia is particularly useful in COPD, in which quite different clinical setups can be seen despite the same basic pathological processes. Moreover, hypoxia exerts a constrictive effect on pulmonary arteries. Hypoxic pulmonary vasoconstriction reduces perfusion in poorly ventilated or nonventilated lung units and diverts it to better ventilated areas, thereby partially restoring PaO_2. The increase of alveolar PO_2 while breathing oxygen inhibits this phenomenon and further deteriorates $\dot{V}_A/\dot{Q}$ mismatch, as shown by increased perfusion to poorly ventilated lung units with low $\dot{V}_A/\dot{Q}$ ratios. This implies that room-air breathing-induced arteriolar constriction contributes to maintain $\dot{V}_A/\dot{Q}$ matching in these units. Similar effects have been observed with drugs that decrease pulmonary vascular tone.

This chapter reviews the current knowledge on pulmonary gas exchange response to different therapeutic interventions in COPD patients, using essentially conventional arterial blood gas studies. We will discuss extensively the gas exchange response to bronchodilators, the cornerstone of COPD therapy [3]. To a much less extent, we will review the role of steroids and that of vasodilators. There are very few data using oxygen saturation measurements, the simplest and least invasive approach to explore the status of pulmonary gas exchange. Unfortunately, the variability of the latter approach makes it unsuitable to have an accurate estimate of the short-term changes in PaO_2 and $PaCO_2$.

II. Bronchodilators

A. β-Adrenergic Agonists

The early studies showed that the administration of β-adrenergics to patients with airways obstruction (essentially, asthma and COPD) results in bronchodilatation and often in a transient decrease in PaO_2 without major changes in $PaCO_2$ [4–11]. These studies were done primarily on asthmatic patients with mild hypoxemia [6,12,13], and the changes were maximal approximately at 5 min to return to baseline by 10–20 min. Isoproterenol (isoprenaline), a relatively short-acting nonselective β-adrenergic with both β_1 and β_2 activities, was the most studied agent. The addition of intravenous practolol, a selective β_1-blocker, to inhaled isoproterenol did not cause hypoxemia [14], suggesting that hypoxemia could be related, at least in part, to its β_1-agonist component. The comparison of isoproterenol and fenoterol, a more selective β_2-agonist, showed that the changes on PaO_2 were more marked after isoproterenol [15].

The transient hypoxemia after β-adrenergic administration, so-called paradoxical hypoxemia, was basically attributed to the potent vasodilator effects of these agents mediated via β_2-receptors releasing hypoxic pulmonary vasoconstriction. By increasing blood flow to altered $\dot{V}_A/\dot{Q}$ areas, $\dot{V}_A/\dot{Q}$ relationships further deteriorated [12,13,16], alveolar–arterial PO_2 difference ($AaPO_2$) increased, and PaO_2 decreased. Subsequently, the use of MIGET in patients with asthma showed that 5 min after inhaled isoproterenol, perfusion to lung areas with low $\dot{V}_A/\dot{Q}$ ratios increased, cardiac output increased, and PaO_2 fell, likely indicating together that release of hypoxic vasoconstriction was the principal mechanism behind further $\dot{V}_A/\dot{Q}$ worsening [13]. These changes returned to baseline 10 min after the inhalation of isoproterenol, while expiratory flow rates continued to improve, suggesting that the increase in perfusion to relatively underventilated regions was greater than the increase in ventilation to these alveoli. Most of the studies describing the effects of β-adrenergics on gas exchange in COPD were published later.

We will describe first the effects of bronchodilators used intravenously, subcutaneously, and orally, as opposed to the recommended inhaled route, to better gain an insight into the pathophysiology of pulmonary gas exchange. The effects of bronchodilators using noninhaled routes, both at the bronchial and cardiovascular levels, are closely dependent on serum levels, while the effects of bronchodilators given by inhalation are related to the amount of drug deposited within the airways. Any serum level depends on the absortion of the medication. Thus, after salbutamol aerosolization, the bronchodilator effect start within seconds, reaching about 80% of its peak in 5 min, its maximal peak in about 60 min, waning a variable time thereafter, lasting between 4 and 7 hr [17]. On the other hand, plasma levels rise to their maximum within 5 min and then decline. In addition, there is a relative β_2-specificity when the drug is given by inhalation. Even a drug with the cardiovascular effect of isoproterenol becomes more β_2-specific when it is administered by aerosol, such that local deposition in the airways maximizes bronchial effects, while cardiac effects due to absorbed drug are minimized. The vast majority of these studies were done in patients with stable COPD, and very few during exacerbations. This may be of importance, since during exacerbations there are substantial transient changes in the status of gas exchange, hemodynamic and pulmonary vascular tone, suggesting that the vasoactive effects of β-agonists may be more relevant, at least during these episodes.

Intravenous β-Adrenergics

Ringstedt et al. [18] studied the pulmonary vascular tone response and gas exchange in a small group of patients with advanced COPD and mild respiratory failure, after a continuous infusion of terbutaline (β_2-agonist). Following terbutaline, cardiac output increased and systemic blood pressure and pulmonary vascular resistance decreased. Moreover, while PaO_2 decreased and mixed venous PO_2 and oxygen delivery increased, $PaCO_2$ did not change. There was further $\dot{V}_A/\dot{Q}$ worsening, as assessed by increases in the perfusion to low $\dot{V}_A/\dot{Q}$ ratios; FEV_1 and minute ventilation increased. Overall, $\dot{V}_A/\dot{Q}$ deterioration could have resulted from an increased pulmonary blood flow to areas with low $\dot{V}_A/\dot{Q}$ ratios, due to the increased cardiac output, not efficiently counterbalanced by the simultaneous increased minute ventilation. However, from these data it was not possible to differentiate between an increased cardiac output, inducing an increase in the amount of $\dot{V}_A/\dot{Q}$ inequalities, or an active reduction in pulmonary vascular tone. In parallel, in another small group of patients with COPD with more airflow obstruction, more hypoxemia, more hypercapnia, and also more pulmonary hypertension, cardiac output increased without pulmonary vascular changes; ventilation increased modestly, but without improving airflow limitation. Nonetheless, PaO_2 and the underlying $\dot{V}_A/\dot{Q}$ mismatching remained unaltered. Despite the fact that terbutaline increased cardiac output and consequently mixed venous PO_2 in a similar way to the other, less affected subset of patients, these more advanced patients did not alter their basal gas-exchange profile after bronchodilator. In these patients, it is possible that hypoxic vasoconstriction could have been weaker or even absent due to more intense chronic alveolar hypoxia and/or to anatomical alterations in the pulmonary vasculature coexisting with areas of lung destruction (emphysema). This is in keeping with the concept that the progressive increase of pulmonary vascular resistance seen in advanced COPD is due not only to irreversible structural vascular lesions but also includes a reversible vascular component [19].

A subsequent study [20] of patients with very severe COPD showed that intravenous terbutaline infusion augmented right ventricular function and confirmed that terbutaline decreased pulmonary vascular resistance without decreasing PaO_2, at rest and during exercise. Previous studies on the effects of intravenous terbutaline on gas exchange in COPD [21–24] are in keeping with these findings: unaltered PaO_2, in patients with the lowest PaO_2 [21,23], and moderate decreases in those with less altered resting PaO_2 [22,24]. Yet one of these studies [23] reported a small increase in PaO_2 without changes in $PaCO_2$ 5 min following intravenous terbutaline into the pulmonary artery, when drug concentrations are likely to achieve the highest peak levels. These unexpected findings could be explained by the transient extrapulmonary changes observed after terbutaline administration: increase in minute ventilation, cardiac output, and metabolic rate. Our group has shown that, in patients with acute severe asthma, the infusion of salbutamol further worsened $\dot{V}A/\dot{Q}$ relationships without modifying PaO_2 because the cardiovascular effects of salbutamol, more specifically the increase in cardiac output, counterbalanced the deleterious effect of $\dot{V}_A/\dot{Q}$ imbalance on PaO_2 [25]. In this [25] and in an another study of patients with stable severe persistent asthma [26], we showed that inhaled salbutamol did not alter $\dot{V}_A/\dot{Q}$ inequality nor PaO_2 15 min after the inhalation of salbutamol, when the early and transient decline in PaO_2 was probably resolved.

Subcutaneous β-Adrenergics

Tschopp et al. [27] showed that subcutaneous terbutaline produced a small but significant decrease in PaO_2 associated with vascular changes suggestive of vasodilatation. This effect was not seen in the most hypoxemic patients.

Oral β-Adrenergics

Marvin et al. [28] studied the effects of oral terbutaline, theophylline, and their combination in COPD patients, and showed that the small improvement in airflow even in the most "irreversible" patients was accompanied by negligible gas exchange responses both at rest and during exercise. Postma et al. [29] showed that oral slow-release terbutaline prevented the nocturnal decrease of FEV_1 and PaO_2 in patients with COPD with large circadian airflow variation.

Short-Acting Inhaled β-Adrenergics

Gross et al. [30] compared the gas exchange response to nebulized metaproterenol (a relatively selective β_2-agonist) versus atropine methonitrate (an anticholinergic bronchodilator) in stable, moderately to severely hypoxemic patients with COPD patients (Fig. 1). The PaO_2 fell discretely but significantly (mean, −5 mmHg) 10–30 min after metaproterenol, returning to baseline by 1 hr. The decrease of PaO_2 was more marked in the patients with the highest basal PaO_2, a finding similar to those seen in asthmatics [12] and in COPD patients treated with intravenous terbutaline [18,21–24]. By contrast, the changes after atropine methonitrate inhalation were negligible.

Viegas et al. [31] compared the short-term effect of nebulized fenoterol, a selective β_2-agonist, against that of ipratropium bromide, on gas exchange in patients with severe COPD with mild to moderate hypoxemia. While fenoterol slightly decreased mean PaO_2 (about 6 mmHg) due to further worsening in the amount of low $\dot{V}_A/\dot{Q}$ regions, gas exchange remained stable after ipratropium (Fig. 2). Pulmonary hemodynamics were not measured. Yet the contention was that the pulmonary vascular tone diminished after fenoterol, hence inducing further $\dot{V}_A/\dot{Q}$ inequalities. The most likely explanation for these effects is that fenoterol has been marketed at a higher relative dose than the other β_2-agonists; in addition, fenoterol may be less selective for β_2-receptors [32].

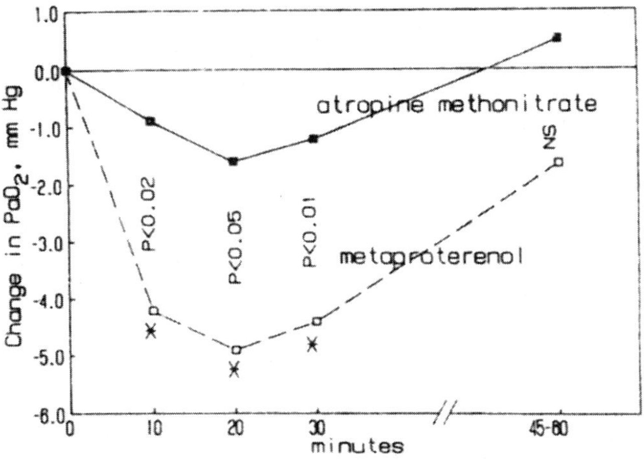

Figure 1 Time course of changes in PaO_2 after metaproterenol and atropine methonitrate in patients with stable COPD. Shown are mean changes in PaO_2 from prebronchodilator levels for each drug. The p values between lines are the significance of the difference between the two agents; NS = not significant. Asterisk indicates significantly different from baseline at $p < 0.01$. (From Ref. 30, with permission.)

Saito et al. [33] compared inhaled fenoterol with oxitropium, another anticholinergic agent, and confirmed the hemodynamic, spirometric, and gas exchange findings seen in the previous study. Additionally, they showed that during exercise both drugs attenuated right heart afterload to a similar degree. The mechanisms by which the two classes of bronchodilators minimized exercise-induced increased pulmonary artery pressure were related indirectly to an improvement in pulmonary mechanics rather than to a direct cardiovascular effect. Carlone et al. [34] observed no change in PaO_2 or in oxygen transport at rest and during exercise, at the time of maximal bronchodilator effect of inhaled fenoterol (60 min).

Karpel et al. [35] compared the effects of inhaled metaproterenol and ipratropium bromide during severe exacerbations not requiring mechanical ventilation. Thirty minutes after dosing, PaO_2 fell by a mean of 6.2 mmHg after metaproterenol, while ipratropium induced a small but significant transient increase in PaO_2 (by 5.8 mmHg). Bernasconi et al. [36] showed that, in COPD patients needing mechanical ventilation, inhaled fenoterol transiently decreased PaO_2, returning to baseline values 2 hr after drug administration. In this study, the PaO_2 was on average 15 mmHg lower than baseline at 30 min after fenoterol.

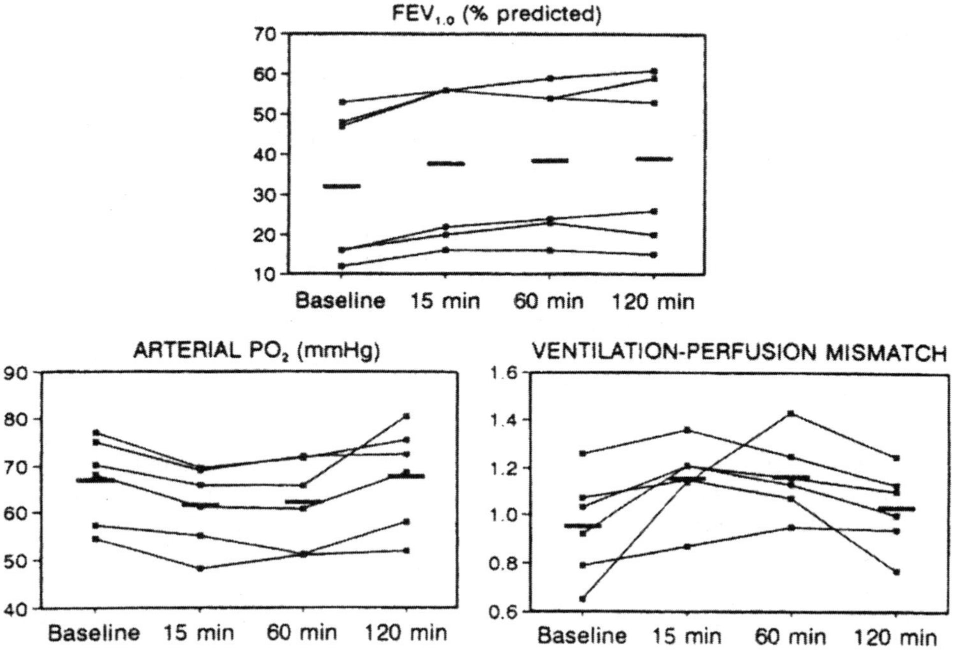

Figure 2 Individual time course of FEV_1, PaO_2, and $\dot{V}_A/\dot{Q}$ mismatch (measured as log SDQ using the multiple inert gas elimination technique) after inhaled fenoterol in stable hypoxemic COPD patients (solid bars = mean). (From Ref. 31, with permission.)

In patients with severe COPD patients, nebulized β-adrenergics may increase minute ventilation, leading to a substantial increase in PaO_2 (by approximately 5%) and a decrease in $PaCO_2$ [37].

During severe COPD exacerbation [38], arterial hypoxemia is more prominent because of the influence of three determinants of gas exchange, namely, worsened $\dot{V}_A/\dot{Q}$ abnormalities, disproportionately increased metabolic demand of oxygen consumption, which in part may be attributable to high doses of β-agonists [39], and a decreased mixed venous PO_2. The latter mechanism amplifies the detrimental effects of $\dot{V}_A/\dot{Q}$ inequalities on gas exchange.

When patients with COPD adopt the supine position, PaO_2 can either increase or decrease [40]. Pinet et al. [41], using a randomized, double-blind, crossover design, demonstrated that the supine position was associated with a decrease in PaO_2 after nebulized salbutamol in moderate to severe hypoxemic

COPD patients. This finding likely suggests further $\dot{V}_A/\dot{Q}$ worsening in that body position. This decrease was of greater magnitude than that caused by salbutamol in the upright position alone. Half of the patients exhibited large PaO_2 decreases (from 9 to 21 mm Hg) 30 min following nebulization, whereas increases or minor decreases occurred in the remainder. Many inpatients usually get their aerosol treatment upright and then resume the supine position after the nebulization. Considering that one cannot predict which particular patient may be at risk, it is recommended that patients be discouraged from lying down immediately after treatment. In addition, it may be prudent to monitor oxygen saturation if available and/or to provide supplemental oxygen where monitoring is unavailable.

Long-Acting Inhaled β-Adrenergics

The gas exchange response to inhaled salmeterol has been studied by Khoukaz et al. [42] (Fig. 3) in a small subset of patients with stable severe COPD, and mild to moderate hypoxemia (PaO_2 range 62–80 mmHg). They compared its short-term effects with those of salbutamol and ipratropium. The authors measured arterial blood gases at baseline and at different intervals until 2 hr after the administration of each drug, and showed small significant PaO_2 decrements following both β-adrenergics. Interestingly, the decline in PaO_2

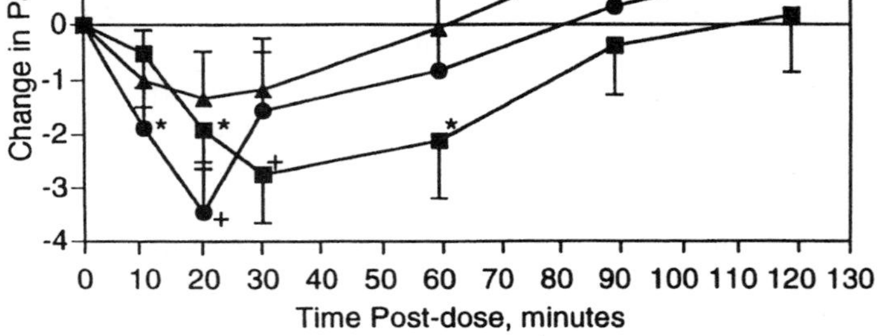

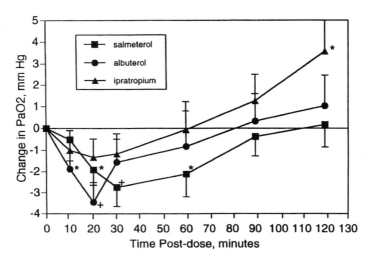

Figure 3 Mean changes in PaO_2 with time after administration of salmeterol, salbutamol (albuterol), and ipratropium. Error bars are SEM (*$p < 0.05$, *$p < 0.005$: statistically significant differences between drug and baseline). Differences among drugs were not statistically significant at any time point. (From Ref. 42, with permission.)

after salmeterol was slower in onset and of lesser magnitude but more prolonged than that observed after salbutamol. These changes are consistent with the chronology of the beneficial effects of these agents on airflow (the greatest mean PaO_2 change after salmeterol was −2.7 mmHg at 30 min, compared to −3.5 mmHg at 20 min after salbutamol). The anticholinergic agent tended to have smaller effects than either of the two adrenergics. Following ipratropium, the corresponding change was not significant (−1.3 mmHg) at 20 min. Akin to previous studies with other bronchodilators [12,18,20–24], the decreases in oxygen saturation tended to be more marked in those patients with the highest basal PaO_2 values. Changes in PaO_2 were reciprocal to those in $AaPO_2$, hence suggesting further $\dot{V}_A/\dot{Q}$ deterioration. The gas exchange responses to β-adrenergics were of shorter duration than the effect on airflow, which characteristically persisted for 4–6 hr following salbutamol and for 12 hr after salmeterol. This could be due to the shorter time constants for agonist–receptor interaction on vascular smooth muscle than those for airway smooth muscle or, alternatively, that unknown adaptive mechanisms come into play when the vascular reflexes that correct for $\dot{V}_A/\dot{Q}$ inequality are overridden by β-adrenergics. The decline in PaO_2 in all study arms was small, transient, and of doubtful clinical significance.

The administration of formoterol at a high dose (cumulative dose of 90 μg) in a series of patients with acute severe bronchoconstriction and mild to moderate hypoxemia (two-thirds having asthma, one-third COPD), admitted to an emergency room, was safe [43]. The control group received inhaled terbutaline. Except for mean pulse rate, higher in the terbutaline arm than in the formoterol group, all the other variables, including arterial blood gases, were not different between the treatment groups.

More recently, Cazzola et al. [44] compared inhaled salbutamol and long-acting formoterol given as needed in mild COPD exacerbations. Formoterol induced a fast bronchodilation that was dose-dependent but not significantly different from that caused by salbutamol. Furthermore, formoterol appeared to be as well tolerated as salbutamol. Neither oxygen saturation by pulse oximetry nor heart rate changed significantly after formoterol or salbutamol. More recently, the same authors showed similar data using total cumulative doses of inhaled salbutamol (400 μg) and salmeterol (100 μg) and the same outcome variables in acute COPD exacerbations [45]. It seems that salmeterol is as effective and safe as salbutamol in the management of COPD exacerbations.

Side Effects

Inhaled β_2-agonists have considerable cardiovascular effects, such as increased heart rate, systolic blood pressure, and contractility, all at the origin of an increase in oxygen consumption of the heart. However, the commonly used doses of inhaled or nebulized salbutamol do not induce acute myocardial ischemia, arrhythmias, or changes in heart rate variability in patients with coronary artery disease and coexistent clinically stable asthma or COPD [46]. This concept has been very recently reinforced by a study in a cohort of more than 12,000 COPD patients taken from the Saskatchewan Health Services databases. It did not appear that short-acting inhaled β-adrenergics used in these patients increased the risk of fatal or near-fatal acute myocardial infarction [47]. However, at doses based on those used in clinical practice, fenoterol causes more adverse effects (increased heart rate and decreased plasma potassium) than salbutamol or terbutaline [32].

Summary

From a gas exchange viewpoint, it can be concluded that in patients with COPD, inhaled β-adrenergics are relatively safe, regardless of the severity of airway obstruction. Both short-acting and long-acting agents may induce small decreases in oxygen saturation that can be easily corrected with supplemental oxygen therapy. These mild to moderate deleterious effects on gas exchange, namely, a decrease in PaO_2 of the order of 5 mmHg as a mean in the vast majority of studies, are clinically well tolerated. As a general rule, these episodes of oxygen desaturation, usually occurring within the first 30 min following the administration of the agents, are always transient, and are more conspicuous in patients with relatively well-preserved PaO_2. Conceivably, this reflects a more intact tone of the underlying pulmonary vasculature, which can be more sensitive to the vasodilatory effect. Accordingly, this would further worsen the ventilation to perfusion imbalance of those lung regions more structurally deranged. Because of the frequent association of increased cardiac output, it is not possible to differentiate between an active pulmonary vasodilation, i.e., release of hypoxic pulmonary vasoconstriction, and/or passive relaxation of the pulmonary vessels, due to an increase in pulmonary blood flow. In more severe advanced COPD, the pulmonary vascular tone is more affected, with the vessels being more rigid and fixed, such that it is less liable to be relaxed (vasodilated) by selective β-agonists.

The detrimental effect on arterial oxygen saturation following treatment with adrenergic agents can be offset, at least in part, by the simultaneous increase in cardiac output through optimization of mixed venous PO_2 or further worsened by parallel increases in oxygen consumption, via a decreased mixed venous PO_2. This overall gas-exchange response in COPD is aggravated when the dose of adrenergic agents is disproportionately high, which may reflect a high bioavailability or more systemic effects of the drug. The effect is more noticeable when the drug is delivered via the nebulized or intravenous route. Except for fenoterol, which is a less selective β-agonist [32], the differences between short-acting β-agonists (salbutamol and terbutaline) are almost negligible. It appears that the same may be true for long-acting adrenergics, although there are fewer data in the literature.

B. Anticholinergics

Several studies have shown that in COPD, inhaled short-acting anticholinergics have a similar [48–51] or even more effective [52–56] bronchodilating action as β-adrenergics, with relatively fewer side effects [53]. We have extensively alluded to different studies comparing short-acting β-adrenergics and anticholinergics. These studies have shown that anticholinergics have relatively small effects on arterial blood gases in either stable COPD [30,31,33,42] or during exacerbations [35]. The only study of the effects of short-acting anticholinergics on $\dot{V}_A/\dot{Q}$ relationship [31] showed that ipratropium did not produce changes in this outcome. Patients with COPD have an increased cholinergic tone, which may be in part responsible for the impaired pulmonary function seen at rest [57]. Anticholinergic agents act specifically on bronchial smooth muscle rather than on pulmonary vessels, hence improving airway resistance without inducing further gas exchange impairment.

The lack of detrimental effects of short-acting anticholinergics on $\dot{V}_A/\dot{Q}$ mismatching, together with their wide therapeutic margin due to their fewer systemic side effects, makes these drugs particularly suitable for the elderly. This represents a substantial subset of the COPD population. Nonetheless, recent data from the Lung Health Study [58] show that there is an unexpected tendency for coronary and cardiovascular disease to be more common among patients treated with ipratropium than with placebo over 5 years. Although it was not possible to demonstrate a dose effect for major disease categories, there was an apparent dose-related preponderance of tachycardia in the anticholinergic arm, suggesting a possible deleterious effect of ipratropium which requires further investigation.

Although no data are available as yet on the gas exchange response to the new long-acting anticholinergic, tiotropium bromide, it may be expected that this should be mild, if any, in keeping with the cumulative evidence of the lack of effects of ipratropium [59].

C. Theophyllines

While some studies have shown a reduction in PaO_2 or an increase in AaPO2 after intravenous aminophylline in patients with stable COPD [4,60,61] or during exacerbations [62], other studies have not documented any changes [63–65]. It was suggested that the mechanism responsible for the reduction in PaO_2 was the inhibition of hypoxic pulmonary vasoconstriction by the drug resulting in further $\dot{V}_A/\dot{Q}$ worsening. This hypothesis was supported by two experimental studies [66,67], but contradicted in another study which reached opposite conclusions [68]. Studies conducted in dogs suggest that the inhibition of hypoxic vasoconstriction by aminophylline takes place only at high plasma concentrations, above the conventional therapeutic range. Barberà et al. [69] studied the effects of intravenous aminophylline and 100% oxygen breathing on $\dot{V}_A/\dot{Q}$ relationships (using the MIGET) in patients recovering from acute exacerbation of COPD. Aminophylline alone increased FVC and FEV_1, but it did not produce changes in blood gases or in $\dot{V}_A/\dot{Q}$ relationships. Oxygen alone caused modest further deterioration of $\dot{V}_A/\dot{Q}$ relationships compared with air breathing, and the simultaneous administration of aminophylline and oxygen also worsened $\dot{V}_A/\dot{Q}$ mismatching. Individual patients with preexisting low $\dot{V}_A/\dot{Q}$ areas showed a deterioration of $\dot{V}_A/\dot{Q}$ inequalities by aminophylline, and these same individuals further worsened $\dot{V}_A/\dot{Q}$ inequality when oxygen was added to aminophylline. The increased $\dot{V}_A/\dot{Q}$ inequality observed while breathing oxygen during the administration of aminophylline suggests that this agent only partially mitigated the hypoxic vasoconstriction. Although therapeutic doses of aminophylline can increase $\dot{V}_A/\dot{Q}$ inequality in some patients, in general the effect is moderate and of little clinical significance. This study suggests that the possible deleterious effect of aminophylline on gas exchange in patients with COPD had been overemphasized. Another study by the same group in patients with acute severe asthma [70] also showed no deterioration of $\dot{V}_A/\dot{Q}$ mismatching after aminophylline. While several studies have observed that oxygen saturation during sleep in COPD patients improves with theophylline [71–73], others have not confirmed these changes [74,75].

III. Glucocorticosteroids

A. Systemic Steroids

Although there have been three important randomized clinical trials assessing the effects of systemic steroids in patients with COPD during exacerbations over the last few years [76–78], only one has fully documented the benefit on pulmonary gas exchange. Thompson et al. [76] included 27 outpatients with COPD exacerbation in a randomized, double-blind, placebo-controlled trial to assess the efficacy of glucocorticosteroids in the treatment of these episodes. Treatment with oral prednisone (tapering 9-day course starting at 60 mg/day), resulted in a more rapid improvement of PaO_2, $AaPO_2$, and of airflow compared with placebo. Compared with baseline, the changes in PaO_2 were significantly greater on day 3 (23%) and day 10 (26%). Besides the accelerated recovery of gas exchange, treatment with oral prednisone was associated with reduced treatment failure rate and improved perception of shortness of breath.

The mechanisms by which glucocorticosteroids accelerate and facilitate a sustained recovery from episodes of COPD exacerbations remain unsettled, but are likely multifactorial. First, bronchodilatation may be enhanced by upregulation of β-adrenergic receptors located in the airway wall and bronchial vessels. Second, airway wall edema may be minimized by the antiexudative effects of steroids together with vasoconstriction of the bronchial circulation. Indeed, in patients with asthma, fluticasone reduces bronchial blood flow 90 min following inhalation [79]. And, third, $\dot{V}_A/\dot{Q}$ imbalance may be reduced, at least in part, by inhibition of the release of inflammatory mediators and cells, inducing vasoconstriction of the pulmonary vasculature and restore $\dot{V}_A/\dot{Q}$ disturbances.

Another controlled study [80] assessed, the efficacy of a 3- versus 10-day course of intravenous methylprednisolone (at the same doses, 0.5 mg/kg q.i.d. for the first 3 days, then tapered and stopped by the 10th day) in severely hypoxemic COPD patients with exacerbations requiring hospitalization. The 10-day treatment was more effective in improving outcome, but did not benefit a reduction of subsequent exacerbation rates.

A recent multicenter study [81] compared the efficacy of nebulized budesonide (2 mg every 6 hr), to that of oral prednisolone (30 mg every 12 hr), or placebo in 199 patients. All received standard treatment with nebulized bronchodilators, antibiotics, and supplemental oxygen. Both budesonide and prednisolone improved the FEV_1 without significant differences between treatment groups. Interestingly, although there were no differences in PaO_2 improvements, $PaCO_2$ decrements were significantly greater in both steroid arms than in the placebo group. Moreover, the proportion of patients showing a considerable decline in $PaCO_2$ (i.e., $\geq$5 mmHg) was substantially larger in the prednisolone than in the budesonide or placebo arms, suggesting that systemic steroids may be more effective than nebulized steroids. This may be relevant to COPD patients with hypercapnic respiratory failure, as it may be plausible that a higher dose of inhaled steroids might provide greater efficacy. The conclusion was that budesonide may constitute an alternative to oral steroids in the management of nonacidotic exacerbations of COPD patients. However, this is a very costly treatment that needs validation.

B. Inhaled Steroids

In addition to the former study [81], the effects of inhaled steroids on gas exchange have been assessed in a 2-month treatment of budesonide (800 μg twice daily) in 19 stable severe COPD patients using a noncontrolled design [82]. Disturbances of $\dot{V}_A/\dot{Q}$ ratios (by MIGET), arterial blood gases, and diffusing capacity for carbon monoxide (DL_{CO}) were all measured, the hypothesis being that each of these indices may reflect the status of the gas exchange zone of the lungs. The only positive finding was a significant increase in DL_{CO} (by 9%) after the treatment period, with increases of order 50% in half of the patients, precisely in those with more moderate $\dot{V}_A/\dot{Q}$ inequalities at baseline. Although the clinical relevance of these data remain unsettled, it was hypothesized that inhaled steroids might improve an increase in volume of inspired air at the alveolar level, without parallel measurable changes of $\dot{V}_A/\dot{Q}$ descriptors.

IV. Vasodilators

A. Systemic Vasodilators

Mild to moderate pulmonary hypertension signals a worse outcome for COPD patients. This is why numerous attempts have been made to manage these patients with vasodilators. However, a major side effect of vasodilators on the pulmonary circulation is the inhibition of hypoxic vasoconstriction. Mélot et al. [83] were the first to demonstrate that the decrease in pulmonary vascular resistance induced by nifedipine was accompanied by a substantial decrease of PaO_2, due to the increase in perfusion of areas with low $\dot{V}_A/\dot{Q}$ ratios in the context of a substantial increase in cardiac output. This suggested that nifedipine had suppressed the beneficial effect of hypoxic vasoconstriction on the underlying $\dot{V}_A/\dot{Q}$ relationships. The deleterious effect of the acute administration of systemic vasodilators on $\dot{V}_A/\dot{Q}$ inequalities in COPD has also been assessed using felodipine [84], prostaglandin E_1 [85], atrial natriuretic factor [86], and acetylcholine [87]. In only one study, using diltiazem, was there no effect on gas exchange [85].

Similar effects of vasodilator treatment have been demonstrated in exercise-induced pulmonary hypertension. Agusti et al. [88] showed that nifedipine dampened the exercise-induced increase in pulmonary vascular resistance while it increased cardiac output. This was associated with further $\dot{V}_A/\dot{Q}$ imbalance and lower arterial oxygenation. These data highlight that the deleterious effect of vasodilators on $\dot{V}_A/\dot{Q}$ balance during exercise and suggest that hypoxic pulmonary vasoconstriction may also be an important mechanism to improve $\dot{V}_A/\dot{Q}$ matching while exercising [88].

B. Selective Vasodilators (Nitric Oxide)

Inhaled nitric oxide (NO) is a selective vasodilator of the pulmonary circulation [89]. The lack of a systemic effect of NO is due to its inactivation when it combines with hemoglobin, for which it has a very high affinity. In patients with acute respiratory distress syndrome (ARDS), the administration of inhaled NO produces significant increases of PaO_2, secondary to reduction of increased intrapulmonary shunting [90]. Subsequently, the effect of inhaled NO in COPD has been evaluated in several studies [87,91–94]. When inhaled NO is administered using low concentrations, it does not appear to exert any effect on gas exchange, whereas it decreases pulmonary arterial pressure in a dose-dependent manner [87]. When given at high doses (40 ppm), the individual response to inhaled NO may be variable [87,92]. In general, PaO_2 decreases in most of the patients [92–94]. This deleterious effect on pulmonary gas exchange is the result of a further $\dot{V}_A/\dot{Q}$ worsening, as shown by a greater proportion of lung units with low $\dot{V}_A/\dot{Q}$ ratios [92]. The negligible increased intrapulmonary shunt of COPD is not modified by inhaled NO [92]. The detrimental effect of inhaled NO on pulmonary blood flow in COPD patients has been attributed to the release of hypoxic pulmonary vasoconstriction in areas with low $\dot{V}_A/\dot{Q}$ ratios, to which the gas has access, producing an effect similar to that of systemic vasodilators [92]. In fact, in healthy subjects, inhaled NO (40 ppm) fully mitigates the increase in pulmonary vascular tone following a hypoxic mixture breathing [95]. Thus, in COPD patients in whom hypoxemia is caused essentially by $\dot{V}_A/\dot{Q}$ imbalance rather than by increased intrapulmonary shunt, inhaled NO worsens gas exchange due to the impairment of the hypoxic regulation of the ventilation to perfusion balance. This may help in predicting which patients with respiratory failure should show a greater improvement of gas exchange with inhaled NO. Patients without preexisting chronic lung disease in which increased intrapulmonary shunt is the principal determinant of hypoxemia (i.e., ARDS, pneumonia) appear to be the most likely candidates to benefit from NO inhalation. This suggestion is supported by experimental studies in dogs [96].

The effects of inhaled NO on gas exchange may be different during exercise than at rest. Roger et al. [93] studied the effects of inhaled NO during exercise in COPD patients. They showed that pulmonary vasodilation occurred both at rest and during exercise. However, whereas PaO_2 decreased during exercise while breathing room air, no change was shown during NO inhalation. Furthermore, at-rest inhalation of NO worsened $\dot{V}_A/\dot{Q}$ inequality. During exercise, $\dot{V}_A/\dot{Q}$ imbalance improved while breathing both room air and NO, such that perfusion of poorly ventilated alveolar units with low $\dot{V}_A/\dot{Q}$ ratios was similar under both conditions [93]. Accordingly, from rest to exercise the proportion of blood flow to low $\dot{V}_A/\dot{Q}$ units decreased significantly with inhaled NO, whereas it remained unchanged while breathing room air. These findings indicate that in COPD, the inhalation of NO during exercise reduces pulmonary hypertension and, at variance with the effects shown at rest, it may prevent the development of further hypoxemia. The latter may be explained by a preferential distribution of NO during exercise to well-ventilated $\dot{V}_A/\dot{Q}$ units with faster time constants, which are more efficient in terms of gas exchange. In clinical terms, these findings may imply that if inhaled NO could be delivered specifically to those alveolar units that are better ventilated and have faster time constants, the beneficial vasodilator effect of NO would not be offset by its deleterious impact on gas exchange. In this regard, the so-called spiked delivery of NO, which is specifically adjusted to deliver the gas at the beginning of inspiration [97,98], might be particularly useful to treat pulmonary hypertension, especially during exercise, in COPD patients.

V. Other Drugs

There have been a few studies assessing the effect of oral almitrine bismesylate, a peripheral chemoreceptor [99,100], in COPD patients with hypercapnic respiratory insufficiency. In a study [99] of patients on mechanical ventilation, conventional and inert gas exchange indices improved, together with a small but significant decrease in cardiac output and a modest increase in pulmonary vascular resistance. In another study [100], arterial blood gases improved slightly but significantly due to $\dot{V}_A/\dot{Q}$ improvement, with a modest increase in pulmonary vascular resistance. In these studies, there was essentially a redistribution of pulmonary blood flow from areas with low $\dot{V}_A/\dot{Q}$ units to regions with normal $\dot{V}_A/\dot{Q}$ relationships. Despite its mild beneficial effects on gas exchange, the small increase in pulmonary artery pressure combined with some important side effects, such as weight loss and peripheral neuropathy, have made almitrine not recommendable in the management of respiratory insufficiency in COPD [3].

References

1. Barberà JA. Chronic obstructive pulmonary disease. In: Roca J, Rodriguez-Roisin R, Wagner PD, eds. Pulmonary and Peripheral Gas Exchange in Health and Disease. New York: Marcel Dekker, 2000:229–261.
2. Roca J, Wagner PD. Contribution of multiple inert gas elimination technique to pulmonary medicine. 1. Principles and information content of the multiple inert gas elimination technique. Thorax 1994; 49:815–824.
3. Pauwels RA, Buist AS, Calverley PM, Jenkins CR, Hurd SS, on behalf of the GOLD Scientific Committee. Global strategy for the diagnosis, management, and prevention of chronic obstructive pulmonary disease. NHLBI/WHO Global Initiative for Chronic Obstructive Lung Disease (GOLD) Workshop Summary. Am J Respir Crit Care Med 2001; 163:1256–1276.
4. Halmagyi DF, Cotes JE. Reduction in systemic blood oxygen as a result of

procedures affecting the pulmonary circulation in patients with chronic pulmonary disease. Clin Sci 1959; 18:475–489.
5. Knudson RJ, Constantine HP. An effect of isoproterenol on ventilation-perfusion in asthmatic versus normal subjects. J Appl Physiol 1967; 22:402–406.
6. Tai E, Read J. Response of blood gas tensions to aminophylline and isoprenaline in patients with asthma. Thorax 1967; 22:543–549.
7. Palmer KN, Diament ML. Spirometry and blood-gas tensions in bronchial asthma and chronic bronchitis. Lancet 1967; 2:383–384.
8. Palmer KN, Legge JS, Hamilton WF, Diament ML. Comparison of effect of salbutamol and isoprenaline on spirometry and blood-gas tensions in bronchial asthma. Br Med J 1970; 2:23–24.
9. Streeton JA, Morgan EB. Salbutamol in status asthmaticus and severe chronic obstructive bronchitis. Postgrad Med J 1971; 47(suppl):125–128.
10. Gazioglu K, Condemi JJ, Hyde RW, Kaltreider NL. Effect of isoproterenol on gas exchange during air and oxygen breathing in patients with asthma. Am J Med 1971; 50:185–190.
11. Harris L. Comparison of the effect on blood gases, ventilation, and perfusion of isoproterenol-phenylephrine and salbutamol aerosols in chronic bronchitis with asthma. J Allergy Clin Immunol 1972; 49:63–71.
12. Ingram RH Jr, Krumpe PE, Duffell GM, Maniscalco B. Ventilation-perfusion changes after aerosolized isoproterenol in asthma. Am Rev Respir Dis 1970; 101:364–370.
13. Wagner PD, Dantzker DR, Iacovoni VE, Tomlin WC, West JB. Ventilation-perfusion inequality in asymptomatic asthma. Am Rev Respir Dis 1978; 118:511–524.
14. Palmer KN, Hamilton WF, Lge JS, Diament ML. Effect of a selective beta-adrenergic blocker in preventing falls in arterial oxygen tension following isoprenaline in asthmatic subjects. Lancet 1969; 2:1092–1094.
15. Ashraf M, Sharp J, Kehoe T, Cugell DW. A comparison of the effects of Th115a (fenoterol) and isoproterenol on spirometry and arterial blood gases. Chest 1978; 73:981.
16. Chick TW, Nicholson DP, Johnson RL Jr. Effects of isoproterenol on distribution of ventilation and perfusion in asthma. Am Rev Respir Dis 1973; 107:869–873.
17. Riding WD, Dinda P, Chatterjee SS. The bronchodilator and cardiac effects of five pressure-packed aerosols in asthma. Br J Dis Chest 1970; 64:37–45.
18. Ringsted CV, Eliasen K, Andersen JB, Heslet L, Qvist J. Ventilation-perfusion distributions and central hemodynamics in chronic obstructive pulmonary disease. Effects of terbutaline administration. Chest 1989; 96:976–983.
19. Peinado VI, Barberà JA, Ramirez J, et al. Endothelial dysfunction in pulmonary arteries of patients with mild COPD. Am J Physiol 1998; 274:L908–L913.
20. Eliasen K, Ringsted C, Munck O, Hjortso E, Heslet L. Pulmonary vasodilatation and augmentation of right ventricular function following terbuta-

line infusion in severe chronic pulmonary disease. Clin Physiol 1991; 11:231–243.
21. Stockley RA, Finnegan P, Bishop JM. Effect of intravenous terbutaline on arterial blood gas tensions, ventilation, and pulmonary circulation in patients with chronic bronchitis and cor pulmonale. Thorax 1977; 32:601–605.
22. Teule GJ, Majid PA. Haemodynamic effects of terbutaline in chronic obstructive airways disease. Thorax 1980; 35:536–542.
23. Jones RM, Stockley RA, Bishop JM. Early effects of intravenous terbutaline on cardiopulmonary function in chronic obstructive bronchitis and pulmonary hypertension. Thorax 1982; 37:746–750.
24. Brent BN, Mahler D, Berger HJ, Matthay RA, Pytlik L, Zaret BL. Augmentation of right ventricular performance in chronic obstructive pulmonary disease by terbutaline: a combined radionuclide and hemodynamic study. Am J Cardiol 1982; 50:313–319.
25. Ballester E, Reyes A, Roca J, Guitart R, Wagner PD, Rodriguez-Roisin R. Ventilation-perfusion mismatching in acute severe asthma: effects of salbutamol and 100% oxygen. Thorax 1989; 44:258–267.
26. Ballester E, Roca J, Ramis L, Wagner PD, Rodriguez-Roisin R. Pulmonary gas exchange in severe chronic asthma. Response to 100% oxygen and salbutamol. Am Rev Respir Dis 1990; 141:558–562.
27. Tschopp JM, Gabathuler J, Righetti A, Junod AF. Comparative effects of acute O_2 breathing and terbutaline in patients with chronic obstructive pulmonary disease. A combined hemodynamic and radionuclide study. Eur J Respir Dis 1985; 67:351–359.
28. Marvin PM, Baker BJ, Dutt AK, Murphy ML, Bone RC. Physiologic effects of oral bronchodilators during rest and exercise in chronic obstructive pulmonary disease. Chest 1983; 84:684–689.
29. Postma DS, Koeter GH, vd Mark TW, Reig RP, Sluiter HJ. The effects of oral slow-release terbutaline on the circadian variation in spirometry and arterial blood gas levels in patients with chronic airflow obstruction. Chest 1985; 87:653–657.
30. Gross NJ, Bankwala Z. Effects of an anticholinergic bronchodilator on arterial blood gases of hypoxemic patients with chronic obstructive pulmonary disease. Comparison with a beta-adrenergic agent. Am Rev Respir Dis 1987; 136:1091–1094.
31. Viegas CA, Ferrer A, Montserrat JM, Barberà JA, Roca J, Rodriguez-Roisin R. Ventilation-perfusion response after fenoterol in hypoxemic patients with stable COPD. Chest 1996; 110:71–77.
32. Wong CS, Pavord ID, Williams J, Britton JR, Tattersfield AE. Bronchodilator, cardiovascular, and hypokalaemic effects of fenoterol, salbutamol, and terbutaline in asthma. Lancet 1990; 336:1396–1399.
33. Saito S, Miyamoto K, Nishimura M, et al. Effects of inhaled bronchodilators on pulmonary hemodynamics at rest and during exercise in patients with COPD. Chest 1999; 115:376–382.
34. Carlone S, Angelici E, Palange P, Serra P, Farber MO. Effects of fenoterol on

oxygen transport in patients with chronic airflow obstruction. Chest 1988; 93: 790–794.
35. Karpel JP, Pesin J, Greenberg D, Gentry E. A comparison of the effects of ipratropium bromide and metaproterenol sulfate in acute exacerbations of COPD. Chest 1990; 98:835–839.
36. Bernasconi M, Brandolese R, Poggi R, Manzin E, Rossi A. Dose-response effects and time course of effects of inhaled fenoterol on respiratory mechanics and arterial oxygen tension in mechanically ventilated patients with chronic airflow obstruction. Intensive Care Med 1990; 16:108–114.
37. Higgins RM, Cookson WO, Chadwick GA. Changes in blood gas levels after nebuhaler and nebulizer administration of terbutaline in severe chronic airway obstruction. Bull Eur Physiopathol Respir 1987; 23:261–264.
38. Barberà JA, Roca J, Ferrer A, et al. Mechanisms of worsening gas exchange during acute exacerbations of chronic obstructive pulmonary disease. Eur Respir J 1997; 10:1285–1291.
39. Amoroso P, Wilson SR, Moxham J, Ponte J. Acute effects of inhaled salbutamol on the metabolic rate of normal subjects. Thorax 1993; 48:882–885.
40. Minh VD, Chun D, Fairshter RD, Vasquez P, Wilson AF, Dolan GF. Supine change in arterial oxygenation in patients with chronic obstructive pulmonary disease. Am Rev Respir Dis 1986; 133:820–824.
41. Pinet C, Ferre R, Tessonnier F, Orehek J. Supine hypoxemia following nebulizated salbutamol in patients with chronic airway obstruction. Lung 2001; 179:259–263.
42. Khoukaz G, Gross NJ. Effects of salmeterol on arterial blood gases in patients with stable chronic obstructive pulmonary disease. Comparison with albuterol and ipratropium. Am J Respir Crit Care Med 1999; 160:1028–1030.
43. Malolepszy J, Boszormenyl G, Nagy O, Selroos P, Larsso R. Safety of formoterol Turbuhaler at cumulative dose of 90 microg in patients with acute bronchial obstruction. Eur Respir J 2001; 18:928–934.
44. Cazzola M, D'Amato M, Califano C, et al. Formoterol as dry powder oral inhalation compared with salbutamol metered-dose inhaler in acute exacerbations of chronic obstructive pulmonary disease. Clin Ther 2002; 24:595–604.
45. Cazzola M, Califano C, DiPerna F, et al. Acute effects of higher than customary doses of salmeterol and salbutamol in patients with acute exacerbation of COPD. Respir Med 2002; 96:790–795.
46. Rossinen J, Partanen J, Stenius-Aarniala B, Nieminen MS. Salbutamol inhalation has no effect on myocardial ischaemia, arrhythmias and heart-rate variability in patients with coronary artery disease plus asthma or chronic obstructive pulmonary disease. J Intern Med 1998; 243:361–366.
47. Suissa S, Assimes T, Ernst P. Inhaled short acting beta agonist use in COPD and the risk of acute myocardial infarction. Thorax 2003; 58:43–46.
48. Klock LE, Miller TD, Morris AH, Watanabe S, Dickman M. A comparative study of atropine sulfate and isoproterenol hydrochloride in chronic bronchitis. Am Rev Respir Dis 1975; 112:371–376.
49. Leitch AG, Hopkin JM, Ellis DA, Merchant S, McHardy GJ. The effect of

aerosol ipratropium bromide and salbutamol on exercise tolerance in chronic bronchitis. Thorax 1978; 33:711–713.
50. Thiessen B, Pedersen OF. Maximal expiratory flows and forced vital capacity in normal, asthmatic and bronchitic subjects after salbutamol and ipratropium bromide. Respiration 1982; 43:304–316.
51. Easton PA, Jadue C, Dhingra S, Anthonisen NR. A comparison of the bronchodilating effects of a beta-2 adrenergic agent (albuterol) and an anti-cholinergic agent (ipratropium bromide), given by aerosol alone or in sequence. N Engl J Med 1986; 315:735–739.
52. Hughes JA, Tobin MJ, Bellamy D, Hutchison DC. Effects of ipratropium bromide and fenoterol aerosols in pulmonary emphysema. Thorax 1982; 37:667–670.
53. Gross NJ, Skorodin MS. Anticholinergic, antimuscarinic bronchodilators. Am Rev Respir Dis 1984; 129:856–870.
54. Passamonte PM, Martinez AJ. Effect of inhaled atropine or metaproterenol in patients with chronic airway obstruction and therapeutic serum theophylline levels. Chest 1984; 85:610–615.
55. Braun SR, McKenzie WN, Copeland C, Knight L, Ellersieck M. A comparison of the effect of ipratropium and albuterol in the treatment of chronic obstructive airway disease. Arch Intern Med 1989; 149:544–547.
56. Chapman KR. The role of anticholinergic bronchodilators in adult asthma and chronic obstructive pulmonary disease. Lung 1990; 168:295–303.
57. Gross NJ. Anticholinergic agents in chronic bronchitis and emphysema. Postgrad Med J 1987; 63:29–34.
58. Anthonisen NR, Connett JE, Enright PL, Manfreda J. Hospitalizations and mortality in the Lung Health Study. Am J Respir Crit Care Med 2002; 166:333–339.
59. Casaburi R, Mahler DA, Jones PW, et al. A long-term evaluation of once-daily inhaled tiotropium in chronic obstructive pulmonary disease. Eur Respir J 2002; 19:217–224.
60. Pain MC, Charlton GC, Read J. Effect of intravenous aminophylline on distribution of pulmonary blood flow in obstructive lung disease. Am Rev Respir Dis 1967; 95:1005–1014.
61. Daly JJ, Howard P. Effect of intravenous aminophylline on the arterial oxygen saturation in chronic bronchitis. Thorax 1965; 20:324–326.
62. Zielinski J, Chatterjee SS. Effect of aminophylline on arterial blood gases in patients with exacerbation of chronic respiratory failure. Bull Physiopathol Respir (Nancy) 1972; 8:797–806.
63. Alexander MR, Dull WL, Kasik JE. Treatment of chronic obstructive pulmonary disease with orally administered theophylline. A double-blind, controlled study. JAMA 1980; 244:2286–2290.
64. Mahler DA, Matthay RA, Snyder PE, Wells CK, Loke J. Sustained-release theophylline reduces dyspnea in nonreversible obstructive airway disease. Am Rev Respir Dis 1985; 131:22–25.
65. Rice KL, Leatherman JW, Duane PG, et al. Aminophylline for acute

exacerbations of chronic obstructive pulmonary disease. A controlled trial. Ann Intern Med 1987; 107:305–309.
66. Hales CA, Kazemi H. Hypoxic vascular response of the lung: effect of aminophylline and epinephrine. Am Rev Respir Dis 1974; 110:126–132.
67. Bisgard GE, Will JA. Glucagon and aminophylline as pulmonary vasodilators in the calf with hypoxic pulmonary hypertension. Chest 1977; 71:263–265.
68. Benumof JL, Trousdale FR. Aminophylline does not inhibit canine hypoxic pulmonary vasoconstriction. Am Rev Respir Dis 1982; 126:1017–1019.
69. Barberà JA, Reyes A, Roca J, Montserrat JM, Wagner PD, Rodriguez-Roisin R. Effect of intravenously administered aminophylline on ventilation/perfusion inequality during recovery from exacerbations of chronic obstructive pulmonary disease. Am Rev Respir Dis 1992; 145:1328–1333.
70. Montserrat JM, Barberà JA, Viegas C, Roca J, Rodriguez-Roisin R. Gas exchange response to intravenous aminophylline in patients with a severe exacerbation of asthma. Eur Respir J 1995; 8:28–33.
71. Berry RB, Desa MM, Branum JP, Light RW. Effect of theophylline on sleep and sleep-disordered breathing in patients with chronic obstructive pulmonary disease. Am Rev Respir Dis 1991; 143:245–250.
72. Mulloy E, McNicholas WT. Theophylline improves gas exchange during rest, exercise, and sleep in severe chronic obstructive pulmonary disease. Am Rev Respir Dis 1993; 148:1030–1036.
73. Man GC, Champman KR, Ali SH, Darke AC. Sleep quality and nocturnal respiratory function with once-daily theophylline (Uniphyl) and inhaled salbutamol in patients with COPD. Chest 1996; 110:648–653.
74. Brander PE, Salmi T. Nocturnal oxygen saturation and sleep quality in patients with advanced chronic obstructive pulmonary disease during treatment with moderate dose CR-theophylline. Eur J Clin Pharmacol 1992; 43:125–129.
75. Martin RJ, Pak J. Overnight theophylline concentrations and effects on sleep and lung function in chronic obstructive pulmonary disease. Am Rev Respir Dis 1992; 145:540–544.
76. Thompson WH, Nielson CP, Carvalho P, Charan NB, Crowley JJ. Controlled trial of oral prednisone in outpatients with acute COPD exacerbation. Am J Respir Crit Care Med 1996; 154:407–412.
77. Davies L, Angus RM, Calverley PM. Oral corticosteroids in patients admitted to hospital with exacerbations of chronic obstructive pulmonary disease: a prospective randomised controlled trial. Lancet 1999; 354:456–460.
78. Niewoehner DE, Erbland ML, Deupree RH, et al. Effect of systemic glucocorticoids on exacerbations of chronic obstructive pulmonary disease. Department of Veterans Affairs Cooperative Study Group. N Engl J Med 1999; 340:1941–1947.
79. Kumar SD, Brieva JL, Danta I, Wanner A. Transient effect of inhaled fluticasone on airway mucosal blood flow in subjects with and without asthma. Am J Respir Crit Care Med 2000; 161:918–921.
80. Sayiner A, Aytemur ZA, Cirit M, Unsal I. Systemic glucocorticoids in severe exacerbations of COPD. Chest 2001; 119:726–730.

81. Maltais F, Ostenelli J, Bourbeau J, et al. Comparison of nebulized budesonide and oral prednisolone with placebo in the treatment of acute exacerbations of chronic obstructive pulmonary disease: a randomized controlled trial. Am J Respir Crit Care Med 2002; 165:698–703.
82. Sandek K, Bratel T, Lagerstrand L. Effects on diffusing capacity and ventilation-perfusion relationships of budesonide inhalations for 2 months in chronic obstructive pulmonary disease (COPD). Respir Med 2001; 95:676–684.
83. Mélot C, Hallemans R, Naeije R, Mols P, Lejeune P. Deleterious effect of nifedipine on pulmonary gas exchange in chronic obstructive pulmonary disease. Am Rev Respir Dis 1984; 130:612–616.
84. Bratel T, Hedenstierna G, Nyquist O, Ripe E. The use of a vasodilator, felodipine, as an adjuvant to long-term oxygen treatment in COLD patients. Eur Respir J 1990; 3:46–54.
85. Guénard H, Castaing Y, Mélot C, Naeije R. Gas exchange during acute respiratory failure in patients with chronic obstructive pulmonary disease. In: Derenne JP, Whitelaw WA, Similowski T, eds. Acute Respiratory Failure in Chronic Obstructive Pulmonary Disease. New York: Marcel Dekker, 1996: 227–266.
86. Andrivet P, Chabrier PE, Defouilloy C, Brun-Buisson C, Adnot S. Intravenously administered atrial natriuretic factor in patients with COPD. Effects on ventilation-perfusion relationships and pulmonary hemodynamics. Chest 1994; 106:118–124.
87. Adnot S, Kouyoumdjian C, Defouilloy C, et al. Hemodynamic and gas exchange responses to infusion of acetylcholine and inhalation of nitric oxide in patients with chronic obstructive lung disease and pulmonary hypertension. Am Rev Respir Dis 1993; 148:310–316.
88. Agustí AG, Barberà JA, Roca J, Wagner PD, Guitart R, Rodriguez-Roisin R. Hypoxic pulmonary vasoconstriction and gas exchange during exercise in chronic obstructive pulmonary disease. Chest 1990; 97:268–275.
89. Pepke-Zaba J, Higenbottam TW, Dinh-Xuan AT, Stone D, Wallwork J. Inhaled nitric oxide as a cause of selective pulmonary vasodilatation in pulmonary hypertension. Lancet 1991; 338:1173–1174.
90. Reyes A, Roca J, Rodriguez-Roisin R, Torres A, Ussetti P, Wagner PD. Effect of almitrine on ventilation-perfusion distribution in adult respiratory distress syndrome. Am Respir Dis 1988; 137:1062–1067.
91. Moinard J, Manier G, Pillet O, Castaing Y. Effect of inhaled nitric oxide on hemodynamics and V_A/Q inequalities in patients with chronic obstructive pulmonary disease. Am J Respir Crit Care Med 1994; 149:1482–1487.
92. Barberà JA, Roger N, Roca J, Rovira I, Higenbottam TW, Rodriguez-Roisin R. Worsening of pulmonary gas exchange with nitric oxide inhalation in chronic obstructive pulmonary disease. Lancet 1996; 347:436–440.
93. Roger N, Barberà JA, Roca J, Rovira I, Gómez FP, Rodriguez-Roisin R. Nitric oxide inhalation during exercise in chronic obstructive pulmonary disease. Am J Respir Crit Care Med 1997; 156:800–806.
94. Katayama Y, Higenbottam TW, Diaz de Atauri MJ, et al. Inhaled nitric oxide

and arterial oxygen tension in patients with chronic obstructive pulmonary disease and severe pulmonary hypertension. Thorax 1997; 52:120–124.

95. Frostell CG, Blomqvist H, Hedenstierna G, Lundberg J, Zapol WM. Inhaled nitric oxide selectively reverses human hypoxic pulmonary vasoconstriction without causing systemic vasodilatation. Anesthesiology 1993; 78:427–435.
96. Hopkins SR, Johnson EC, Richardson RS, Wagner H, De Rosa M, Wagner PD. Effects of inhaled nitric oxide on gas exchange in lungs with shunt or poorly ventilated areas. Am J Respir Crit Care Med 1997; 156:484–491.
97. Katayama Y, Higenbottam TW, Cremona G, et al. Minimizing the inhaled dose of NO with breath-by-breath delivery of spikes of concentrated gas. Circulation 1998; 98:2429–2432.
98. Siddons TE, Asif M, Higenbottam T. Does the method of delivery of inhaled nitric oxide influence oxygenation and V_A/Q patterns in severe COPD? (abstr). Eur Respir J 2000; 16:267s.
99. Castaing Y, Manier G, Varene N, Guenard H. Effects of oral almitrine on the distribution of VA/Q ratio in chronic obstructive lung diseases. Bull Eur Physiopathol Respir 1981; 17:917–932.
100. Mélot C, Naeije R, Rothschild T, Mertens P, Mols P, Hallemans R. Improvement in ventilation-perfusion matching by almitrine in COPD. Chest 1983; 83:528–533.

7

Genetics of COPD

JIAN-QING HE, IKUMA KASUGA, and PETER D. PARÉ

St. Paul's Hospital
Vancouver, British Columbia, Canada

I. Introduction

Chronic obstructive pulmonary disease (COPD) is characterized by progressive development of airflow obstruction that is not fully reversible. The airflow obstruction is caused by a combination of small-airway narrowing and fibrosis and parenchymal destruction due to an exaggerated inflammatory response to noxious particles and gases. Although cigarette smoking is by far the most important risk factor, only 10–20% of smokers develop symptomatic COPD and <15% of the variation in lung function among smokers can be explained by the extent and duration of cigarette smoking. Therefore, differences in susceptibility to COPD in smokers must exist. Environmental risk factors, such as air pollution, occupational dusts and chemicals, and childhood viral respiratory infection have been identified as contributors to this variation. In this chapter we review evidence of genetic risk for COPD and genetic factors that might influence the response to therapy.

II. Evidence of Genetic Risk

Since 1963, severe α_1-antitrypsin (α_1-AT) deficiency, which follows a simple Mendelian pattern of inheritance, has remained the only proven genetic risk factor for COPD [1]. However, compelling evidence of other genetic factors for COPD has been provided by epidemiological studies. There is an increased risk of COPD within the families of COPD probands but without clear Mendelian inheritance [2]. Lower forced expiratory volume in 1 sec (FEV_1), chronic bronchitis, and COPD are more prevalent among the first-degree relatives and siblings of cases, after correction for other risk factors such as smoking habits, and α_1-AT deficiency [3]. The prevalence of COPD and similarity in lung function decrease with increased genetic distance [4].

Although familial clustering of COPD may be due to shared environmental factors, there is more evidence to support a genetic basis; twin studies have found estimates of heritability for FEV_1 that range from 0.5 to 0.8 (i.e., 50–80% of the variability in lung function can be attributed to genes) [5,6].

Models for a genetic contribution to COPD indicate that, with the exception of α_1-AT, it is a complex genetic disease [7]. It is likely that several genes, each with relatively small effects, mediate the genetic susceptibility to COPD, and different combinations of susceptibility genes may lead to similar phenotypes. This speculation is consistent with our knowledge of the pathogenesis of COPD, which involves several cell types, and many enzymes and inflammatory mediators, interacting in an intricate manner to influence the development of airway inflammation and parenchymal destruction.

III. Methods to Identify Susceptibility Genes

There are several approaches to identifying susceptibility genes for disease. The two main strategies used to identify COPD susceptibility genes are genomic scans and association studies.

A. Genomic Scans

The genomic scan approach involves searching the entire human genome for regions that harbor disease-causing genes. Traditionally, it has been performed by studying families using a technique known as linkage analysis. It requires affected families of at least two generations. Each family member is typed for DNA markers such as dinucleotide repeats and single nucleotide polymorphisms (SNPs), which are scattered throughout the genome. Linkage analysis determines whether any of the markers are inherited with the disease more than predicted by chance. If so, that disease is said to be "linked" to that marker on a certain chromosome. The next step is to identify candidate genes near that marker. The advantage of a genomic scan is that novel genes can be identified and implicated in the pathogenesis of a disease. However, the disadvantage is the requirement for families with several affected members in whom accurate phenotypic data are available. This is difficult in COPD due to its late age of onset and the importance of cigarette smoking in the pathogenesis. By the time patients present with COPD, their parents are likely to have died and their children may be too young to manifest significant airflow obstruction. In addition, it is difficult to identify families in which each member has a similar level of exposure to cigarette smoke.

Silverman et al. tested the power of linkage to detect COPD susceptibility genes by studying 28 α_1-AT-deficient families containing 155 individuals [8]. They performed linkage analysis between protease inhibitor (PI) type and serum α_1-AT level and spirometry-related phenotypes. They found that qualitative phenotypes provided stronger evidence for linkage than quantitative phenotypes. As qualitative phenotypes they used mild or moderate COPD, defined as an FEV_1 <80% predicted and <60% predicted, respectively, in combination with a FEV_1/FVC (forced vital capacity) ratio less than 90% predicted.

There is only one group that has used linkage analysis in COPD [8–10]. Silverman and his associates enrolled 72 individuals who had severe, early-onset COPD (without α_1-AT deficiency) and 585 of their relatives. They performed classical linkage analysis using quantitative spirometric phenotypes as well as categorical phenotypes of airway obstruction and chronic bronchitis. The probands in these studies had an FEV_1 less than 40% predicted and were less than 53 years old. The qualitative phenotypes included mild and moderate COPD, as defined above, and a clinical diagnosis of chronic bronchitis. Using these qualitative phenotypes they found suggestive evidence for linkage (LOD score >1.21) on chromosomes 12, 19, and 22. The highest LOD score for chronic bronchitis was 1.37 on chromosome 22. The highest two-point LOD score (3.14) was seen when the analysis was restricted to smokers and when mild obstruction was the phenotype. For the quantitative phenotypes, FEV_1, FVC, and FEV_1/FVC, multipoint variance-component linkage analysis was performed and the highest LOD score was 4.12 for FEV_1/FVC on chromosome 2q with suggestive evidence for linkage on chromosomes 1 and 17. The highest LOD score for FEV_1 was 2.43 on chromosome 12 in the same region that was linked in the qualitative study. Interleukin-8 (IL-8) receptor α is located within the linked locus on chromosome 2 and microsomal glutathione S-transferase, a xenobiotic metabolizing enzyme involved in detoxification of toxic substances in cigarette smoke, is located on chromosome 12 in the linked region.

The other type of genomic scan method, affected sib-pair analysis, is suitable for complex diseases such as COPD. A multicenter consortium is in the process of identifying ~1000 affected sib pairs with COPD [11]. Using this method, greater than expected sharing of alleles at a locus by the affected sibs suggests that the locus contains, or is near, a disease-causing gene.

B. Association Studies

The association study approach involves choosing candidate genes that are implicated in the pathogenesis of COPD. The next step is to identify polymorphisms within or close to the gene, especially ones that could affect its regulation or function. Finally, one examines whether the polymorphisms occur more frequently in individuals who have COPD than in an appropriate control population. A disadvantage of association studies is that only known genes can be examined.

The two basic designs of association studies are prospective cohort studies and respective case-control studies. To date most association studies in COPD have been case-control studies, which involve unrelated individuals. Although this approach circumvents many of the problems associated with family studies, there is a risk of false positive results due to population admixture. This and small sample size has led to lack of reproducibility between studies.

Part of the lack of reproducibility could be because the genetic basis of COPD may not be the same in different populations. Recently, Weiss et al. listed 10 specific issues that should be addressed in any case-control association study of a candidate gene [12]. First, the selection and matching of cases and controls is very important, since false negative or false positive results may arise from population admixture. Second, a large sample size and relatively high allele frequency are necessary to power studies sufficiently, since each gene polymorphism is likely to have a small effect. An important issue in any association study is the recognition that the polymorphic allele being studied may directly affect the expression of the phenotype, or more likely, the polymorphic allele may be in linkage disequilibrium with another allele at a nearby locus that is the true susceptibility allele. Linkage disequilibrium relates to the tendency for polymorphic alleles that are located in the same chromosomal region to be inherited together over many generations. Other issues discussed by Weiss include observational bias, multivariate analysis, and multiple comparisons.

IV. Phenotypes

For years, clinician, physiologists, pathologists, and epidemiologists have struggled with the definition of COPD. For research purposes, clinicians,

Table 1 COPD Phenotypes in Genetic Studies

Chronic bronchitis—defined on the basis of persistent cough and sputum, weakly related to airflow obstruction.
Emphysema—defined pathologically or by CT scanning.
COPD—defined functionally, usually on the basis of reduced FEV_1 % predicted and FEV_1/FVC ratio. No universally accepted cutoff values are available.
Lung function—various measures of lung function can be used as quantitative traits in genetic studies.
Rate of change of lung function—accelerated decline in lung function in response to cigarette smoking is believed to be the most important pathophysiological event in COPD. This is a powerful phenotype.
Rate of lung growth, maximum achieved lung function, or age at onset of decline of lung function—there could be genetic influence on the maximal achieved lung function or the rate of decline of lung function. These phenotypes require study of longitudinal cohorts.

epidemiologists, and pathologists have created terminology based on a variety of criteria. In Table 1 we briefly summarize those phenotypes. Among them, the most common phenotypes in COPD genetic studies are the presence and degree of airflow obstruction and its rate of change over time. It has long been recognized that airflow obstruction can occur on the basis of either of two very different pathophysiological processes in the lung: inflammation of the parenchyma, resulting in a proteolytic process and loss of lung recoil (emphysema), and inflammation and fibrotic narrowing of the small airways. In any individual patient one of these processes may predominate, although both usually coexist. Recently, Nakano et al. [13] have shown that the relative contribution of airway and parenchymal disease can be separated in smokers who have COPD by using high-resolution computed tomography (HRCT). Although it has not yet been demonstrated that these phenotypic subsets are heritable, it is likely that they are under separate genetic control. This suggests that they should be measured and analyzed separately in any future genetic studies.

V. Candidate Genes in COPD

Two major hypotheses have dominated our thinking in the pathogenesis of smoke-related COPD [14]. One is the protease–antiprotease hypothesis, which states that various proteases break down connective tissue components, particularly elastin, in the lung parenchyma to produce emphysema. This theory is believed to explain the mechanism of development of COPD in α_1-AT deficiency. The other hypothesis is related to the oxidant–antioxidant balance, which proposes that oxidant stress and reactive oxygen species (ROS), derived from cigarette smoke and inflammatory cells, alter the oxidant/antioxidant balance, resulting in cellular damage. The possible mechanisms include oxidative inactivation of antiproteases, alveolar epithelial injury, increased sequestration of neutrophils in the pulmonary microvasculature, and increased expression of proinflammatory mediators [15]. The genes involved, or potentially involved, in the pathogenesis of COPD are summarized in Fig. 1.

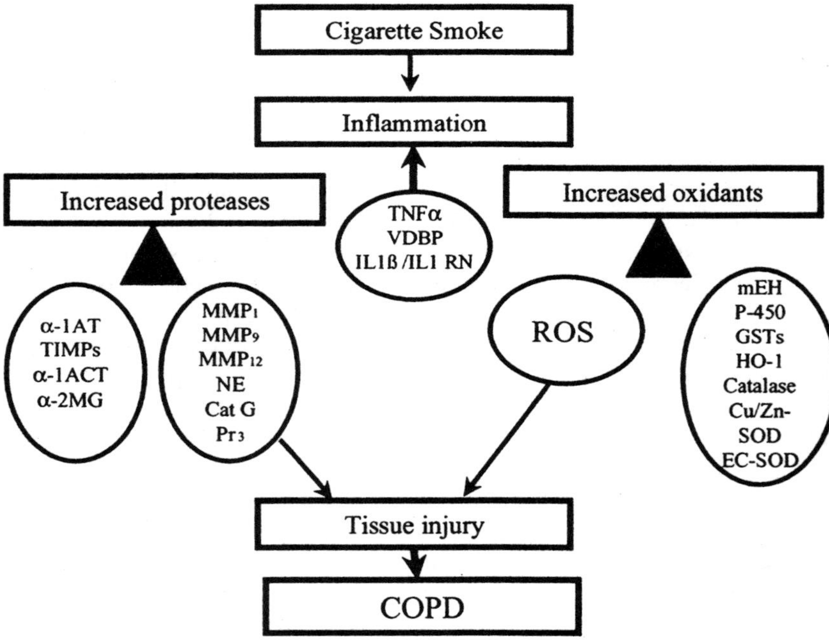

Figure 1 Summary of pathways and possible candidate genes involved in the pathogenesis of COPD. α_1-AT = α_1-antitrypsin; TIMP = tissue inhibitors of metalloproteinases; α_1-ACT = α_1-antichymotrypsin; α_2-MG = α_2-macroglobulin; TNF-α = tumor necrosis factor-α; VDBP = vitamin D-binding protein; IL1b/IL1RN = interleukin-1β/interleukin-1β receptor-antagonist; mEH = microsomal expoide hydrolase; P450 = cytochrome P450; GST = glutathione-S-transferase; HO-1 = heme oxygenase-1; Cu/Zn-SOD = copper-zinc superoxide dismutase; EC-SOD = extracellular SOD; MMPs = matrix metalloproteinases; NE = neutrophil elastase; CatG = cathepsin G; Pr3 = proteinase 3.

A. Antiproteinase Genes

α_1-Antitrypsin (α_1-AT)

The α_1-AT, gene on chromosome 14q32.1, is the major plasma protease inhibitor of neutrophil elastase. The PI locus is polymorphic; in the Caucasian population, the frequencies of M, S, and Z alleles are >95%, 2–3%, and 1%, respectively. They are associated with normal, mildly reduced, and severely reduced antitrypsin levels. A small percentage of subjects inherit a null allele, which leads to complete absence of α_1-AT production.

Individuals with two Z alleles or one Z and one null allele are referred as PI Z. PI Z individuals have approximately 15% of normal plasma antitrypsin levels and occur with prevalence of about 1/3000 in the United States [16]. The levels are low because 85% of the synthesized mutant Z α_1-AT is retained as polymers within hepatocytes [17]. The prevalence of heterozygous PI MS and MZ genotypes in Caucasian populations is about 10% and 3%, respectively; individuals with MS and MZ genotypes have ~80% and 60% of normal α_1-AT levels, respectively. Heterozygous PI SZ is rare, and individuals with this genotype have α_1-AT levels ~40% of normal.

In 1963 Laurell et al. first showed that individuals who had extremely low levels of α_1-AT had increased prevalence of emphysema [18]. Two years later, it was shown that α_1-AT deficiency was usually associated with the Z isoform of α_1-AT [19]. Since then, many association studies have been done. Table 2 summarizes the association studies of α_1-AT genotypes and phenotypes of COPD.

In addition to the S and Z polymorphisms, which affect the level of α-1 antitrypsin, there are two SNPs in the 3′ untranslated region of the gene which have been associated with COPD. The 3′ Taq-1 and Hand-III polymorphisms are not associated with alterations in α_1-AT levels. However, the Taq-1 polymorphism may be in a regulatory sequence and could affect the acute-phase increase in α_1-AT gene expression [29]. In an in-vitro study it was associated with reduced production of α_1-AT in response to the inflammatory cytokine interleukin-6 (IL-6) [35], but had no effect on the α_1-AT levels or on the rise in α_1-AT levels in vivo during the inflammatory response [36]. Thus, the true role of the 3′ polymorphisms in the pathogenesis of COPD remains to be determined.

Other Antiprotease Genes

Tissue Inhibitors of Metalloproteinases (TIMPs)

TIMPs are inhibitors of the matrix metalloproteinases (MMPs). Four members of the TIMP family (TIMP1-4) interact with the active form of MMPs to inhibit their activities. TIMP1 and 2 have the potential to participate in

Table 2 Associations of Antiprotease Gene Polymorphisms and COPD

α_1-antitypsin (α_1-AT)
• ZZ genotype:
Increase prevalence of emphysema [20]
Accelerated rate of decline of lung function [21]
Early onset of COPD [20]
• MS and MZ genotypes:
MZ genotype frequency increased in COPD, MS genotype not consistent [22]
Lung function: decreased [23]; no association [24]
• SZ genotype:
Increase prevalence of COPD [25]
• 3′ Taq-1 polymorphism:
Increased frequency in emphysema [26] and COPD [27]
No association with COPD [28]
• 3′ Hind-III polymorphism:
Increased frequency in COPD [29]
Other antiprotease genes
TIMP-2: association with COPD [30]
α_1-ACT: association with COPD [31,32]; no association with COPD [33]
α_2-MG: associated with COPD [34]

pulmonary diseases such as emphysema. TIMP1 is secreted by alveolar macrophages and plays a major role in modulating the activity of MMP1 as well as a number of other metalloproteinases. Alveolar macrophages from smokers secrete less TIMP1 than nonsmokers [37]. The sequence of the TIMP1 gene is known, and it has been localized to chromosome Xp11.4-p11.1. The gene contains two polymorphisms, although the functional consequences of the alleles are unknown [38], and no associations between the SNPs and COPD have been reported. TIMP2 is a more effective inhibitor of MMP2 and MMP9 than MMP1 [39]. There is some evidence to suggest that the membrane-type MMP1 (MT1MMP)/MMP2/TIMP2 system plays a role in the formation of pulmonary emphysema [40]. A recent study in a Japanese population identified two polymorphisms (−418G/C, +853G/A) in the TIMP2 gene. +853G was significantly more prevalent in 88 COPD patients than in 40 controls (94.9% in COPD versus 77.5% in control; $p < 0.0001$) [30]. However, the sample size was small, and there was no functional information for the polymorphisms reported.

α_1-Antichymotrypsin (α_1-ACT)

α_1-ACT belongs to the serine protease inhibitor family and is expressed in alveolar macrophages and airway epithelia. Poller [31] reported that the

Leu55Pro and Pro229Ala substitutions caused lower than normal α_1-ACT levels and were associated with COPD. Recently, Ishii reported that the α_1-ACT Ala-15Thr polymorphism in the signal peptide was associated with COPD [32].

α_2-Macroglobulin (α_2-MG)

α_2-MG is a major human plasma protease inhibitor. Its association with COPD was described more than 10 years ago [34], but the evidence that contributes to susceptibility of COPD is weak, and there have been no further positive reports.

B. Proteinase Genes

Matrix Metalloproteinases (MMPs)

MMPs comprise a structurally and functionally related family of at least 20 proteolytic enzymes that play an essential role in tissue remodeling. Overexpression of human MMP1 results in emphysema in transgenic mice [41], and deletion of MMP12 in mice prevents smoking-related emphysema [42]. MMP9 and MMP12 account for most of the macrophage-derived elastase activity in smokers [43]. MMPs have been shown to play a role in the pathogenesis of pulmonary emphysema in humans [40,44]. In a recent study, Russell et al. showed that the alveolar macrophages from smokers who had COPD secreted more MMP9 in response to lipopolysaccharide (LPS), interleukin-1β (IL-1β), and cigarette smoke conditioned media than nonsmokers and smokers without COPD [37]. A polymorphism in the promoter region of MMP9 (−1562C/T) has been associated with increased promoter activity [45], and in a recent study the T allele frequency was higher in Japanese subjects with distinct emphysema on chest CT scan ($n = 45$) than in those without emphysema ($n = 65$) (0.244 versus 0.123, $p = 0.02$) [46]. However, Joos et al. did not find an association between this polymorphism and the rate of lung function decline in a cohort of 590 Caucasian patients from the Lung Health Study. On the other hand, they did report that MMP1 G-1607GG and haplotypes consisting of this allele and a MMP12 Asn357Ser polymorphism were associated with rate of decline of lung function ($p=$ 0.02 and 0.0007, respectively) [47].

Neutrophil Serine Proteinases

Neutrophil serine proteinases include neutrophil elastase (NE), cathepsin G (CatG), and proteinase 3 (Pr3), all of which are stored within the azurophilic granules of neutrophils. The fact that α_1-AT is the major inhibitor of neutrophil serine proteinases prompted the hypothesis that serine proteinases could be involved in the pathogenisis for COPD. Although there is compelling evidence that serine proteinases, especially NE, are major mediators in the development of emphysema in animal experiments, there is only indirect evidence in humans [48]. Recently, polymorphisms in the NE, Pr3, and CatG genes have been identified, and their association with severe congenital neutropenia, Wegener's granulomatosis, and cardiovascular disease were reported separately [49–51]. There have been no reports of association of these polymorphisms with COPD.

C. Antioxidant Genes

Heme Oxygenase-1 (HMOX1)

HMOX1 is a key enzyme in heme catabolism and functions as an antioxidant enzyme, since its catabolic product bilirubin works as an efficient scavenger of ROS. The *HMOX1* gene (GT)n dinucleotide repeat in the 5′-flanking region shows length polymorphism, and specific alleles are associated with the level of gene transcription during thermal stress. Recently, it has been reported to be associated with pulmonary emphysema in Japanese smokers [52]. There is also in-vitro evidence that a high number of (GT)n repeats may reduce HMOX1 inducibility by ROS in cigarette smoke [52]. However, He et al. could not confirm an association of this polymorphism with rate of lung function decline in Caucasian smokers chosen from the Lung Health Study [53].

Catalase, Copper-Zinc Superoxide Dismutase (Cu/Zn-SOD), and Extracellular Superoxide Dismutase (EC-SOD)

Catalase, Cu/Zn-SOD, and EC-SOD are well-known antioxidant enzymes. Catalase is found in all aerobic cells and catalyzes the decomposition of hydrogen peroxide to oxygen and water [54]. Cu/Zn-SOD catalyzes the dismutation of superoxide to hydrogen peroxide and oxygen in the cytoplasmic space and may protect DNA and intracellular organelles from injury caused by ROS [55]. EC-SOD is the extracellular Cu/Zn-SOD and metabolizes superoxide radicals into hydrogen and oxygen [55]. Polymorphisms in catalase, Cu/Zn-SOD, and EC-SOD have been identified, but they have not been associated with COPD [56–58].

D. Xenobiotic Metabolizing Enzymes

There are four enzyme families of primary importance in the metabolism of xenobiotics; they are microsomal epoxide hydrolases (mEHs), glutathione-S-transferases (GSTs), cytochrome P450s, and N-acetyltransferases (NATs). Several polymorphisms that affect xenobiotic metabolism by these enzymes have been identified. Polymorphisms in three enzyme genes (mEH, GST, cytochrome P450) have been reported to be involved in the pathogenesis of COPD. Polymorphisms of these candidate genes are summarized in Table 3.

Microsomal Epoxide Hydrolase

Microsomal epoxide hydrolase (mEH) metabolizes polycyclic aromatic hydrocarbons, which are carcinogens found in cigarette smoke and cooked meat. In the lung, mEH is expressed in bronchial epithelial cells and plays an important role in regulating the entry of xenobiotics into the body. The function of mEH is the irreversible hydration of reactive epoxides and their immediate excretion from the body. Therefore, the action of mEH is generally thought as detoxification.

Two polymorphisms that produce amino acid variations have been described in the coding region of the mEH gene: $Tyr^{113} \rightarrow His^{113}$ (T-to-C transition; exon 3) and $His^{139} \rightarrow Arg^{139}$ (A-to-G transition; exon 4) [63]. These polymorphisms alter the enzyme activity and have been implicated in several disorders [63,64]. The change from Tyr^{113} to His^{113} causes reduced enzyme activity to at least 50% (slow allele), and His^{139} to Arg^{139} causes increased enzyme activity by at least 25% (fast allele). Recently, it was found that individuals who were homozygous for the slow mEH activity allele were significantly more frequent in a COPD and emphysema group than in a control group [59]. Sandford et al. showed that homozygosity for the His^{113}-His^{139} haplotype was significantly associated with a rapid decline in lung function among smokers and interacted with a family history of COPD [23].

Glutathione-S-Transferases

Although human glutathione-S-transferases (GSTs) are generally recognized as detoxifying enzymes since they metabolize the conjugation of xenobiotic

Table 3 Gene Variation of Xenobiotic Metabolizing Enzymes in COPD

Enzyme	Isoform	Genetic variation/activity	Risk of COPD	References
mEH		$Tyr^{113} \rightarrow His^{113}/\downarrow$	↑	[23,59]
		$His^{139} \rightarrow Arg^{139}/\uparrow$	↓	
GST	GST-M1	$M1(+) \rightarrow M1(-)/\downarrow$	↑	[60]
	GST-P1	$Ile^{105} \rightarrow Val^{105}/\uparrow$	↓	[61]
Cytochrome P450	CYP1A1	$Ile^{462} \rightarrow Val^{462}/\uparrow$	↑	[62]

compounds with glutathione, they may also be involved in activation of carcinogens. One of the genes of this superfamily, GST-M1, is polymorphic because of a partial gene deletion. In the lung, GST-M1 is expressed in the bronchiolar epithelium, alveolar macrophages, and pneumocytes. The lack of GST-M1 has been associated with an increased risk of lung cancer in the presence of COPD [65], and homozygosity for the null GST-M1 allele has been associated with a high risk of COPD [60]. Approximately 50% of Caucasians have a null GST-M1 genotype.

GST-P1, which is expressed in the same cell types as GST-M1, has a polymorphism within exon 5 (A to G) that induces an amino acid change from isoleucine to valine ($Ile^{105} \rightarrow Val^{105}$). The isoleucine GST-P1 isoform has been found to be less active than the valine isoform in vitro [66]. In a Japanese population, homozygosity for the *Ile* allele was significantly increased in COPD patients compared with controls [61]. A recent study suggested that the combination of a low-activity GST-P1 (homozygous Ile^{105}) genotype with a high-activity mEH (homozygous Tyr^{113}) genotype may increase lung cancer risk among smokers [67].

Cytochrome P4501A1

The polycyclic aromatic hydrocarbon-metabolizing cytochrome P450 isoform, P4501A1 (CYP1A1), is an enzyme that metabolizes exogenous compounds to enable them to be excreted in the urine or bile. This enzyme is found throughout the lung and is highly inducible. The most common allelic variants of CYP1A1 are the MspI recognition site located in the 3′-flanking region, the I462V ($Ile^{462} \rightarrow Val^{462}$) site located in exon 7, and the −459 C-to-T site located in the promoter. Among these polymorphisms, the CYP1A1 Val^{462} variant results in increased CYP1A1 activity in vivo [68]. This high-activity allele was associated with susceptibility to centriacinar emphysema in patients who had lung cancer [62]. However, the polymorphism was not associated with lung cancer in the absence of emphysema. Recently, the relationship between pulmonary expression of CYPA1 and polymorphic genotypes was investigated, and it was shown that individual variation of CYP1A1 levels in smokers' lung tissue could not be explained by any of the polymorphisms [69].

E. Inflammatory Mediators

The inflammatory response clearly plays an important role in the pathogenesis of COPD. The genes involved in the regulation of inflammation are increasingly being considered as candidate genes for COPD. Several genetic polymorphisms of inflammatory mediator genes have been implicated in the susceptibility to COPD.

Tumor Necrosis Factor-Alpha

Tumor necrosis factor-alpha (TNF-α) is a proinflammatory cytokine; its production is elevated in the airways of COPD patients, especially during acute exacerbations [70]. The expression of TNF-α can be regulated at the transcriptional level. The TNF-α gene contains several polymorphisms including a guanine-to-adenine transition at position −308 of the promoter (TNF-αG-308A). The rare allele, TNF-α-308A, has been associated with higher baseline and induced expression of TNF-α [71]. Several researchers have investigated disease susceptibility associated with this polymorphism and have found positive associations for asthma [72] and COPD [73]. In one study, patients who were homozygous for the A allele had less reversibility of airflow obstruction and a worse prognosis [73]. On the other hand, no association has been found between this polymorphism and COPD in some studies [74]. Therefore, the role of this polymorphism in COPD has not yet been elucidated.

Vitamin D-Binding Protein

Vitamin D-binding protein (VDBP) binds vitamin D, but also functions as a modulator of inflammation because it enhances the neutrophil chemotactic activity of complement component 5a (C5a) and can act as a potent macrophage-activating factor. The VDBP gene is located on chromosome 4, and three major isoforms occur due to two separate point mutations. Both of these mutations result in a single amino acid substitution, and the isoforms are named 1F, 1S, and 2 [75]. In the Caucasian population, the allele frequencies are 0.16-1F, 0.56-1S, and 0.28-2 [76]. The prevalence of 1F homozygotes was significantly increased in a sample of COPD patients [77,78]. In contrast, individuals who have at least one 2 allele appear to be protected from developing COPD [77]. The biological explanation for the association is unknown; there were no significant differences between the VDBP isoforms in their ability to enhance chemotaxis of neutrophils to C5a [76], but there have been no studies of the differential ability of the isoforms to act as a macrophage-activating factor. Thus, the biological mechanism of VDBP in the development to COPD is not sufficiently clarified.

IL-I Complex

Interleukins are important mediators in immune responses and inflammatory processes. The balance between levels of cytokines, their receptors, and specific inhibitors controls the inflammatory process. The IL-1 family consists of proinflammatory cytokines (IL-1α, IL-1β) and an anti-inflammatory agent, IL-1 receptor antagonist (IL1RN). IL-1α and IL-1β originate from different genes; IL-1α is primarily cell-associated, whereas IL-1β is released from cells. Both cytokines share a common receptor. IL1RN competitively inhibits the binding of IL-1α and IL-1β to its receptor but does not induce any intracellular response [79]. IL1RN is coded by the IL-1 gene which, like the genes for IL-1α and IL-1β, is located on chromosome 2. There is an amino acid-changing SNP at position +4845 in exon 5 of the IL-1 gene, resulting in an Ala^{114}-to-Ser^{114} substitution [80]. There are also polymorphisms within the IL-1β gene: in the promoter region (C-551T) [81] and in exon 5 (position +3953) [82]. The gene coding IL1RN has a six-allelic, 86-bp tandem repeat in intron 2 [83], corresponding to 2, 3, 4, 5, 6, and 8 repeats [84]. Several investigators have shown that allele 2 of IL1RN is associated with enhanced IL-1RN production [85] and with chronic inflammatory and autoimmune diseases [86,87]. The IL-1β C-551T polymorphism has also been associated with inflammatory bowel disease [86]. Joos et al. recently found no association of either the IL-1β or IL-1RN genotypes when studied alone with rate of decline in lung function, but they did report that specific IL-1β/IL1RN haplotypes are associated with an accelerated rate of decline in smokers [84].

F. Mucocilliary Clearance

Mucocillary clearance is an important respiratory defense mechanism protecting the lung from microorganisms and toxic inhaled particles. The rate at which particulate matter is cleared from the lung is highly variable among individuals. Thirty-years ago, a twins study was performed to investigate the intertwin correlation in clearance rate [88]. This study demonstrated that monozygotic twins have a significantly higher correlation of clearance rate than dizygotic twins, suggesting that genetic factors influence mucocilliary clearance.

Cystic Fibrosis Transmembrane Regulator

The cystic fibrosis transmembrane conductance regulator (CFTR) forms a chloride channel at the apical surface of airway epithelial cells and is involved in the control of airway secretions. In 1989, mutations in the CFTR gene were identified as the cause of cystic fibrosis (CF). Homozygous deficiency or defective function of this protein results in CF, characterized by early-onset obstructive lung disease secondary to chronic bacterial infection and bronchiectasis. CF heterozygotes had increased bronchial reactivity to methacholine [89] and an increased incidence of wheeze accompanied by decreased FEV_1 and FEF_{25-75} [90]. The most frequent CF-causing variant is the ΔF508 mutation, though more than 500 different disease-associated alleles of the CFTR gene have been detected. Heterozygosity of this mutation has been reported more frequently than predicted in patients who have disseminated bronchiectasis [91], and in patients who had bronchial hypersecretion [92], whereas its prevalence was not increased in patients with chronic bronchitis [91].

Another CFTR mutation is located on a variable-length thymine repeat (IVS8) in intron 8. The IVS8-5T allele results in less accurate splicing, therefore increases amount of aberrant transcript, but decreases normal, and has been associated with an increased risk for pulmonary emphysema [93], diffuse bronchiectasis, but not COPD [94]. Recently, the Met allele of the M470V polymorphism was found more frequently in COPD patients than in the controls [95]. However, the reason for the association is unclear, since the Met^{470} allele increases the CFTR chloride channel activity compared with the Val variant [96].

G. Other Genes

Table 4 summarizes additional genes that may associate with COPD. Among them, the β_2-adrenergic receptor is a candidate for allergy and asthma. The "Dutch hypothesis," which was formulated in 1961, proposes that there are common genetic factors that underlie the development of asthma and cigarette smoke-induced airway disease [107]. Apart from the β_2-adrenergic receptor, there are as yet no overlapping susceptibility genes, although the IL-13 gene that is clearly important in the atopic phenotype has also been proposed as a COPD susceptibility gene [108].

Table 4 Other Genes That May be Associated with COPD

Blood group:
ABO and Lewis blood group:
Association of blood group A with COPD [97] or accelerated lung function decline [98]
Lewis negative associated with poor lung function [99]
No association of ABO blood group with COPD or lung function [100]
Blood group antigen secretor status:
Association of nonsecretor with COPD and accelerated lung function decline [101,102]
No association of secretor status with lung function [103]
HLA status:
Association with lung function [101] or diffuse panbronchiolitis [104]
Immunoglobulin deficiency:
Association between selective IgA deficiency and COPD [105]
β_2-Adrenergic receptor:
Associations of Gly16 with COPD [106] and Gln27 with COPD severity [106]

VI. Therapeutic Implications of COPD Genetics

One potential application of the study of the genetics of COPD is the potential to develop individualized therapeutic strategies that target the predominant pathogenesis in individual patients. For example, antioxidant therapy might benefit individuals who have decreased antioxidant defenses [109]. Inhibitors of metalloproteinases might benefit individuals who have overexpression of metalloproteinases (MMPs) [110], such as has been done in individuals who are homozygous for α_1-AT deficiency alleles [111].

The results of replacement therapy for α_1-antitrypsin have been modest. After 3.5–7 years of follow-up of a U.S. registry, there was no difference in mortality or rate of decline of FEV_1 between 277 α_1-AT-deficient individuals who never received replacement therapy and 650 deficient individuals who did receive intravenous therapy. However, among the 763 subjects with an initial FEV_1 <50% predicted, mortality was significantly higher ($p \leqslant 0.001$) in the 162 subjects who did not, as opposed to the 601 who did receive augmentation therapy [112]. In Europe, 198 severe α_1-AT-deficient German individuals who did receive replacement therapy were compared to 97 Danish patients who did not. Only those whose initial FEV_1 between 31% and 65% predicted showed a significant decrease in the rate of decline of FEV_1 during therapy [113].

To date the only placebo-controlled trial was reported in 1999 [114]. The Danish-Dutch study group included 28 patients in each arm, who were followed for up to 5 years. There was no difference on the annual change of FEV_1, however, the loss of lung tissue measured by CT was 2.6 ± 0.41 g/L/yr for placebo as compared with 1.5 ± 0.41 g/L/yr for α_1-AT infusion ($p = 0.07$). Recently, a multicenter, retrospective study including 96 patients with severe α_1-AT deficiency was reported [115]. Lung function data were followed up for a minimum of 12 months, both before and during α_1-AT treatment. The results showed that for the group as a whole, the decline of FEV_1 was significantly lower during the treatment period (34.2 mL/yr versus 49.3 mL/yr, $p = 0.019$). In patients whose initial FEV_1 was >65%, α_1-AT treatment reduced the decline in FEV_1 by 73.6 mL/yr ($p = 0.045$). The loss in FEV_1 was reduced from 256 mL/yr to 53 mL/yr ($p = 0.001$) in seven individuals who had a rapid decline of FEV_1 before treatment. This result indicates that certain subsets of patients may benefit from augmentation therapy.

VII. Pharmacogenetics of COPD

Pharmacological therapy of COPD is used to prevent and control symptoms and reduce the frequency and severity of exacerbations. To date no existing therapy for COPD has been shown to modify the long-term decline in lung function. Bronchodilators (such as β_2-agonists, anticholinergics and theophyllines) are used for symptom control in COPD. Glucocoticosteroids have limited role in COPD management. The pharmacogenetics of β_2-agonist, anticholinergic, theophylline, and glucocoticosteroid therapy were recently reviewed in detail [116]. Although polymorphisms in the β_2-adrenergic receptor (β_2AR) gene influence responsiveness to β_2-agonist, the power of these associations has not proven great enough to influence individualized dosage or drug selection. No polymorpisms have been detected which influence the response to anticholinergic agents or theophylline. Corticosteroids can shorten the symptomatic period during acute exacerbations of COPD and may decrease the frequency of exacerbations, but once again, no genetic determinants of this responsiveness has been reported.

VIII. Conclusion

In this chapter we have reviewed the evidence of a genetic contribution to the pathogenesis of COPD and described the candidate genes. Due to the difficulty of ascertaining large families with multiple affected individuals and the lack of large studies of affected sib pairs, almost all of the studies have been case-control association studies. The disadvantage of this approach is that only known genes can be tested. In addition, in most studies individual single nucleotide polymorphisms (SNPs) have been studied in and around a candidate gene. Negative results do not rule out an association involving other nearby SNPs; positive results do not mean the discovery of the causal SNP, since the result may simply reflect linkage disequilibrium (LD), with a true causal SNP located some distance away [117]. The recent linkage studies of Silverman et al. are the first systematic approach to the identification of novel genes involved in the disease and offer exciting future prospects [9,10].

For genetically complex diseases such as COPD, emphasis has been focused on the common disease–common variant hypothesis, which states that disease susceptibility gene polymorphisms are expected to be relatively common in the human population and enriched in the coding and regulatory sequence of genes [118]. Haplotypes defined by common SNPs have attracted recent interest [117,119,120]. With sufficient LD, haplotypes may be useful in association studies to map common alleles that may influence susceptibly to complex diseases. Discrete haplotype blocks, each with a limited diversity, have been demonstrated in the human genome [117,119]. Once the haplotype blocks are defined, the next step will be to define a subset of SNPs that uniquely distinguish the common haplotypes in each block. This allows the common variants in a gene to be tested exhaustively for associations with disease.

In the future, more information on the genetics of COPD will be provided by large-scale family studies and genome-wide association studies using haplotype blocks. It is anticipated that the study of the genetics of COPD will lead to the discovery of new mechanisms, new predictors, and new therapeutic opportunities.

References

1. Silverman EK. Genetics of chronic obstructive pulmonary disease. Novartis Found Symp 2001; 234:45–58 (discussion 58–64).
2. Lebowitz MD, Knudson RJ, Burrows B. Family aggregation of pulmonary function measurements. Am Rev Respir Dis 1984; 129(1):8–11.
3. McCloskey SC, Patel BD, Hinchliffe SJ, Reid ED, Wareham NJ, Lomas DA. Siblings of patients with severe chronic obstructive pulmonary disease have a significant risk of airflow obstruction. Am J Respir Crit Care Med 2001; 164(8 pt 1):1419–1424.
4. Tager I, Tishler PV, Rosner B, Speizer FE, Litt M. Studies of the familial aggregation of chronic bronchitis and obstructive airways disease. Int J Epidemiol 1978; 7(1):55–62.
5. Redline S, Tishler PV, Lewitter FI, Tager IB, Munoz A, Speizer FE. Assessment of genetic and nongenetic influences on pulmonary function: a twin study. Am Rev Respir Dis 1987; 135(1):217–222.
6. McClearn GE, Svartengren M, Pedersen NL, Heller DA, Plomin R. Genetic and environmental influences on pulmonary function in aging Swedish twins. J Gerontol 1994; 49(6):264–2648.
7. Givelber RJ, Couropmitree NN, Gottlieb DJ, Evans JC, Levy D, Myers RH, O'Connor GT. Segregation analysis of pulmonary function among families in the Framingham Study. Am J Respir Crit Care Med 1998; 157(5 pt 1):1445–1451.
8. Silverman EK, Mosley JD, Rao DC, Palmer LJ, Province MA, Elston RC, Weiss ST, Campbell EJ. Linkage analysis of alpha 1-antitrypsin deficiency: lessons for complex diseases. Hum Hered 2001; 52(4):223–232.
9. Silverman EK, Palmer LJ, Mosley JD, Barth M, Senter JM, Brown A, Drazen JM, Kwiatkowski DJ, Chapman HA, Campbell EJ, Province MA, Rao DC, Reilly JJ, Ginns LC, Speizer FE, Weiss ST. Genomewide linkage analysis of quantitative spirometric phenotypes in severe early-onset chronic obstructive pulmonary disease. Am J Hum Genet 2002; 70(5):1229–1239.
10. Silverman EK, Mosley JD, Palmer LJ, Barth M, Senter JM, Brown A, Drazen JM, Kwiatkowski DJ, Chapman HA, Campbell EJ, Province MA, Rao DC, Reilly JJ, Ginns LC, Speizer FE, Weiss ST. Genome-wide linkage analysis of severe, early-onset chronic obstructive pulmonary disease: airflow

obstruction and chronic bronchitis phenotypes. Hum Mol Genet 2002; 11(6): 623–632.
11. Lomas DA, Silverman EK. The genetics of chronic obstructive pulmonary disease. Respir Res 2001; 2(1):20–26.
12. Weiss ST, Silverman EK, Palmer LJ. Case-control association studies in pharmacogenetics. Pharmacogenom J 2001; 1:157–158.
13. Nakano Y, Muro S, Sakai H, Hirai T, Chin K, Tsukino M, Nishimura K, Itoh H, Pare PD, Hogg JC, Mishima M. Computed tomographic measurements of airway dimensions and emphysema in smokers. Correlation with lung function. Am J Respir Crit Care Med 2000; 162(3 pt 1):1102–1108.
14. Sethi JM, Rochester CL. Smoking and chronic obstructive pulmonary disease. Clin Chest Med 2000; 21(1):67–86, viii.
15. MacNee W. Oxidants/antioxidants and COPD. Chest 2000; 117(5 suppl 1): 303S–317S.
16. Silverman EK, Miletich JP, Pierce JA, Sherman LA, Endicott SK, Broze GJ Jr, Campbell EJ. Alpha-1-antitrypsin deficiency. High prevalence in the St. Louis area determined by direct population screening. Am Rev Respir Dis 1989; 140(4):961–966.
17. Mahadeva R, Chang WS, Dafforn TR, Oakley DJ, Foreman RC, Calvin J, Wight DG, Lomas DA. Heteropolymerization of S, I, and Z alpha1-antitrypsin and liver cirrhosis. J Clin Invest 1999; 103(7):999–1006.
18. Laurell CC, Eriksson S. The electrophorectic $alpha_1$-globulin pattern of serum in $alpha_1$-antitrypsin deficiency. Scand J Clin Lab Invest 1963; 15:132–140.
19. Axelsson U, Laurell CB. Hereditary variants of serum alpha-1-antitrypsin. Am J Hum Genet 1965; 17(6):466–472.
20. Larsson C. Natural history and life expectancy in severe alpha1-antitrypsin deficiency, Pi Z. Acta Med Scand 1978; 204(5):345–351.
21. Piitulainen E, Eriksson S. Decline in FEV1 related to smoking status in individuals with severe alpha1-antitrypsin deficiency (PiZZ). Eur Respir J 1999; 13(2):247–251.
22. Sandford AJ, Weir TD, Spinelli JJ, Paré PD. Z and S mutations of the α_1-antitrypsin gene and the risk of chronic obstructive pulmonary disease. Am J Respir Cell Molec Biol 1999; 20(2):287–291.
23. Sandford AJ, Chagani T, Weir TD, Connett JE, Anthonisen NR, Paré PD. Susceptibility genes for rapid decline of lung function in the Lung Health Study. Am J Respir Crit Care Med 2001; 163(2):469–473.
24. Morse JO, Lebowitz MD, Knudson RJ, Burrows B. Relation of protease inhibitor phenotypes to obstructive lung diseases in a community. N Engl J Med 1977; 296(21):1190–1194.
25. Turino GM, Barker AF, Brantly ML, Cohen AB, Connelly RP, Crystal RG, Eden E, Schluchter MD, Stoller JK. Clinical features of individuals with PI*SZ phenotype of α_1-antitrypsin deficiency. α_1-Antitrypsin Deficiency Registry Study Group. Am J Respir Crit Care Med 1996; 154(6 pt 1):1718–1725.
26. Kalsheker NA, Hodgson IJ, Watkins GL, White JP, Morrison HM, Stockley

RA. Deoxyribonucleic acid (DNA) polymorphism of the α_1-antitrypsin gene in chronic lung disease. Br Med J 1987; 294(6586):1511–1514.
27. Poller W, Meisen C, Olek K. DNA polymorphisms of the α_1-antitrypsin gene region in patients with chronic obstructive pulmonary disease. Eur J Clin Invest 1990; 20(1):1–7.
28. Sandford AJ, Spinelli JJ, Weir TD, Paré PD. Mutation in the 3′ region of the α_1-antitrypsin gene and chronic obstructive pulmonary disease. J Med Genet 1997; 34(10):874–875.
29. Kalsheker NA, Watkins GL, Hill S, Morgan K, Stockley RA, Fick RB. Independent mutations in the flanking sequence of the α_1-antitrypsin gene are associated with chronic obstructive airways disease. Dis Markers 1990; 8(3):151–157.
30. Hirano K, Sakamoto T, Uchida Y, Morishima Y, Masuyama K, Ishii Y, Nomura A, Ohtsuka M, Sekizawa K. Tissue inhibitor of metalloproteinases-2 gene polymorphisms in chronic obstructive pulmonary disease. Eur Respir J 2001; 18(5):748–752.
31. Poller W, Faber JP, Scholz S, Weidinger S, Bartholome K, Olek K, Eriksson S. Mis-sense mutation of α_1-antichymotrypsin gene associated with chronic lung disease. Lancet 1992; 339(8808):1538.
32. Ishii T, Matsuse T, Teramoto S, Matsui H, Hosoi T, Fukuchi Y, Ouchi Y. Association between alpha-1-antichymotrypsin polymorphism and susceptibility to chronic obstructive pulmonary disease. Eur J Clin Invest 2000; 30(6): 543–548.
33. Sandford AJ, Chagani T, Weir TD, Paré PD. α_1-Antichymotrypsin mutations in patients with chronic obstructive pulmonary disease. Dis Markers 1998; 13(4):257–260.
34. Poller W, Barth J, Voss B. Detection of an alteration of the alpha 2-macroglobulin gene in a patient with chronic lung disease and serum alpha 2-macroglobulin deficiency. Hum Genet 1989; 83(1):93–96.
35. Morgan K, Scobie G, Marsters P, Kalsheker NA. Mutation in an α_1-antitrypsin enhancer results in an interleukin-6 deficient acute-phase response due to loss of cooperativity between transcription factors. Biochim Biophys Acta 1997; 1362(1):67–76.
36. Sandford AJ, Chagani T, Spinelli JJ, Paré PD. α_1-Antitrypsin genotypes and the acute-phase response to open heart surgery. Am J Respir Crit Care Med 1999; 159:1624–1628.
37. Russell RE, Culpitt SV, DeMatos C, Donnelly L, Smith M, Wiggins J, Barnes PJ. Release and activity of matrix metalloproteinase-9 and tissue inhibitor of metalloproteinase-1 by alveolar macrophages from patients with chronic obstructive pulmonary disease. Am J Respir Cell Mol Biol 2002; 26(5):602–609.
38. Aldred MA, Wright AF. PCR detection of existing and new polymorphism at the TIMP locus. Nucleic Acids Res 1991; 19(5):1165.
39. Howard EW, Bullen EC, Banda MJ. Preferential inhibition of 72- and 92-kDa gelatinases by tissue inhibitor of metalloproteinases-2. J Biol Chem 1991; 266(20):13070–13075.
40. Ohnishi K, Takagi M, Kurokawa Y, Satomi S, Konttinen YT. Matrix me-

talloproteinase-mediated extracellular matrix protein degradation in human pulmonary emphysema. Lab Invest 1998; 78(9):1077–1087.
41. D'Armiento J, Dalal SS, Okada Y, Berg RA, Chada K. Collagenase expression in the lungs of transgenic mice causes pulmonary emphysema. Cell 1992; 71(6): 955–961.
42. Hautamaki RD, Kobayashi DK, Senior RM, Shapiro SD. Requirement for macrophage elastase for cigarette smoke-induced emphysema in mice. Science 1997; 277(5334):2002–2004.
43. Shapiro SD. Elastolytic metalloproteinases produced by human mononuclear phagocytes. Potential roles in destructive lung disease. Am J Respir Crit Care Med 1994; 150(6 pt 2):S160–S164.
44. Imai K, Dalal SS, Chen ES, Downey R, Schulman LL, Ginsburg M, D'Armiento J. Human collagenase (matrix metalloproteinase-1) expression in the lungs of patients with emphysema. Am J Respir Crit Care Med 2001; 163(3 Pt 1):786–791.
45. Zhang BP, Ye S, Herrmann SM, Eriksson P, de Maat M, Evans A, Arveiler D, Luc G, Cambien F, Hamsten A, Watkins H, Henney AM. Functional polymorphism in the regulatory region of gelatinase B gene in relation to severity of coronary atherosclerosis. Circulation 1999; 99(14):1788–1794.
46. Minematsu N, Nakamura H, Tateno H, Nakajima T, Yamaguchi K. Genetic polymorphism in matrix metalloproteinase-9 and pulmonary emphysema. Biochem Biophys Res Commun 2001; 289(1):116–119.
47. Joos L, He JQ, Shepherdson MB, Connett JE, Anthonisen NR, Pare PD, Sandford AJ. The role of matrix metalloproteinase polymorphisms in the rate of decline in lung function. Hum Mol Genet 2002; 11(5):569–576.
48. Stockley RA. Proteases and antiproteases. Novartis Found Symp 2001; 234:189–199 (discussion 199–204).
49. Ancliff PJ, Gale RE, Liesner R, Hann IM, Linch DC. Mutations in the ELA2 gene encoding neutrophil elastase are present in most patients with sporadic severe congenital neutropenia but only in some patients with the familial form of the disease. Blood 2001; 98(9):2645–2650.
50. Gencik M, Meller S, Borgmann S, Fricke H. Proteinase 3 gene polymorphisms and Wegener's granulomatosis. Kidney Int 2000; 58(6):2473–2477.
51. Herrmann SM, Funke-Kaiser H, Schmidt-Petersen K, Nicaud V, Gautier-Bertrand M, Evans A, Kee F, Arveiler D, Morrison C, Orzechowski HD, Elbaz A, Amarenco P, Cambien F, Paul M. Characterization of polymorphic structure of cathepsin G gene: role in cardiovascular and cerebrovascular diseases. Arterioscler Thromb Vasc Biol 2001; 21(9):1538–1543.
52. Yamada N, Yamaya M, Okinaga S, Nakayama K, Sekizawa K, Shibahara S, Sasaki H. Microsatellite polymorphism in the heme oxygenase-1 gene promoter is associated with susceptibility to emphysema. Am J Hum Genet 2000; 66(1): 187–195.
53. He JQ, Ruan J, Connett J, Anthonisen N, Paré P, Sandford A. Antioxidant gene polymorphisms and susceptibility to a rapid decline in lung function in smokers. Am J Respir Crit Care Med 2002; 166(3):323–328.

54. Deisseroth A, Dounce AL. Catalase: physical and chemical properties, mechanism of catalysis, and physiological role. Physiol Rev 1970; 50(3):319–375.
55. Nilsson J. Extracellular sodium dismutase: does it have a role in cardiovascular disease? J Intern Med 1997; 242(1):1–3.
56. Ukkola O, Erkkila PH, Savolainen MJ, Kesaniemi YA. Lack of association between polymorphisms of catalase, copper-zinc superoxide dismutase (SOD), extracellular SOD and endothelial nitric oxide synthase genes and macroangiopathy in patients with type 2 diabetes mellitus. J Intern Med 2001; 249(5):451–459.
57. Forsberg L, Lyrenas L, de Faire U, Morgenstern R. A common functional C-T substitution polymorphism in the promoter region of the human catalase gene influences transcription factor binding, reporter gene transcription and is correlated to blood catalase levels. Free Radic Biol Med 2001; 30(5):500–505.
58. Chistyakov DA, Savost'anov KV, Zotova EV, Nosikov VV. Polymorphisms in the Mn-SOD and EC-SOD genes and their relationship to diabetic neuropathy in type 1 diabetes mellitus. BMC Med Genet 2001; 2(1):4.
59. Smith CA, Harrison DJ. Association between polymorphism in gene for microsomal epoxide hydrolase and susceptibility to emphysema. Lancet 1997; 350(9078):630–633.
60. Baranova H, Perriot J, Albuisson E, Ivaschenko T, Baranov VS, Hemery B, Mouraire P, Riol N, Malet P. Peculiarities of the GSTM1 0/0 genotype in French heavy smokers with various types of chronic bronchitis. Hum Genet 1997; 99(6):822–826.
61. Ishii T, Matsuse T, Teramoto S, Matsui H, Miyao M, Hosoi T, Takahashi H, Fukuchi Y, Ouchi Y. Glutathione S-transferase P1 (GSTP1) polymorphism in patients with chronic obstructive pulmonary disease. Thorax 1999; 54(8):693–696.
62. Cantlay AM, Lamb D, Gillooly M, Norrman J, Morrison D, Smith CAD, Harrison DJ. Association between the CYP1A1 gene polymorphism and susceptibility to emphysema and lung cancer. J Clin Pathol: Mol Pathol 1995; 48:M210–M214.
63. Hassett C, Aicher L, Sidhu JS, Omiecinski CJ. Human microsomal epoxide hydrolase: genetic polymorphism and functional expression in vitro of amino acid variants. Hum Mol Genet 1994; 3(3):421–428.
64. Wang X, Wang M, Niu T, Chen C, Xu X. Microsomal epoxide hydrolase polymorphism and risk of spontaneous abortion. Epidemiology 1998; 9(5):540–544.
65. Harrison DJ, Cantlay AM, Rae F, Lamb D, Smith CA. Frequency of glutathione S-transferase M1 deletion in smokers with emphysema and lung cancer. Hum Exp Toxicol 1997; 16(7):356–360.
66. Sundberg K, Johansson AS, Stenberg G, Widersten M, Seidel A, Mannervik B, Jernstrom B. Differences in the catalytic efficiencies of allelic variants of glutathione transferase P1-1 towards carcinogenic diol epoxides of polycyclic aromatic hydrocarbons. Carcinogenesis 1998; 19(3):433–436.
67. To-Figueras J, Gene M, Gomez-Catalan J, Pique E, Borrego N, Corbella J.

Lung cancer susceptibility in relation to combined polymorphisms of microsomal epoxide hydrolase and glutathione S-transferase P1. Cancer Lett 2001; 173(2):155–162.
68. Cosma G, Crofts F, Taioli E, Toniolo P, Garte S. Relationship between genotype and function of the human CYP1A1 gene. J Toxicol Environ Health 1993; 40(2–3):309–316.
69. Anttila S, Tuominen P, Hirvonen A, Nurminen M, Karjalainen A, Hankinson O, Elovaara E. CYP1A1 levels in lung tissue of tobacco smokers and polymorphisms of CYP1A1 and aromatic hydrocarbon receptor. Pharmacogenetics 2001; 11(6):501–509.
70. Aaron SD, Angel JB, Lunau M, Wright K, Fex C, Le Saux N, Dales RE. Granulocyte inflammatory markers and airway infection during acute exacerbation of chronic obstructive pulmonary disease. Am J Respir Crit Care Med 2001; 163(2):349–355.
71. Wilson AG, Symons JA, McDowell TL, McDevitt HO, Duff GW. Effects of a polymorphism in the human tumor necrosis factor alpha promoter on transcriptional activation. Proc Natl Acad Sci USA 1997; 94(7):3195–3199.
72. Chagani T, Paré PD, Zhu S, Weir TD, Bai TR, Behbehani NA, FitzGerald JM, Sandford AJ. Prevalence of tumour necrosis factor-α and angiotensin converting enzyme polymorphisms in mild/moderate and fatal/near-fatal asthma. Am J Respir Crit Care Med 1999; 160:278–282.
73. Keatings VM, Cave SJ, Henry MJ, Morgan K, O'Connor CM, FitzGerald MX, Kalsheker N. A polymorphism in the tumor necrosis factor-alpha gene promoter region may predispose to a poor prognosis in COPD. Chest 2000; 118(4):971–975.
74. Ishii T, Matsuse T, Teramoto S, Matsui H, Miyao M, Hosoi T, Takahashi H, Fukuchi Y, Ouchi Y. Neither IL-1beta, IL-1 receptor antagonist, nor TNF-alpha polymorphisms are associated with susceptibility to COPD. Respir Med 2000; 94(9):847–851.
75. Kamboh MI, Ferrell RE. Ethnic variation in vitamin D-binding protein (GC): a review of isoelectric focusing studies in human populations. Hum Genet 1986; 72(4):281–293.
76. Schellenberg D, Paré PD, Weir TD, Spinelli JJ, Walker BA, Sandford AJ. Vitamin D binding protein variants and the risk of COPD. Am J Respir Crit Care Med 1998; 157(3 pt 1):957–961.
77. Horne SL, Cockcroft DW, Dosman JA. Possible protective effect against chronic obstructive airways disease by the GC 2 allele. Hum Hered 1990; 40(3): 173–176.
78. Ishii T, Keicho N, Teramoto S, Azuma A, Kudoh S, Fukuchi Y, Ouchi Y, Matsuse T. Association of Gc-globulin variation with susceptibility to COPD and diffuse panbronchiolitis. Eur Respir J 2001; 18(5):753–757.
79. Arend WP, Malyak M, Guthridge CJ, Gabay C. Interleukin-1 receptor antagonist: role in biology. Annu Rev Immunol 1998; 16:27–55.
80. van den Velden PA, Reitsma PH. Amino acid dimorphism in IL1A is detectable by PCR amplification. Hum Mol Genet 1993; 2(10):1753.

81. di Giovine FS, Takhsh E, Blakemore AI, Duff GW. Single base polymorphism at −511 in the human interleukin-1 beta gene (IL1 beta). Hum Mol Genet 1992; 1(6):450.
82. Pociot F, Molvig J, Wogensen L, Worsaae H, Nerup J. A TaqI polymorphism in the human interleukin-1 beta (IL-1 beta) gene correlates with IL-1 beta secretion in vitro. Eur J Clin Invest 1992; 22(6):396–402.
83. Tarlow JK, Blakemore AI, Lennard A, Solari R, Hughes HN, Steinkasserer A, Duff GW. Polymorphism in human IL-1 receptor antagonist gene intron 2 is caused by variable numbers of an 86-bp tandem repeat. Hum Genet 1993; 91(4):403–404.
84. Joos L, McIntyre L, Ruan J, Connett JE, Anthonisen NR, Weir TD, Pare PD, Sandford AJ. Association of IL-1beta and IL-1 receptor antagonist haplotypes with rate of decline in lung function in smokers. Thorax 2001; 56(11): 836–863.
85. Wilkinson RJ, Patel P, Llewelyn M, Hirsch CS, Pasvol G, Snounou G, Davidson RN, Toossi Z. Influence of polymorphism in the genes for the interleukin (IL)-1 receptor antagonist and IL-1beta on tuberculosis. J Exp Med 1999; 189(12):1863–1874.
86. Nemetz A, Nosti-Escanilla MP, Molnar T, Kope A, Kovacs A, Feher J, Tulassay Z, Nagy F, Garcia-Gonzalez MA, Pena AS. IL1B gene polymorphisms influence the course and severity of inflammatory bowel disease. Immunogenetics 1999; 49(6):527–531.
87. Whyte M, Hubbard R, Meliconi R, Whidborne M, Eaton V, Bingle C, Timms J, Duff G, Facchini A, Pacilli A, Fabbri M, Hall I, Britton J, Johnston I, Di Giovine F. Increased risk of fibrosing alveolitis associated with interleukin-1 receptor antagonist and tumor necrosis factor-alpha gene polymorphisms. Am J Respir Crit Care Med 2000; 162(2 pt 1):755–758.
88. Camner P, Philipson K, Friberg L. Tracheobronchial clearance in twins. Arch Environ Health 1972; 24(2):82–87.
89. Davis PB. Autonomic and airway reactivity in obligate heterozygotes for cystic fibrosis. Am Rev Respir Dis 1984; 129(6):911–914.
90. Davis PB, Vargo K. Pulmonary abnormalities in obligate heterozygotes for cystic fibrosis. Thorax 1987; 42(2):120–125.
91. Gervais R, Lafitte JJ, Dumur V, Kesteloot M, Lalau G, Houdret N, Roussel P. Sweat chloride and ΔF508 mutation in chronic bronchitis or bronchiectasis. Lancet 1993; 342(8877):997.
92. Dumur V, Lafitte JJ, Gervais R, Debaecker D, Kesteloot M, Lalau G, Roussel P. Abnormal distribution of cystic fibrosis ΔF508 allele in adults with chronic bronchial hypersecretion. Lancet 1990; 335(8701):1340.
93. Bombieri C, Benetazzo M, Saccomani A, Belpinati F, Gile LS, Luisetti M, Pignatti PF. Complete mutational screening of the CFTR gene in 120 patients with pulmonary disease. Hum Genet 1998; 103(6):718–722.
94. Pignatti PF, Bombieri C, Benetazzo M, Casartelli A, Trabetti E, Gile LS, Martinati LC, Boner AL, Luisetti M. CFTR gene variant IVS8-5T in disseminated bronchiectasis. Am J Hum Genet 1996; 58(4):889–892.

95. Tzetis M, Efthymiadou A, Strofalis S, Psychou P, Dimakou A, Pouliou E, Doudounakis S, Kanavakis E. CFTR gene mutations—including three novel nucleotide substitutions—and haplotype background in patients with asthma, disseminated bronchiectasis and chronic obstructive pulmonary disease. Hum Genet 2001; 108(3):216–221.
96. Cuppens H, Lin W, Jaspers M, Costes B, Teng H, Vankeerberghen A, Jorissen M, Droogmans G, Reynaert I, Goossens M, Nilius B, Cassiman JJ. Polyvariant mutant cystic fibrosis transmembrane conductance regulator genes. The polymorphic (Tg)m locus explains the partial penetrance of the T5 polymorphism as a disease mutation. J Clin Invest 1998; 101(2):487–496.
97. Cohen BH, Diamond EL, Graves CG, Kreiss P, Levy DA, Menkes HA, Permutt S, Quaskey S, Tockman MS. A common familial component in lung cancer and chronic obstructive pulmonary disease. Lancet 1977; 2(8037):523–526.
98. Beaty TH, Menkes HA, Cohen BH, Newill CA. Risk factors associated with longitudinal change in pulmonary function. Am Rev Respir Dis 1984; 129(5): 660–667.
99. Kauffmann F, Frette C, Pham QT, Nafissi S, Bertrand JP, Oriol R. Associations of blood group-related antigens to FEV_1, wheezing, and asthma. Am J Respir Crit Care Med 1996; 153(1):76–82.
100. Vestbo J, Hein HO, Suadicani P, Sorensen H, Gyntelberg F. Genetic markers for chronic bronchitis and peak expiratory flow in the Copenhagen Male Study. Danish Med Bull 1993; 40(3):378–380.
101. Kauffmann F, Kleisbauer JP, Cambon-De-Mouzon A, Mercier P, Constans J, Blanc M, Rouch Y, Feingold N. Genetic markers in chronic air-flow limitation: a genetic epidemiologic study. Am Rev Respir Dis 1983; 127(3):263–269.
102. Horne SL, Cockcroft DW, Lovegrove A, Dosman JA. ABO, Lewis and secretor status and relative incidence of airflow obstruction. Dis Markers 1985; 3:55–62.
103. Abboud RT, Yu P, Chan-Yeung M, Tan F. Lack of relationship between ABH secretor status and lung function in pulp-mill workers. Am Rev Respir Dis 1982; 126(6):1089–1091.
104. Keicho N, Tokunaga K, Nakata K, Taguchi Y, Azuma A, Bannai M, Emi M, Ohishi N, Yazaki Y, Kudoh S. Contribution of HLA genes to genetic predisposition in diffuse panbronchiolitis. Am J Respir Crit Care Med 1998; 158(3):846–850.
105. Webb DR. Selective IgA deficiency and chronic obstructive pulmonary disease—a family study. Adv Exp Med Biol 1974; 45(0):437–439.
106. Ho LI, Harn HJ, Chen CJ, Tsai NM. Polymorphism of the beta(2)-adrenoceptor in COPD in Chinese subjects. Chest 2001; 120(5):1493–1499.
107. Vestbo J, Prescott E. Update on the "Dutch hypothesis" for chronic respiratory disease. Thorax 1998; 53(suppl 2):S15–S19.
108. Zhu Z, Homer RJ, Wang Z, Chen Q, Geba GP, Wang J, Zhang Y, Elias JA. Pulmonary expression of interleukin-13 causes inflammation, mucus hypersecretion, subepithelial fibrosis, physiologic abnormalities, and eotaxin production. J Clin Invest 1999; 103(6):779–788.

109. MacNee W. Oxidants/antioxidants and chronic obstructive pulmonary disease: pathogenesis to therapy. Novartis Found Symp 2001; 234:169–185. Discussion 185–188.
110. Cawston T, Carrere S, Catterall J, Duggleby R, Elliott S, Shingleton B, Rowan A. Matrix metalloproteinases and TIMPs: properties and implications for the treatment of chronic obstructive pulmonary disease. Novartis Found Symp 2001; 234:205–218. Discussion 218–228.
111. McElvaney NG, Stoller JK, Buist AS, Prakash UB, Brantly ML, Schluchter MD, Crystal RD. Baseline characteristics of enrollees in the National Heart, Lung and Blood Institute Registry of α_1-antitrypsin deficiency. α_1-Antitrypsin Deficiency Registry Study Group. Chest 1997; 111(2):394–403.
112. The a1-Antitrypsin Deficiency Registry Study Group. Survival and FEV_1 decline in individuals with severe deficiency of α_1-antitrypsin. Am J Respir Crit Care Med 1998; 158(1):49–59.
113. Seersholm N, Wencker M, Banik N, Viskum K, Dirksen A, Kok-Jensen A, Konietzko N. Does α_1-antitrypsin augmentation therapy slow the annual decline in FEV_1 in patients with severe hereditary α_1-antitrypsin deficiency? Wissenschaftliche Arbeitsgemeinschaft zur Therapie von Lungenerkrankungen (WATL) α_1-AT study group. Eur Respir J 1997; 10(10):2260–2263.
114. Dirksen A, Dijkman JH, Madsen F, Stoel B, Hutchison DC, Ulrik CS, Skovgaard LT, Kok-Jensen A, Rudolphus A, Seersholm N, Vrooman HA, Reiber JH, Hansen NC, Heckscher T, Viskum K, Stolk J. A randomized clinical trial of alpha(1)-antitrypsin augmentation therapy. Am J Respir Crit Care Med 1999; 160(5 pt 1):1468–1472.
115. Wencker M, Fuhrmann B, Banik N, Konietzko N. Longitudinal follow-up of patients with alpha(1)-protease inhibitor deficiency before and during therapy with IV alpha(1)-protease inhibitor. Chest 2001; 119(3):737–744.
116. He JQ, Joos L, Sandford AJ. Recent developments in the genetics of asthma. Pharmacogenomics 2001; 2(4):329–339.
117. Daly MJ, Rioux JD, Schaffner SF, Hudson TJ, Lander ES. High-resolution haplotype structure in the human genome. Nat Genet 2001; 29(2):229–232.
118. Collins FS, Guyer MS, Charkravarti A. Variations on a theme: cataloging human DNA sequence variation. Science 1997; 278(5343):1580–1581.
119. Patil N, Berno AJ, Hinds DA, Barrett WA, Doshi JM, Hacker CR, Kautzer CR, Lee DH, Marjoribanks C, McDonough DP, Nguyen BT, Norris MC, Sheehan JB, Shen N, Stern D, Stokowski RP, Thomas DJ, Trulson MO, Vyas KR, Frazer KA, Fodor SP, Cox DR. Blocks of limited haplotype diversity revealed by high-resolution scanning of human chromosome 21. Science 2001; 294(5547):1719–1723.
120. Weiss KM, Clark AG. Linkage disequilibrium and the mapping of complex human traits. Trends Genet 2002; 18(1):19–24.

8

Dyspnea

DONALD A. MAHLER

Dartmouth Medical School
Lebanon, New Hampshire, U.S.A.

I. Introduction

There are at least three reasons for measuring breathlessness in symptomatic patients with chronic obstructive pulmonary disease (COPD). First, although dyspnea is a warning signal, it also limits activities (e.g., patients stop to rest during housework, carrying packages, or climbing stairs in order to minimize dyspnea). This was confirmed by a telephone survey of over 3000 patients with COPD in North America and Europe [1]. Of patients less than 65 years of age, 56% reported shortness of breath during normal physical activities, and 42% described breathlessness while doing household chores. These experiences commonly lead patients to seek medical attention.

Second, patients with COPD generally experience a gradual progression of dyspnea over time. For example, Mahler et al. [2] reported that there was a significant decrease (-0.7 ± 2.9 units; $p = 0.04$) in the Transition Dyspnea Index (TDI) over a two-year time period in 76 male patients who had stable COPD at the time of enrollment into the study. In a randomized clinical trial comparing tiotropium, a once-a-day inhaled anticholingeric medication, and placebo, Casaburi et al. [3] found that there was decline of ~ 0.3 in the TDI over one year in the 325 patients with COPD who received placebo therapy. These consistent results illustrate that the severity of breathlessness generally worsens over time in patients with COPD. This is likely due to a combination of progression of airflow obstruction, possible weight gain, and any deconditioning.

Third, the measurement of dyspnea is important in order to evaluate an individual's response to therapy. In April 2001 the Global Obstructive Lung Disease (GOLD) Initiative, a joint effort of the World Health Organization and the National Heart, Lung, and Blood Institute, emphasized that the treatment of COPD should be directed *toward relief of symptoms* [4]. As smoking cessation is the only treatment that slows the decline in lung function, the GOLD committee recommended that all other therapeutic strategies should focus on treating the symptoms. Thus, dyspnea needs to be measured initially, as a baseline, and after an intervention in order to determine whether a specific treatment is efficacious.

II. The Measurement of Dyspnea

Like any sensation, dyspnea can be quantified using a stimulus–response relationship [5]. Although the precise stimuli and the exact mechanisms for dyspnea have not been completely identified, it is possible to consider probable stimuli for provoking dyspnea as measured by different approaches (Table 1). For example, the addition of resistive or elastic loads to breathing in a laboratory experiment has been used to study the mechanisms contributing to breathing difficulty. However, this approach has little if any relevance to the daily problem of dyspnea experienced by patients with COPD [6].

Table 1 Proposed Stimulus → Response Relationships for the Measurement of Dyspnea

Stimulus		Instruments for measuring the dyspnea response
Added respiratory loads	→	Open magnitude scale (zero → infinity) Visual analog scale 0–10 category-ratio scale
Activities of daily living	→	Baseline and Transition Dyspnea Indexes Dyspnea component of CRQ
Exercise testing	→	Visual analog scale 0–10 category-ratio scale

CRQ = Chronic Respiratory Questionnaire.

The Medical Research Council (MRC) breathlessness questionnaire was one of the initial instruments developed to quantify dyspnea [7]. This questionnaire includes five grades based on physical activities. The individual patient selects a grade that most closely matches his or her severity of breathlessness. Although this instrument continues to be used for discriminative purposes (to determine the severity of dyspnea in an individual), it is relatively insensitive to detect changes with an intervention.

A. Multidimensional Clinical Instruments

Multidimensional instruments use *activities of daily living* as the putative stimulus in order to quantify the severity of dyspnea. This approach has been considered as an "indirect" measure of breathlessness, as it relies on the individual patient to provide information based on recall.

In 1984 the Baseline Dyspnea Index (BDI) and the Transition Dyspnea Index (TDI) were published, which included three components—functional impairment, magnitude of task, and magnitude of effort—that provoke breathing difficulty (Table 2) [8]. The BDI, a discriminative instrument, describes specific criteria for each of the three components at a single point in time. The TDI, an evaluative instrument, includes specific criteria for each of the three components to measure *changes from the baseline state*.

In 1987 the Chronic Respiratory Questionnaire (CRQ) was published to measure health status in patients with lung disease [9]. Dyspnea was one of four dimensions included in the CRQ (Table 2). The individual patient is required to select or identify the five most important activities that caused breathlessness over the past two weeks. The severity of dyspnea for each activity is then graded by the patient on 1 ("extremely short of breath") to 7 ("not at all short of breath") scale. By dividing the total score of 5 to 35 by the number of activities selected (usually 5), an overall score of 1 to 7 is obtained. The CRQ was developed as an evaluative instrument to measure *changes over time*.

Other published instruments proposed to measure dyspnea include the University of California San Diego (UCSD) Shortness of Breath Questionnaire [10] and the Dyspnea Questionnaire [11]. The UCSD questionnaire is a 24-item instrument that assesses self-reported shortness of breath as related to a variety of activities of daily living. The Dyspnea Questionnaire provides a general rating of dyspnea as well as the intensity using a numerical scale from 0 (none) to 10 (very severe) for each of 79 activities. However, the responsiveness of these two questionnaires has not been examined to evaluate pharmacotherapy in patients with COPD and therefore requires prospective testing.

Table 2 Characteristics of Two Multidimensional Instruments for Measuring Dyspnea Based on Activities of Daily Living

Characteristic	BDI/TDI	Dyspnea component of CRQ
Components	1. Functional impairment 2. Magnitude of task 3. Magnitude of effort	Five activities selected by the patient that cause dyspnea (specific to the individual)
Interviewer	Required	Required
Grading scale	Specific criteria for different grades for each component	1 ("extremely short of breath") to 7 ("not at all short of breath") for each activity
Range of score for each component/activity	0 to 4 (BDI) −3 to +3 (TDI)	1 to 7
Range of total score	0 to 12 (BDI) −9 to +9 (TDI)	5 to 35 (1 to 7 if total score is divided by the number of activities, typically 5)
Time to complete (min)	4 to 5	10 to 20 (initially) 5 to 10 (follow-up)
MID	Δ 1 unit on the TDI	Δ 0.5 for the dyspnea component

BDI = Baseline Dyspnea Index; TDI = Transition Dyspnea Index; CRQ = Chronic Respiratory Questionnaire; MID = minimal important difference.

B. Dyspnea Ratings During Exercise

Incremental Exercise

Cardiopulmonary exercise testing has been a traditional method to examine an individual's exercise capacity. In the past decade the intensity of dyspnea has been routinely measured as part of the exercise testing protocol [5,12]. As an example, patients give ratings of dyspnea on either a category or visual analog scale during the exercise task. Guidelines for the assessment of dyspnea and other symptoms during cardiopulmonary exercise testing are provided in Table 3.

Initial studies instructed subjects to rate dyspnea at the end of the exercise test (peak values). Both healthy individuals and patients with cardiorespiratory disease report "symptom limitation," or stop exercise, at ratings between 5 (severe) and 8 on the 0–10 category-ratio (CR-10) scale

Table 3 Guidelines for the Assessment of Dyspnea During Cardiopulmonary Exercise Testing

Measurement
1. Based on discussion with the individual patient, select one (dyspnea) or two symptoms for patient to rate:
   (a) Dyspnea and leg discomfort are appropriate symptoms for patients with respiratory disease.
   (b) Chest pain and dyspnea are appropriate symptoms for patients with cardiovascular disease.
2. Provide written instructions for the patient to use for selecting an intensity on the 0–10 category-ratio scale or the visual analog scale (typically, patients are asked to indicate a rating each minute of the incremental exercise test).
3. Review the instrument with the patient prior to the exercise test.
4. Ask the patient at the end of the test, "What stopped or limited you from doing more exercise?"

Analysis
1. Compare dyspnea ratings before and after an intervention at comparable work loads or time periods.
2. Examine the stimulus → response relationship (e.g., VO_2 → dyspnea) for the entire continuum of the exercise test by calculating the slope and intercept.

Interpretation
1. Integrate the physiological and perceptual results.
2. Approximately 10% of individuals have difficulty rating any sensation (i.e., "poor raters").
3. The intensity of dyspnea obtained from a cardiopulmonary exercise test may be used as a "target" for prescription of exercise intensity.

developed by Borg [13]. However, peak dyspnea ratings have provided limited information, particularly when evaluating the effect of an intervention. Consequently, the "next step" was to instruct patients to give ratings each minute throughout an incremental or ramp exercise test. In this procedure the subject is instructed to provide ratings "on cue" each minute; thus, a series of discrete dyspnea ratings are obtained throughout exertion. In general, the slope of the regression between power output, or oxygen consumption, on the cycle ergometer and dyspnea ratings is higher in patients with respiratory disease compared with healthy individuals of comparable age [12].

In 1993 Harty et al. [14] described the methodology and results of the continuous measurement of dyspnea during exercise. Six healthy subjects used a potentiometer to give ratings on a visual analog scale displayed on a monitor. In 2001 Mahler and colleagues [15] reported on a continuous method in which subjects moved a computer mouse (positioned on a platform attached to the handle bars of a cycle ergometer) throughout exercise to indicate the current intensity of perceived dyspnea on the CR-10 scale displayed on a monitor. This approach enabled the subject to provide ratings *spontaneously* and *continuously* while performing the exercise test, without waiting for a cue or request from the physician or technician.

The major advantages of the continuous method are:

1. Subjects can report the actual intensity of breathlessness as it changes throughout the entire course of exercise rather than only at arbitrary 1-min time intervals.
2. Subjects provide substantially more dyspnea ratings compared with the discrete method (ratings each minute)—the standard method currently used in most laboratories. As many patients with cardiopulmonary diseases can exercise for only 4 or 5 min, only 4 or 5 dyspnea ratings can be obtained with the discrete method. Statistical accuracy is a concern when performing regression analysis with such a small number of data points [15].
3. Additional statistical metrics can be calculated with the continuous method, such as an absolute threshold, "just noticeable differences" (JNDs), and the Weber fraction.

Further testing will determine whether these "new" measures prove more responsive to assess the efficacy of pharmacotherapy for relief of dyspnea during cardiopulmonary exercise testing.

Submaximal Exercise

Submaximal steady-state exercise more closely simulates daily physical activities compared with incremental exercise to exhaustion. Franco and colleagues [16] observed a gradual increase in dyspnea ratings reported by patients with COPD on the CR-10 scale at intensities of both 55% and 77% of peak oxygen consumption (VO_2) during minutes 6–10, while heart rate and VO_2 remained constant. O'Donnell et al. [17] also demonstrated that patients increase their ratings of breathlessness up to at least 8 min of exercise at 50–60% of the maximum work rate.

In an investigation of three different exercise tests to evaluate the effects of inhaled oxitropium bromide, Oga et al. [18] reported that cycle endurance testing at 80% of the maximal workload "was the most sensitive in detecting" the benefits of bronchodilator therapy. The data by O'Donnell et al. [17] and by Oga et al. [18] suggest that submaximal exercise may be a more appropriate exercise stimulus to examine the benefits of bronchodilator therapy in patients with COPD.

III. Responsiveness

From a clinical perspective, the major interest for measuring dyspnea is to determine the *responsiveness* of an evaluative instrument. Responsiveness refers to an instrument's ability to detect change. For example, if a treatment results in an important difference in dyspnea, the physician wants to be confident that the difference can be detected even if it is small. Ideally, a statistically significant difference in dyspnea scores should also be clinically important.

Jaeschke et al. [19] defined a minimal clinically important difference as "the smallest difference in measured health status that signifies an important rather than trivial difference in patient symptoms."

A. Transition Dyspnea Index (TDI)

The minimal important difference for the TDI is a change of 1 unit [7,20]. A 1-unit increase in the TDI focal score corresponds to "slight improvement" for each component of the instrument. For example, a change of 1 unit in the functional impairment domain describes a patient who either *was able to return to work or resumes some customary activities with more vigor due to an improvement in breathlessness*. This improvement is likely quite meaningful to the affected individual. In addition, Witek and Mahler [20] used an anchor-based approach and showed that a change in the TDI focal score of 1 unit corresponded to a definite change in the physician's global evaluation.

A variety of interventions, including bronchodilator therapy, exercise training, inspiratory muscle training, and lung volume reduction surgery, have been shown to reduce dyspnea as measured with the TDI [5]. Various randomized controlled trials have shown $\geq$1 unit improvements in the TDI focal score with tiotropium [3,21], formoterol (only at 18 μg dose) [22], salmeterol [23], theophylline [23,24], inhaled fluticasone [25], and the combination of fluticasone and salmeterol [25] in patients with COPD (Table 4). In the study by Vincken et al. [26], tiotropium provided greater relief of dyspnea than ipratropium bromide as measured by the difference in the TDI focal score (0.9 ± 0.3; $p = 0.001$) at 1 year.

B. Dyspnea Component of the CRQ

The minimal important difference for the dyspnea component of the CRQ is 0.5 [19,27]. Although the CRQ has been used to measure health status in a variety of randomized clinical trials involving patients with COPD, in most of these studies the actual scores for the dyspnea component have not been reported [28–30]. However, Rutten-van Molken et al. [31] examined responsiveness of the dyspnea component of the CRQ with three treatments: sal-

Table 4 Responsiveness of the TDI in Randomized Controlled Trials Evaluating Pharmacotherapy in Patients with COPD[a]

	TDI focal score				
Intervention/author	Treatment group		Placebo group		p Value
Anticholinergic					
Ipratropium bromide					
Mahler [29]—12 weeks		Δ 0.8[b]			<0.05
Tiotropium					
Casaburi [3]—1 year		Δ 1.1 ± 0.2			<0.001
Vincken [26]—1 year		Δ 0.9 ± 0.3 (compared with ipratropium bromide)			0.001
Donohue [21]—6 months		Δ 1.0			0.01
Donohue [21]—6 months		Δ 0.8 (compared with salmeterol)			<0.05
β-Agonist					
Formoterol					
Aalbers [22]—12 weeks		Δ 0.7	Δ 0.5	Δ 1.2	
	Dose (BID)	4.5 μg	9 μg	18 μg	
	p Value	ns	ns	0.002	
Salmeterol		Δ 0.2[c]			
Mahler [29]—12 weeks					>0.05
ZuWallack [23]—12 weeks	+1.3 ± 0.2		No placebo group		NP
Mahler [25]—6 months		Δ 0.5			>0.05
Donohue [21]—6 months		Δ 0.2			0.56
Theophylline					
Kirsten [34]—2–3 days[d]	−0.9 ± 1.9		+0.4 ± 2.6		<0.05
Mahler [24]—4 weeks	+2.4 ± 2.8		−0.7 ± 3.4		<0.05
ZuWallack [23]—12 weeks	+1.1 ± 0.2		No placebo group		NP
Inhaled corticosteroid					
Fluticasone					
Mahler [25]—6 months		Δ 1.0			0.002
Inhaled corticosteroid and long-acting β-agonist					
Fluticasone and salmeterol combination					
Mahler [25]—6 months		Δ 1.7			<0.001

[a] NP = not provided; NS = not significant; Δ refers to difference in TDI between treatment and placebo groups, unless otherwise stated.
[b] At weeks 2, 4, 6, 8, 10, and 12 versus placebo, $p < 0.05$.
[c] At weeks 2, 4, 8, and 10 versus placebo, $p < 0.05$.
[d] The treatment group had theophylline withdrawn which caused a decrease in the TDI (i.e., more breathlessness), while the control group continued to receive theophylline.

meterol and placebo ($n = 43$); salmeterol and ipratropium bromide ($n = 45$); and placebo ($n = 45$). There were no significant differences for the dyspnea component of the CRQ among the three treatment groups ($p = 0.37$) [31].

C. Dyspnea Ratings During Exercise

Improvements in dyspnea ratings during exercise (6-min walking test or cardiopulmonary exercise testing) have been demonstrated with anticholinergic agents, β-agonists, and theophylline (Table 5). For example, O'Donnell

Table 5 Responsiveness of Patient Ratings of Dyspnea During Exercise Testing[a]

Intervention	Dyspnea ratings: Treatment group	Dyspnea ratings: Placebo group	p Value
Anticholinergic			
Ipratropium bromide			
Tsukino [38]—one dose	NP[d]	NP[d]	<0.05
O'Donnell [17]—4 weeks	Δ−0.5 ± 0.2[c] during CPET		<0.01
Oxitropium bromide			
Teramoto [37]—one dose	15.4 ± 1.4[d] (during CPET)	29.7 ± 2.8[d] (during CPET)	<0.05
Teramoto [39]—one dose	Decreased[d] (compared with pre-inhalation)	No change[d] (compared with pre-inhalation)	NP
β-Agonist			
Albuterol			
Belman [32]—one dose	Δ−1.4 ± 0.5[c] during CPET		<0.05
Guyatt [28]—2 weeks	3.9 (at end of 6MW)	2.4 (at end of 6MW)	NP
Salmeterol			
Grove [35]—4 weeks	[b]0.5[c]	[b]1.0[c]	0.004
Mahler [29]—12 weeks	3.1 ± 0.2[c] (at end of 6MW)	3.1 ± 0.1[c] (at end of 6MW)	>0.05
Boyd [36]—16 weeks	Fewer pts reported scores <3 (at end of 6MW)		0.004
Theophylline			
Guyatt [28]—2 weeks	3.6 (at end of 6MW)	2.4 (at end of 6MW)	NP
Tsukino [38]—one dose	NP[d]	NP[d]	<0.05

[a] NP = not provided.
[b] Median values.
[c] On 0–10 Borg scale.
[d] Values are slope of Borg ratings–VO_2.

et al. [18] reported that 500 μg of ipratropium bromide reduced dyspnea ratings by 0.5 ± 0.2 units on the Borg scale during steady-state cycle ergometry compared with placebo ($p < 0.01$) after 4 weeks of therapy in patients with COPD. Belman et al. [32] showed that the acute administration of 300 μg of albuterol contributed to a reduction of 1.4 ± 0.5 units on the Borg scale at equivalent levels of work intensity on the cycle ergometer compared to placebo ($p < 0.05$) in 13 patients with COPD. In both of these studies the improvements in exertional dyspnea were significantly correlated with reductions in measures of dynamic hyperinflation during exercise [18,32]. In a comparative trial, Ayers et al. [33] studied the acute administration of 42 μg (2 puffs) of salmeterol versus 72 μg (4 puffs) of ipratropium bromide during steady-state exercise and found similar effectiveness (ratings of dysnea ~2 on the Borg scale) with each medication.

IV. Summary

Although difficulty breathing has always been one of the major concerns of patients with COPD, dyspnea has been increasingly recognized as an important outcome measure in evaluating therapy. Two approaches have been used to quantify dyspnea:

1. Clinical ratings based on activities of daily living
2. Ratings during exercise

These different methods provide unique yet complimentary information about the severity of breathlessness in affected individuals (Tables 2 and 3).

Various randomized controlled trials have demonstrated that anticholinergic agents, β-agonists, and theophylline provide relief of dyspnea in symptomatic patients with COPD (Tables 4 and 5). The interest of clinicians as well as the requirements of regulatory agencies ensure that the measurement of dyspnea will continue to be an important outcome variable in the assessment and management of patients with respiratory disease.

References

1. Rennard S, Decramer M, Calverly PM, Pride NB, Soriano JB, Vermeire PA, Vestbo J. The impact of COPD in North America and Europe in 2000: the subjects' perspective of the Confronting COPD International Survey. Eur Respir J. In press.
2. Mahler DA, Tomlinson D, Olmstead EM, Tosteson ANA, O'Connor GT. Changes in dyspnea, health status, and lung function in chronic airway disease. Am J Respir Crit Care Med 1995; 151:61–65.

3. Casaburi R, Mahler DA, Jones PW, Wanner A, San Pedro G, Zu Wallack RL, Menjoge SS, Serby CW, Witek T Jr. A long-term evaluation of once-daily inhaled tiotropium in chronic obstructive pulmonary disease. Eur Respir J 2002; 19:217–224.
4. Pauwels RA, Buist AS, Calverley PMA, Jenkins CR, Hurd SS. Global strategy for the diagnosis, management, and prevention of chronic obstructive pulmonary disease. NHLBI/WHO Global Initiative for Chronic Obstructive Lung Disease (GOLD) workshop summary. Am J Respir Crit Care Med 2001; 163:1256–1276.
5. Mahler DA, Jones PW, Guyatt GH. Clinical measurement of dyspnea. In: Mahler DA, ed. Dyspnea. New York: Marcel Dekker, 1998:149–198.
6. Mahler DA, Rosiello RA, Harver A, Lentine T, McGovern JF, Daubenspeck JA. Comparison of clinical dyspnea ratings and psychophysical measurements of respiratory sensation in obstructive airway disease. Am Rev Respir Dis 1987; 135:1229–1233.
7. Fletcher CM, Elmes PC, Wood CH. The significance of respiratory symptoms and the diagnosis of chronic bronchitis in a working population. Br Med J 1959; 2:257–266.
8. Mahler DA, Weinberg DH, Wells CK, Feinstein AR. The measurement of dyspnea: contents, interobserver agreement, and physiologic correlates of two new clinical indexes. Chest 1984; 85:751–758.
9. Guyatt GH, Berman LB, Townsend M, Pugsley SO, Chambers LW. A measure of quality of life for clinical trials in chronic lung diseases. Thorax 1987; 42:773–778.
10. Eakin EG, Resnikoff PM, Prewitt LM, Ries AL, Kaplan RM. Validation of a new dyspnea measure: the UCSD shortness of breath questionnaire. Chest 1998; 113:619–624.
11. Lareau SC, Carrieri-Kohlman V, Janson-Bjerklie S, Ross PJ. Development and testing of the Pulmonary Functional Status and Dyspnea Questionnaire. Heart Lung 1994; 23:242–250.
12. Jones NL, Killian KJ. Exercise limitation in health and disease. N Engl J Med 2000; 343:632–640.
13. Borg GAV. Psychophysical bases of perceived exertion. Med Sci Sports Exer 1982; 14:377–381.
14. Harty HR, Heywood P, Adams L. Comparison between continuous and discrete measurements of breathlessness during exercise in normal subjects using a visual analogue scale. Clin Sci 1993; 85:229–236.
15. Mahler DA, Mejia-Alfaro R, Ward J, Baird JC. Continuous measurement of breathlessness during exercise: validity, reliability, and responsiveness. J Appl Physiol 2001; 90:2188–2196.
16. Franco MJ, Olmstead EM, Tosteson ANA, Lentine T, Ward J, Mahler DA. Comparison of dyspnea ratings during submaximal constant work exercise with incremental testing. Med Sci Sports Exerc 1998; 30:479–482.
17. O'Donnell DE, Lam M, Webb KA. Measurement of symptoms, lung hyperinflation, and endurance during exercise in chronic obstructive pulmonary disease. Am J Respir Crit Care Med 1998; 158:1557–1565.

18. Oga T, Nishimura K, Tsukino M, Hajiro T, Ikeda A, Izumi T. The effects of oxitropium bromide on exercise performance in patients with stable chronic obstructive pulmonary disease. Am J Respir Crit Care Med 2000; 161:1897–1901.
19. Jaeschke R, Singer J, Guyatt GH. Measurement of health status. Ascertaining the minimal clinically important difference. Controlled Clin Trials 1989; 10: 407–415.
20. Witek TJ Jr, Mahler DA. Meaningful effect size and patterns of response of the Transition Dyspnea Index. J Clin Epidemol 2003; 56:248–255.
21. Donohue JF, van Noord JA, Bateman ED, Langley SJ, Lee A, Witek TJ, Kesten S, Towse L. A 6-month, placebo-controlled study comparing lung function and health status changes in COPD patients treated with tiotropium or salmeterol. Chest 2002; 122:47–55.
22. Aalbers R, Ayres J, Backer V, Decramer M, Lier PA, Magyar P, Malolepszy J, Ruffin R, Sybrecht GW. Formoterol in patients with chronic obstructive pulmonary disease: a randomized, controlled, 3-month trial. Eur Respir J 2002; 19:936–943.
23. ZuWallack RL, Mahler DA, Reilly, Church N, Emmett A, Rickard K, Knobil K. Salmeterol plus theophylline combination therapy in the treatment of COPD. Chest 2001; 119:628–630.
24. Mahler DA, Matthay RA, Snyder PE, Wells CK, Loke J. Sustained-release theophylline reduces dyspnea in nonreversible obstructive airway disease. Am Rev Respir Dis 1985; 131:22–25.
25. Mahler DA, Wire P, Horstman D, Clifford D, Chang C, Yates J, Fischer T, Shah T. Effectiveness of fluticasone propionate and salmeterol delivered via the diskus device in the treatment of COPD. Am J Respir Crit Care Med 2002; 166:1084–1091.
26. Vincken W, van Noord JA, Greefhorst APM, Bantje TA, Kesten S, Korducki L, Cornelissen PJG. Improved health outcomes in patients with COPD during 1 yr's treatment with tiotropium. Eur Respir J 2002; 19:209–216.
27. Jones PW. Interpreting thresholds for a clinically significant change in health status in asthma and COPD. Eur Respir J 2002; 19:398–404.
28. Guyatt GH, Townsend M, Pugsley SO, Keller JL, Short HD, Taylor DW. Newhouse MT. Bronchodilators in chronic airflow limitation. Am Rev Respir Dis 1987; 135:1069–1074.
29. Mahler DA, Donohue JF, Barbee RA, Goldman MD, Gross NJ, Wisniewski ME, Yancey SW, Zakes BA, Rickard KA, Anderson WH. Efficacy of salmeterol xinafoate in the treatment of COPD. Chest 1999; 115:957–965.
30. Rennard SI, Anderson W, ZuWallack R, Broughton J, Bailey W, Friedman M, Wisniewski M, Rickard K. Use of a long-acting inhaled β2-adrenergic agonist, salmeterol xinafoate, in patients with chronic obstructive pulmonary disease. Am J Respir Crit Care Med 2001; 163:1087–1092.
31. Rutten-van Molken M, Roos B, van Noord JA. An empirical comparison of the St George's Respiratory Questionnaire (SGRQ) and the Chronic Respiratory Disease Questionnaire (CRQ) in a clinical trial setting. Thorax 1999; 54: 995–1003.

32. Belman MJ, Botnick WC, Shin JW. Inhaled bronchodilators reduce dynamic hyperinflation during exercise in patients with chronic obstructive pulmonary disease. Am J Respir Crit Care Med 1996; 153:967–975.
33. Ayers ML, Mejia R, Ward J, Lentine T, Mahler DA. Effectiveness of salmeterol versus ipratropium bromide on exertional dyspnoea in COPD. Eur Respir J 2001; 17:1132–1137.
34. Kirsten DK, Wegner RE, Jorres RA, Magnussen H. Effects of theophylline withdrawl in severe chronic obstructive pulmonary disease. Chest 1993; 104: 1101–1107.
35. Grove A, Lipworth BJ, Reid P, Smith RP, Ramage L, Ingram CG, Jenkins RJ, Winter JH, Dhillon DP. Effects of regular salmeterol on lung function and exercise capacity in patients with chronic obstructive airways disease. Thorax 1996; 51:689–693.
36. Boyd G, Morice AH, Pounsford JC, Siebert M, Peslis N, Crawford C. An evaluation of salmeterol in the treatment of chronic obstuctive pulmonary disease (COPD). Eur Respir J 1997; 10:815–821.
37. Teramoto S, Fukuchi Y, Orimo H. Effects of inhaled anticholinergic drug on dyspnea and gas exchange during exercise in patients with chronic obstructive pulmonary disease. Chest 1993; 103:1774–1782.
38. Tsukino M, Nishimura K, Ikeda A, Hajiro T, Koyama H, Izumi T. Effects of theophylline and ipratropium bromide on exercise performance in patients with stable chronic obstructive pulmonary disease. Thorax 1998; 53:269–273.
39. Teramoto S, Fukuchi Y. Improvements in exercise capacity and dyspnoea by inhaled anticholinergic drug in elderly patients with chronic obstructive pulmonary disease. Age and Ageing 1995; 24:278–282.

9

Exacerbations of COPD

JADWIGA A. WEDZICHA

St. Bartholomew's Hospital
London, England

I. Definition of a COPD Exacerbation

Exacerbations of chronic obstructive pulmonary disease (COPD) are now recognised to be an important cause of the considerable morbidity and mortality found in COPD and an important cause of impaired health status [1,2]. An exacerbation of COPD is described as an acute worsening of respiratory symptoms associated with a variable degree of physiological deterioration. However, some symptoms are more important in the description of an exacerbation than others, and Anthonisen and colleagues pointed out some years ago that the most common exacerbation symptoms were increased dyspnea, sputum purulence, and increased sputum volume [3]. Other symptoms associated with exacerbation include upper airway symptoms or those associated with cold, increased cough, and wheeze [2].

Exacerbations are associated with increased health care utilization and definitions of exacerbations have also been proposed based on health care utilization, e.g., unscheduled physician visits, changes or increases in medication, use of oral steroids at exacerbation, and hospital admission [4]. However, health care utilization in COPD is very variable, depending on an individual's access to health care, and thus there may be considerable difficulty standardizing such a definition. In addition, many exacerbations are not reported to health care professionals and are either self-treated or left untreated [2].

COPD exacerbations are also associated with increased airway inflammatory changes [5] that are caused by a variety of factors such as respiratory viruses, especially the rhinovirus (the cause of the common cold) [6], bacteria, and common pollutants [7]. COPD exacerbations are more common in the winter months [8], when respiratory viral infections are common, and there may be important interactions between cold temperatures and exacerbations caused by viruses or pollutants. The inflammatory changes at COPD exacerbation are very variable, and this may be related to the etiological agent. Exacerbations associated with symptomatic colds or respiratory viral infections are more severe, with greater physiological deterioration, longer recovery times, and increased airway inflammatory markers [5,9]. Thus, pharmacological therapy needs to be particularly targeted at these viral exacerbations, though to date there are no available antirhinovirus therapies. Pharmacological therapies are available for influenza, though with the availability of influenza vaccination, influenza has become a less frequent cause of COPD exacerbation.

II. Exacerbation Frequency

Recent prospective studies have shown that exacerbations are more common than was previously recognized. The tendency of patients to underreport exacerbations may explain the higher total rate of exacerbation in these studies at around 2.7 per patient per year [2,7], which is higher than previously reported by Anthonisen and co-workers at 1.1 per patient per year [3]. However, in the latter study, exacerbations were diagnosed from patients' recall of symptoms, and daily monitoring of symptoms to detect exacerbation was not carried out.

Some patients are prone to frequent exacerbations from year to year, and these frequent exacerbators (exacerbation frequency of three or more per year) have worse quality of life than patients with less frequent exacerbation. These patients with a history of frequent exacerbations have increased airway inflammatory markers compared to patients with infrequent exacerbations [5]. Factors predictive of frequent exacerbations include daily cough and sputum, and frequent exacerbations in the previous year [2]. A previous study of acute infective exacerbations of chronic bronchitis also found that one of the factors predicting exacerbation was also the number of exacerbations in the previous year [8], though this study was limited to exacerbations presenting with purulent sputum and no physiological data were available during the study. Thus exacerbation frequency is an important target for pharmacological therapy, and reduction of exacerbation frequency will have important effects on health status in COPD patients.

III. Goals of Exacerbation Therapy

The aim of pharmacological therapy in COPD is to treat the individual exacerbation with the goal of reducing its severity and consequences, including hospitalization and death. Pharmacological therapy is also used with the intention of reducing exacerbation frequency and thus improving the impaired quality of life of these COPD patients.

Although in the studies of Fletcher and Peto it was initially considered that COPD exacerbations had no effect on disease progression [1], two studies have recently shown that COPD exacerbations can affect decline in forced expiratory volume in 1 sec (FEV_1) [11,12]. One study has suggested that in patients who are smokers, exacerbations are associated with greater lung function decline [9]. In another study, Donaldson and colleagues showed that patients with a history of frequent exacerbations had a faster decline of FEV_1 compared to patients with a history of infrequent exacerbations [10]. Thus reduction of exacerbation frequency may have an effect on disease progression in COPD.

One of the reasons for the association between exacerbation frequency and disease progression may be that exacerbations do not completely recover to baseline. Seemungal and colleagues have shown that, after the exacerbation, a significant number of patients show incomplete recovery of symptoms or lung function [7]. The reasons for the incomplete recovery of symptoms and lung function are not clear, but may involve inadequate treatment or persistence of the causative agent. This incomplete physiological recovery after an exacerbation could contribute to the decline in lung function with time in patients with COPD. To date there is no evidence that patients with incomplete recovery of their exacerbation have a greater decline in lung function. However, it is important that COPD exacerbations be monitored, and if recovery is determined to be incomplete, then further pharmacological intervention seems to be warranted.

IV. Therapy of the Acute Exacerbation

A. Inhaled Bronchodilator Therapy

Short-acting bronchodilators (β_2-agonists and anticholinergic agents) are frequently used in the treatment of acute exacerbations of COPD. They may be used as sole therapy in patients with relatively mild COPD who have developed a mild exacerbation, or they may be used and increased in dosage in conjunction with other therapy in patients with more severe exacerbations. In patients with stable COPD, symptomatic benefit can be obtained with bronchodilator therapy in COPD, even without significant changes in spirometry. This is probably due to a reduction in dynamic hyperinflation that is characteristic of COPD and hence leads to a decrease in the sensation of dyspnea, especially during exertion [13].

Short-acting bronchodilators are usually combined for exacerbations in clinic practice. Although there is evidence of benefit in patients with stable COPD [14], there is little evidence for the combination in patients at exacerbation. There is also little evidence of benefit of one type of bronchodilator against another at COPD exacerbation [15–18]. Moayyedi and colleagues randomized COPD patients at exacerbation to either the β_2-agonist salbulatomol or salbutamol in combination with the anticholinergic agent ipratropium bromide and found no advantage of the combination on length of hospital stay or on FEV_1 at 1, 3, 7, 14 days or discharge [15]. Karpel et al. compared salbutamol and ipratropium in a crossover trial and showed no difference in outcomes between the two therapies [16]. Rebuck evaluated the effect of fenoterol and ipratropium single and in combination and showed no differences among the three treatments [18].

Methylxanthines such as theophylline are sometimes used in the management of acute exacerbations of COPD. There is some evidence that theophyllines are useful in COPD, though the main limiting factor is the frequency of toxic side effects. The therapeutic action of theophylline is thought to be due to its inhibition of phosphodiesterase, which breaks down cyclic AMP, an intracellular messenger, thus facilitating bronchodilatation, though further studies are required on this point. However, studies of intravenous aminophylline therapy in acute exacerbations of COPD have shown no significant beneficial effect over and above conventional therapy, though the studies reported have been relatively small and performed some years ago [19,20]. In addition, the main outcome was changes in FEV_1 at exacerbation, which we now know can be relatively small, and exacerbations were variably defined. Larger well-designed studies are now required of the role of intravenous aminophylline in COPD patients with severe exacerbations who are hospitalized. When aminophylline is administered, care must be taken so that the appropriate dose is provided to obtain serum levels not to exceed 15 mg/dL, because the therapeutic threshold is very close to that associated with significant toxicity.

B. Corticosteroids

Oral corticosteroids are widely used for COPD exacerbation, and the requirement for corticosteroids for exacerbation has been regarded as a marker of exacerbation severity. Only about 10–15% of patients with stable COPD show an FEV_1 response to oral corticosteroids [21] and, unlike the situation in asthma, steroids have variable effect on airway inflammatory markers in patients with COPD [22,23]. Thus there was previously some skepticism about their role in exacerbations, but there is now evidence from randomized controlled trials of their beneficial role in acute situations [24–29].

A number of early studies have investigated the effects of corticosteroid therapy for COPD exacerbation. In an early controlled trial in patients with COPD exacerbations and acute respiratory failure, Albert and coworkers found that there were larger improvements in pre- and postbronchodilator FEV_1 when patients were treated for the first 3 days of the hospital admission with intravenous methylprednislone than in those treated with placebo [24]. Another trial found that a single dose of methylprednisolone given within 30 min of arrival in the accident and emergency department produced no improvement after 5 hr in spirometry, and also had no effect on hospital admission, though another study showed reduced readmissions [25,26]. In a study by Thompson and colleagues, a 9-day course of prednisolone or placebo was randomly prescribed to outpatients presenting with acute exacerbations of COPD [27]. Unlike the previous studies, these patients were either recruited from outpatients or from a group who were preenrolled and who self-reported the exacerbation to the study team. In this study, patients with exacerbations associated with acidosis or pneumonia were excluded, so exacerbations of moderate severity were generally included. Patients in the steroid-treated group showed a more rapid improvement in PaO_2, alveolar-arterial oxygen gradient, FEV_1, and peak expiratory flow rate. There was a trend toward a more rapid improvement in dyspnea in the steroid-treated group.

In a recent cohort study by Seemungal and colleagues, the effect of therapy with prednisolone on COPD exacerbations diagnosed and treated in the community was studied, though this particular study did not set out to evaluate the role of steroids in exacerbations and the study was not controlled [9]. Exacerbations treated with steroids were more severe and associated with larger falls in peak flow rate. The treated exacerbations also had a longer recovery time to baseline for symptoms and peak flow rate. However, the rate of peak flow rate recovery was faster in the prednisolone-treated group, though not the rate of symptom score recovery. Another interesting finding in this study was that steroids significantly prolonged the median time from the day of onset of the initial exacerbation to the next exacerbation, from 60 days in the group not treated with prednisolone to 84 days in the patients treated with prednisolone. In contrast, antibiotic therapy had no effect on the time to the next exacerbation. If short-course oral steroid therapy at exacerbation does prolong the time to the next exacerbation, then this could be an important way to reduce exacerbation frequency in COPD patients [9].

Davies and colleagues randomized patients admitted to hospital with COPD exacerbations to prednisolone or placebo [28]. In the prednisolone group, the FEV_1 rose faster until day 5, when a plateau was observed in the steroid-treated group (Fig. 1). Changes in the prebronchodilator and postbronchodilator FEV_1 were similar, suggesting that this is not just an effect on bronchomotor tone, but involves faster resolution of airway inflammatory changes or airway wall edema with exacerbation. Analysis of length of hospital stay showed that patients treated with prednisolone had a significantly shorter length of stay. Six weeks later, there were no differences in spirometry between the patient groups, and health status was similar to that measured at 5 days after admission. Thus the benefits of steroid therapy at exacerbation are most obvious during the early period of the exacerbation. A similar proportion of the patients, approximately 32% in both study groups, required further treatment for exacerbations within 6 weeks of follow-up, emphasizing the high exacerbation relapse rate in these patients.

In another randomized study, Niewoehner and colleagues performed a controlled trial of either a 2-week or an 8-week intravenous methyl prednisolone course at exacerbation compared to placebo, in addition to other exacerbation therapy [29]. The primary endpoint was a first treatment fail-

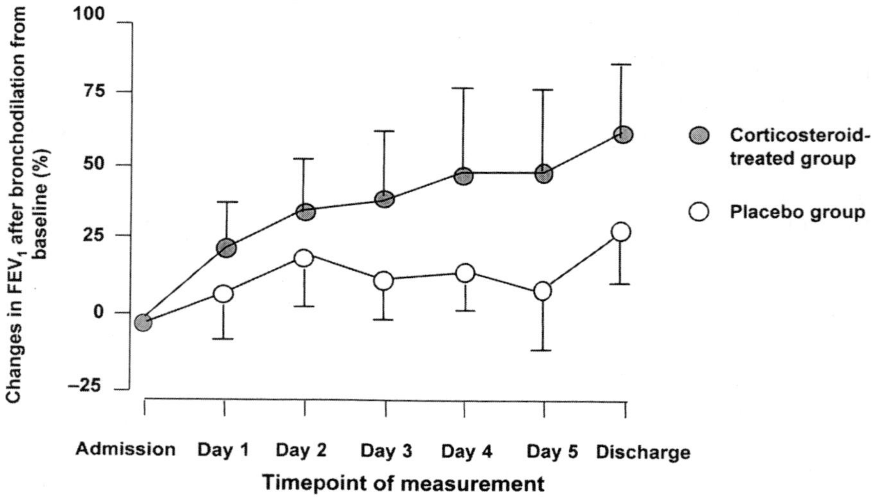

Figure 1 Change in lung function at COPD exacerbation after treatment with corticosteroid or placebo. (Reproduced from Ref. 28, with permission.)

ure, including death, need for intubation, readmission, or intensification of therapy. There was no difference in the results using the 2- or 8-week treatment protocol. The rates of treatment failure were higher in the placebo group at 30 days, compared to the combined 2- and 8-week prednislone groups. As in the study by Davies and colleagues, FEV_1 improved faster in the prednisolone-treated group, though there were no differences by 2 weeks. Niewoehner and colleagues performed a detailed evaluation of steroid complications and found considerable evidence of hyperglycemia in the steroid-treated patients, which it is likely was due to the higher steroid doses used. Thus steroids should be used at COPD exacerbation in short courses of no more than 2 weeks' duration to avoid risk of complications.

C. Antibiotics

Acute exacerbations of COPD often present with increased sputum purulence and volume, and antibiotics have traditionally been used as first-line therapy in such exacerbations. However, viral infections may be the triggers in a significant proportion of acute infective exacerbations in COPD, and antibiotics used for the consequences of secondary infection. The other problem in the use of antibiotics is that bacteria are found in the airways of COPD patients, not only at exacerbation but also when they are stable. This airway bacterial colonisation has been found in approximately 30% of COPD patients, and colonisation has been shown to be related to the degree of airflow obstruction and current cigarette smoking status [30]. Although bacteria such as *Haemophilus influenzae* and *Streptococcus pneumoniae* have been associated with COPD exacerbation, some studies have shown increasing bacterial counts during exacerbation, while others have not confirmed these findings [31,32]. Hill and colleagues, in a larger study, showed that the airway bacterial load was related to inflammatory markers [33], and Patel and colleagues have shown that colonization is related to exacerbation frequency [34]. To date, however, there have been no recent studies evaluating the effect of bacterial eradication with long-term antibiotics on exacerbation frequency and airway inflammation. Recently, a study has suggested that isolation of a new bacterial strain was associated with an increased risk of an exacerbation, though this does not prove conclusively that bacteria are direct causes of exacerbations [35].

A study investigating the benefit of antibiotics in over 300 acute exacerbations demonstrated a greater treatment success rate in patients treated with antibiotics, especially if their initial presentation was with symptoms of increased dyspnoea, sputum volume, and purulence [3]. Patients with mild COPD obtained less benefit from antibiotic therapy. A randomized placebo-controlled study investigating the value of antibiotics in patients with mild obstructive lung disease in the community concluded that antibiotic therapy did not accelerate recovery or reduce the number of relapses [36]. A meta-analysis of trials of antibiotic therapy in COPD identified only nine studies of significant duration and concluded that antibiotic therapy offered a small but significant benefit in outcome in acute exacerbations [37]. Thus the advice is given that antibiotics are indicated in COPD exacerbations when the exacerbation is associated with cough and sputum production. However, with the future introduction of novel antibiotics with a more specific activity profile against airway bacteria, the effects of antibiotics may be greater at COPD exacerbation.

V. Prevention of COPD Exacerbation

One of the most important goals of therapy for COPD is the need to prevent exacerbations, as any therapy that can prevent exacerbations will have important health economic benefits and improve health status.

As upper respiratory tract infections are common factors in causing exacerbation, influenza and pneumococcal vaccinations are recommended for all patients with significant COPD. A study that reviewed the outcome of influenza vaccination in a cohort of elderly patients with chronic lung disease found that influenza vaccination is associated with significant health benefits, with fewer outpatient visits, fewer hospitalisations, and a reduced mortality [38]. Long-term antibiotic therapy has been used in patients with very frequent exacerbations, though there is little evidence of effectiveness. There has been one report of the effects of an immunostimulatory agent in patients with COPD exacerbations, with reduction in severe complications and hospital admissions in the actively treated group [39]. However, there has been no recent progress with such interventions, and further study is required of the immunological mechanisms of exacerbations before the role of these agents in COPD can be defined.

The use of mucolytic agents in COPD is controverial, though their use worldwide is very variable, with little use in the UK and Australia and more prescriptions written in Europe. A recent meta-analysis was published that assessed the effects of oral mucolytics in COPD [40]. A total of 23 randomized controlled trials were identified, and the main outcome was that there was a 29% reduction in exacerbations with mucolytic therapy. The number of patients who had no exacerbations was greater in the mucolytic group, and days of illness were also reduced, though there was no effect on lung function. The drug that contributed most to the beneficial results in the review was N-acetylcysteine, though the mechanism of action of N-acetylcysteine is not entirely clear and it may act through a combination of mucolytic and antioxidative effects. Further large studies on the effects of antioxidants are in progress, and the results will be available in the next few years.

As exacerbations are associated with increased airway inflammation, there has been much interest in the use of inhaled steroids to reduce exacerbation frequency. In the ISOLDE study, in which COPD patients with moderate to severe COPD were treated with the inhaled steroid fluticasone for a period of 3 years, a reduction in exacerbation frequency of around 25% was found [41]. This study also found that inhaled steroid significantly slowed the deterioration in quality-of-life scores that occurs over time in patients with the disease. However, the overall exacerbation frequency was relatively low in that study, and this was probably due to a retrospective assessment of exacerbation [41]. The effect of inhaled steroids was greater in patients with more impaired lung function, suggesting that this is the group most likely to benefit from long-term inhaled steroid therapy. In the Lung Health Study, the group treated with the inhaled steroid triamcinolone had significantly fewer visits to a physician due to respiratory illness, suggesting that triamcinolone reduced exacerbations [42]. Another, earlier study by Paggiaro and colleagues suggested that the severity of exacerbations may be reduced with inhaled steroid therapy, though again the exacerbation frequency in that study was relatively small [43]. An observational study from the ISOLDE multicenter study showed that exacerbations were increased following withdrawal of inhaled steroids during the run in to the major study, though the inhaled steroid withdrawal was not placebo controlled [44].

A number of recent studies have also shown that small reductions in exacerbations can be achieved with bronchodilator therapy, though both studies involved relatively short periods of therapy of 12 weeks [45–48]. Mahler and colleagues found that the time to the first exacerbation was longer with therapy with the long-acting β-agonist salmeterol, though the overall number of exacerbations during the study was relatively small [45]. In another study comparing salmeterol to ipratropium and placebo over a 12-week period, there was no difference in the effect of either treatment arm on exacerbation frequency [46]. Van Noord and colleagues, in a similar study, suggested that the combination of salmeterol and ipratropium was most effective in reducing of exacerbation [47]. Rossi and colleagues compared over 12 months two different dosages of the inhaled bronchodilator formoterol with placebo or theophylline in a randomized double-blind study [48]. Formoterol reduced the number of hospitalizations, and thus severe exacerbations, compared to placebo, and also significantly reduced the number of "bad days" compared to placebo or treatment with theophylline [48].

Recently, in a randomized trial, the new long-acting anticholinergic agent tiotropium was compared to ipratropium. Over 1 year, treatment with tioropium reduced exacerbations by 24% compared to ipratropium [49].

a)

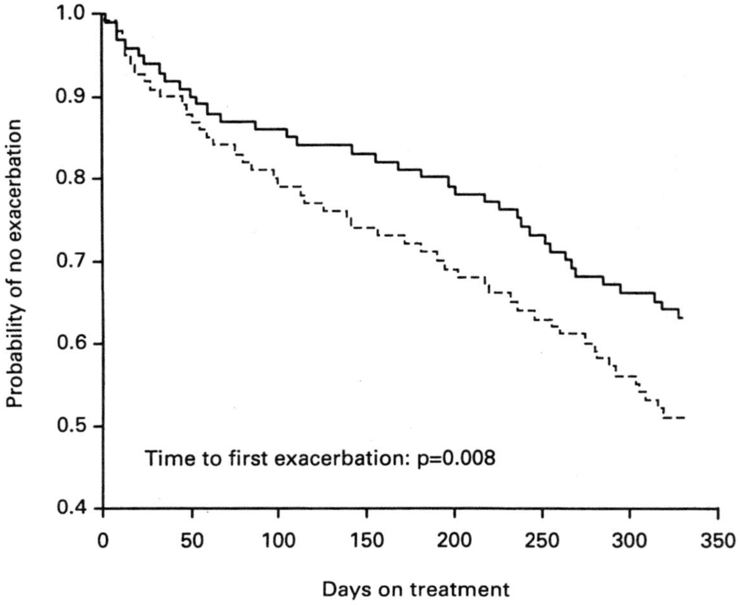
Probability of no exacerbation
1.0
0.9
0.8
0.7
0.6
0.5
0.4
Time to first exacerbation: p=0.008
0
50
100
150
200
250
300
350
Days on treatment

b)

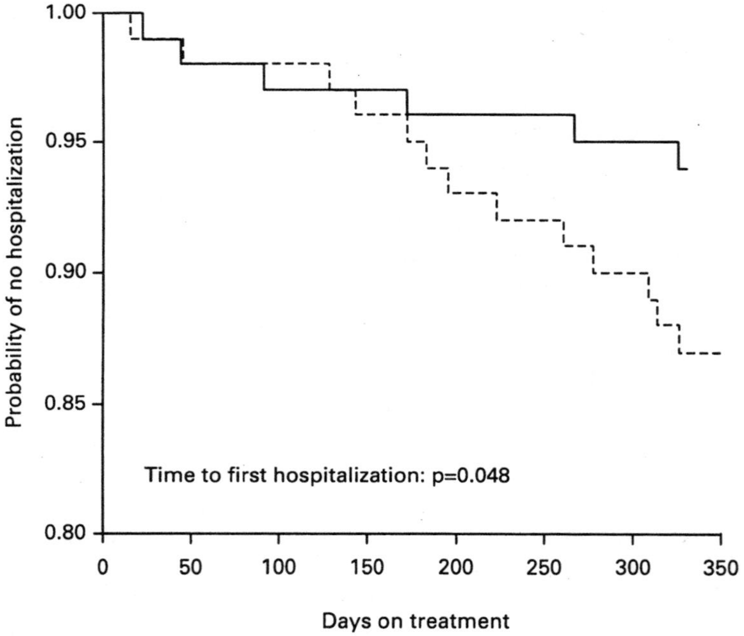
Probability of no hospitalization
1.00
0.95
0.90
0.85
0.80
Time to first hospitalization: p=0.048
0
50
100
150
200
250
300
350
Days on treatment

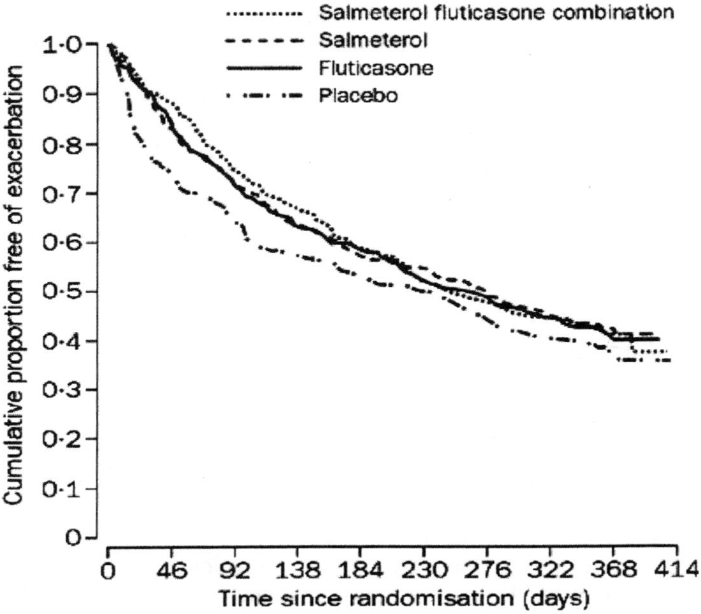

Figure 3 Cumulatve risk of acute exacerbations for the four treatment groups. (Reproduced from Ref. 50, with permission.)

There was also an increased time to the next exacerbation and increased time to first hospitalization (Fig. 2). It is interesting that both long-acting β-agonists and long-acting anticholinergic agents all have some effect on reducing exacerbation frequency and probably also reduce exacerbation severity. Calverley and colleagues have recently reported a 12-month randomized study of the effect of inhaled fluticasone, salmeterol, or the combination compared to placebo [50]. All the active treatments reduced exacerbation frequency compared to placebo and the number of exacerbations that required therapy with oral corticosteroids. Patients with more severe COPD (i.e., FEV_1 less than 50% predicted) showed a greater effect of the active

---

Figure 2 Kaplan-Meier estimates for the probability of (a) no exacerbation, p = 0.008 for time to first exacerbation, and (b) no hospitalization, p = 0.048 for time to first hospitalization due to a COPD exacerbation for the tiotropium (———) and ipratropium (– – – –) groups during the 1-year study. (Reproduced from Ref. 49, with permission.)

treatments on exacerbations than patients with an FEV_1 above 50% predicted. Figure 3 shows the cumulative risk of exacerbations in the placebo and active treatment groups.

Further large controlled studies performed over a longer period of time, e.g., 3–5 years, are required to evaluate exacerbation frequency as the primary outcome. These studies will need to evaluate the effect of inhaled long-acting bronchodilators and corticossteroids, alone and in combination, on exacerbation frequency and severity, and also they will need to compare the outcome of these various pharmacological interventions.

VI. Conclusion

COPD exacerbations are an important cause of morbidity, health-related quality of life, and mortality in COPD. Exacerbations also have significant health economic consequences and affect disease progression and thus deserve attention. Oral corticosteroids are effective in hastening recovery from moderate to severe exacerbations, though antibiotics have been shown to be effective only in exacerbations with sputum purulence or increased sputum volume. Newer antibiotics may be found to be more effective at exacerbation. Pharmacological interventions to reduce exacerbation frequency urgently need to be developed and evaluated further in well-designed and adequately powered randomized controlled trials. The aim of therapy is to reduce significantly the morbidity associated with COPD exacerbations and improve the quality of life of our patients with this disabling condition.

References

1. Fletcher CM, Peto R, Tinker CM, Speizer FE. Natural History of Chronic Bronchitis and Emphysema. Oxford, UK: Oxford University Press, 1976.
2. Seemungal TA, Donaldson GC, Paul EA, Bestall JC, Jeffries DJ, Wedzicha JA. Effect of exacerbation on quality of life in patients with chronic obstructive pulmonary disease. Am J Respir Crit Care Med 1998; 151:1418–1422.
3. Anthonisen NR, Manfreda J, Warren CPW, Hershfield ES, Harding GKM, Nelson NA. Antibiotic therapy in exacerbations of chronic obstructive pulmonary disease. Ann Intern Med 1987; 106:196–220.
4. Rodriguez-Roisin R. Towards a consesnus definition for COPD exacerbations. Chest 2000; 117:398S–401S.
5. Bhowmik A, Seemungal TAR, Sapsford RJ, Wedzicha JA. Relation of sputum inflammatory markers to symptoms and physiological changes at COPD exacerbations. Thorax 2000; 55:114–200.
6. Seemungal TAR, Harper-Owen R, Bhowmik A, Moric I, Sanderson G, Mes-

sage S, MacCallum P, Meade TW, Jeffries DJ, Johnston SL, Wedzicha JA. Respiratory viruses, symptoms and inflammatory markers in acute exacerbations and stable chronic obstructive pulmonary disease. Am J Respir Crit Care Med 2001; 164:1618–1623.
7. Anderson HR, Limb ES, Bland JM, Ponce de Leon A, Strachan DP, Bower JS. Health effects of an air pollution episode in London, December 1991. Thorax 1995; 50:1188–1193.
8. Donaldson GC, Seemungal T, Jeffries DJ, Wedzicha JA. Effect of environmental temperature on symptoms, lung function and mortality in COPD patients. Eur Respir J 1999; 13:844–849.
9. Seemungal TAR, Donaldson GC, Bhowmik A, Jeffries DJ, Wedzicha JA. Time course and recovery of exacerbations in patients with chronic obstructive pulmonary disease. Am J Respir Crit Care Med 2000; 161:1608–1613.
10. Ball P, Harris JM, Lowson D, Tillotson G, Wilson R. Acute infective exacerbations of chronic bronchitis. Q J Med 1995; 88:61–68.
11. Kanner RE, Anthonisen NR, Connett JE. Lower respiratory illnesses promote FEV1 decline in current smokers but not ex-smokers with mild chronic obstructive lung disease: results from the Lung Health Study. Am J Respir Crit Care Med 2001; 164:358–364.
12. Donaldson GC, Seemungal TAR, Bhowmik A, Wedzicha JA. The relationship between exacerbation frequency and lung function decline in chronic obstructive pulmonary disease. Thorax 2002; 57:847–852.
13. Belman MJ, Botnick WC, Shin JW. Inhaled bronchodilators reduce dynamic hyperinflation during exercise in patients with chronic obstructive pulmonary disease. Am J Respir Crit Care Med 1996; 153:967–975.
14. Combivent Inhalation Aerosol Study GroupIn chronic obstructive pulmonary disease, a combination of ipratropium and albuterol is more effective than either agent alone. Chest 1994; 105:1411–1419.
15. Moayyedi P, Congleton J, Page RL, Pearson SB, Muers MF. Comparison of nebulised salbutamol and ipratropium bromide with salbutamol alone in the treatment of chronic obstructive pulmonary disease. Thorax 1995; 50:834–837.
16. Karpel JP, Pesin J, Greenberg D, Gentry E. A comparison of the effects of ipratropium bromide and etaproterenol sulfate in acute exacerbations of COPD. Chest 1990; 98:835–839.
17. O'Driscoll BR, Taylor RJ, Horsley MG, Chambers DK, Bernstein A. Nebulized salbutamol with and without ipratropium bromide in acute airflow obstruction. Lancet 1989; 1418–1420.
18. Rebuck AS, Chapman KR, Abboud R, et al. Nebulized anticholinergic and sympathomimetic treatment of asthma and chronic obstructive airways disease in the emergency room. Am J Med 1987; 82:59–64.
19. Rice KL, Leatherman JW, Duane PG, Snyder LS, Harmon KR, Abel J, Niewoehner DE. Aminophylline for acute exacerbations of chronic obstructive pulmonary disease. A controlled trial. Ann Intern Med 1987; 107:305–309.
20. Barr RG, Rowe BH, Camargo CA. Methyxanthines for Exacerbations of COPD (Cochrane Review). Oxford, UK: The Cochrane Library, 2002:3.

21. Callahan CM, Cittus RS, Katz BP. Oral corticosteroid therapy for patients with stable chronic obstructive pulmonary disease: a meta-analysis. Ann Intern Med 1991; 114:216–223.
22. Keatings VM, Jatakanon A, Worsdell Y, Barnes PJ. Effects of inhaled and oral glucocorticoids on inflammatory indices in asthma and COPD. Am J Respir Crit Care Med 1997; 155:542–548.
23. Culpitt SV, Maziak W, Loukidis S, et al. Effects of high dose inhaled steroids on cells, cytokines and proteases in induced sputum in chronic obstructive pulmonary disease. Am J Respir Crit Care Med 1999; 160:1635–1639.
24. Albert RK, Martin TR, Lewis SW. Controlled clinical trial of methylprednisolone in patients with chronic bronchitis and acute respiratory insufficiency. Ann Intern Med 1980; 92:753–758.
25. Emerman CL, Connors AF, Lukens TW, May ME, Effron D. A randomised controlled trial of methylprednisolone in the emergency treatment of acute exacerbations of chronic obstructive pulmonary disease. Chest 1989; 95:563–567.
26. Bullard MJ, Liaw SJ, Tsai YH, Min HP. Early corticosteroid use in acute exacerbations of chronic airflow limitation. Am J Emerg Med 1996; 14:139–143.
27. Thompson WH, Nielson CP, Carvalho P, et al. Controlled trial of oral prednisolone in outpatients with acute COPD exacerbation. Am J Respir Crit Care Med 1996; 154:407–412.
28. Davies L, Angus RM, Calverley PMA. Oral corticosteroids in patients admitted to hospital with exacerbations of chronic obstructive pulmonary disease: a prospective randomised controlled trial. Lancet 1999; 354:456–460.
29. Niewoehner DE, Erbland ML, Deupree RH, et al. Effect of systemic glucocorticoids on exacerbations of chronic obstuctive pulmonary disease. N Engl J Med 1999; 340:1941–1947.
30. Zalacain R, Sobradillo V, Amilibia J, et al. Predisposing factors to bacterial colonization in chronic obstructive pulmonary disease. Eur Respir J 1999; 13:343–348.
31. Monso E, Rosell A, Bonet G, et al. Risk factors for lower airway bacterial colonization in chronic bronchitis. Eur Respir J 1999; 13:338–342.
32. Wilson R. Bacterial infection and chronic obstructive pulmonary disease. Eur Respir J 1999; 13:233–235.
33. Hill AT, Campbell EJ, Hill SL, Bayley DL, Stockley RA. Association between airway bacterial load and markers of airway inflammation in patients with chronic bronchitis. Am J Med 2000; 109:288–295.
34. Patel IS, Seemungal TAR, Wilks M, Lloyd Owen S, Donaldson GC, Wedzicha JA. Relationship between bacterial colonisation and the frequency, character and severity of COPD exacerbations. Thorax 2002; 57:759–764.
35. Sethi S, Evans N, Grant BJB, Murphy TF. New strains of bacteria and exacerbations of chronic obstructive pulmonary disease. N Engl J Med 2002; 347:465–471.
36. Sachs APE, Koeter GH, Groenier KH, Van der Waaij D, Schiphuis J, Meyboom-de Jong B. Changes in symptoms, peak expiratory flow and sputum flora

during treatment with antibiotics of exacerbations in patients with chronic obstructive pulmonary disease in general practice. Thorax 1995; 50:758–763.
37. Saint S, Bent S, Vittinghoff E, Grady D. Antibiotics in chronic obstructive pulmonary disease exacerbations. A meta-analysis. JAMA 1995; 273:957–960.
38. Nichol KL, Baken L, Nelson A. Relation between influenza vaccination and out patient visits, hospitalisation and mortality in elderly patients with chronic lung disease. Ann Intern Med 1999; 130:397–403.
39. Collet JP, Shapiro S, Ernst P, et al. Effect of an immunostimulating agent on acute exacerbations and hospitalization in COPD patients. Am J Respir Crit Care Med 1997; 156:1719–1724.
40. Poole PJ, Black PN. Oral mucolytic drugs for exacerbations of chronic obstructive pulmonary disease:systematic review. Br Med J 2001; 322:1271–1274.
41. Burge PS, Calverley PMA, Jones PW, et al. Randomised, double blind, placebo controlled study of fluticasone propionate in patients with moderate to sever chronic obstructive pulmonary disease: the ISOLDE trial. Br Med J 2000; 320:1297–1303.
42. The Lung Health Study Research GroupEffect of inhaled triamcinolone on the decline in pulmonary function in chronic obstructive pulmonary disease. N Engl J Med 2000; 343:1902–1909.
43. Paggiaro PL, Dahle R, Bakran I, Frith L, Hollingworth K, Efthimiou J. Multicentre randomised placebo-controlled trial of inhaled fluticasone propionate in patients with chronic obstructive pulmonary disease. Lancet 1998; 351:773–780.
44. Jarad N, Wedzicha JA, Burge PS, Calverley PMA. An observational study of inhaled corticosteroid withdrawal in patients with stable chronic obstructive pulmonary disease. Respir Med 1999; 93:161–166.
45. Mahler DA, Donohue JF, Barbee RA, et al. Efficacy of salmeterol xinafoate in the treatment of COPD. Chest 1999; 115:957–965.
46. Rennard S, Anderson W, ZuWallack R, et al. Use of long-acting inhaled beta2 adrenergic agonist salmeterol xinafoate in patients with COPD. Am J Respir Crit Care Med 2001; 163–169.
47. Van Noord JA, de Munck DRAJ, Bantje ThA, et al. Long-term treatment of chronic obstructive pulmonary disease with salmeterol and the additive effect of ipratropium. Eur Respir J 2000; 15:878–885.
48. Rossi A, Kristufek P, Levine B, et al. Comparison of the efficacy, tolerability and safety of formoterol dry powder and oral slow-release theophylline in treatment of COPD. Chest 2002; 121:1058–1069.
49. Vincken W, van Noord JA, Greefhorst APM. Improved health outcomes in patients with COPD during 1 year treatment with tiotropium. Eur Respir J 2002; 19:209–216.
50. Calverley P, Pauwels R, Vestbo J, et al. Combined salmeterol and fluticasone in the treatment of chronic obstructive pulmonary disease: a randomised controlled trial. Lancet 2003; 361:449–456.

10

Health Status Measurement in COPD

PAUL W. JONES

St. George's Hospital Medical School
London, England

I. Introduction: The Multifactorial Nature of COPD

Chronic obstructive pulmonary disease (COPD) is a multisystem disorder with its primary effects in the lungs but with significant functional consequences in other systems. Even in the lungs there are a number of different pathophysiological processes, each of which may be present to a varying degree. Breathlessness is the characteristic symptom of COPD. It is associated with inspiration and has a complex etiology that is linked to the work of breathing [1]. With increasing lung volume a greater respiratory effort is needed to maintain tidal breathing. Bronchodilator-induced reductions in breathlessness at rest have been shown to correlate better with changes in forced inspiratory flow than with changes in forced expiratory volume (FEV_1) [2]. Static lung volumes are increased in COPD, although this is only moderately correlated with worsening expiratory airflow limitation [3], There is a further rise in functional residual capacity at exercise onset, otherwise known as dynamic hyperinflation. The reduction in breathlessness during exercise following bronchodilators correlates better with improvement in inspiratory capacity during exercise than improvement in FEV_1 [4,5].

Leg fatigue is as important as breathlessness in limiting peak exercise performance in some patients [6]. Patients rate it to be a more important problem than breathlessness, although they do not indicate its importance unless asked about it directly [7]. Muscle weakness is a feature of COPD, particularly of the legs [8], but also the arms [9]. This may not be due entirely to disuse atrophy, since nutritional depletion also occurs [10] and there is evidence of circulating inflammatory cytokines in COPD [11]. COPD also causes functional disturbances other than impaired exercise tolerance and decreased mobility. In particular, sleep disturbance appears to be a common feature. A recent survey carried out by the British Lung Foundation found that half of the respondents had regular sleep disturbance. Disorders of mood state occur in COPD [12], although this may be confined to subgroups within a COPD population who appear to have especially high scores for anxiety and depression [13]. Exacerbations are an important feature of COPD and their frequency increases with disease severity [14], although patients appear to underreport exacerbations [15]. In patients with moderate–severe COPD, prospective data collection with diary cards revealed a median exacerbation rate of 3 per year with a range of 1–8 per year [15]. Lung function can take several weeks to recover following an exacerbation [16], so exacerbation frequency is clearly an important factor in this disease.

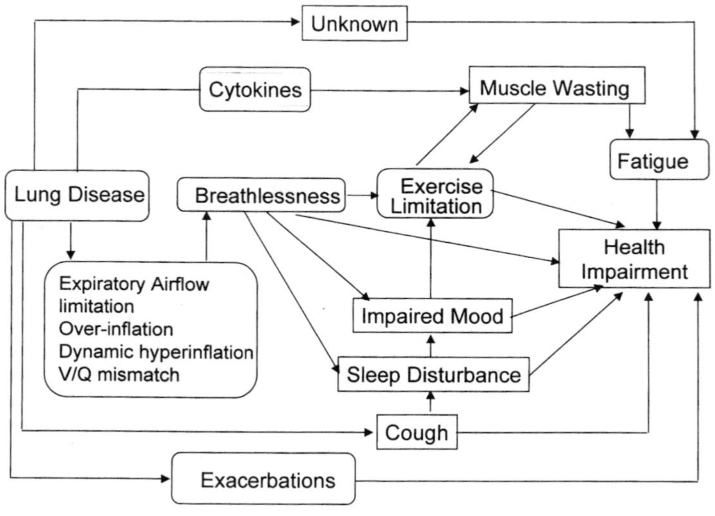

Figure 1 Some of the pathways between lung disease and impaired health.

II. Measuring the Overall Effect of Treatment

It is clear that there are multiple pathways by which COPD can result in impaired health (Fig. 1). This means that there are also multiple points at which pharmacological agents may have an effect. None of these effects may be very large, but they may be cumulative, particularly since they could have an impact of a number of different pathways. For example, long-acting bronchodilators may improve lung function, reduce breathlessness during exercise, improve sleep, and reduce the frequency of exacerbations. There is no single or composite summary measure of impaired lung function, although the FEV_1 has provided this function in the absence of anything better. Exercise performance is the best overall measure of physiological dysfunction, but does not reflect sleep disturbance, the effect of exacerbations, or any effect on mood state. There is clearly a need for a measure that can aggregate into a single score the summed effect of the multiple pathophysiological processes that involve different organs and different systems. This is the role of health status measurement—to provide a comprehensive estimate of the primary and secondary effects of the disease.

III. Health Status Questionnaires

There are a number of instruments that may be described as COPD-specific health status questionnaires. These include the Chronic Respiratory Questionnaire (CRQ) [17], the St George's Hospital Questionnaire (SGRQ), which is for both asthma and COPD [18], and the QOL-RIQ [19]. There are also two functions limitation questionnaires that are similar in many respects to health status instruments: the modified Pulmonary Functional Status and Dyspnea Questionnaire (PFSDQ-M) [20] and the Pulmonary Functional Status Scale (PFSS) [21]. These questionnaires all have a degree of complexity that makes them rather unsuitable for routine use. Simpler questionnaires include the Breathing Problems Questionnaire (BPQ) [22,23], and AQ20, which is a 20-item instrument that takes 2–3 min to complete and score. This questionnaire is suitable for both asthma [24] and COPD [25,26]. A UK study concluded that the BPQ provided more valid assessments of health status than the CRQ [27], although a Japanese group reached the opposite conclusion—that the CRQ and SGRQ discriminated between patients with different degrees of severity better than the BPQ [28]. In terms of responsiveness, there is one report that the BPQ was not as sensitive as the CRQ in detecting change following a pulmonary rehabilitation program [29]. The other short questionnaire (the AQ20) appeared to discriminate between patients as well as the CRQ and SGRQ and also to be responsive to changes following pulmonary rehabilitation [25].

A. Disease Factors Associated with Impaired Health

There is now a large body of data to show that health status scores are significantly associated with abnormalities in a wide range of markers of impaired health, although it is inappropriate to expect high correlations with any specific aspect of COPD, since the questionnaires are designed to address a wide range of different effects of the disease. Poorer health status is correlated with impaired exercise performance [13,18,30,31] and breathless-induced disability in daily life [18,30,32,33]. The presence of daily symptoms [18] and a high exacerbation frequency are other important factors [15]. Emotional factors have been shown to be important and common in COPD patients [7], so it is not surprising that anxiety and depression are quite consistent correlates of impaired health [18,30,31]. A number of factors may have interactive effects on health status. For example, COPD patients with a low lean body mass had much worse SGRQ scores than those in whom it was normal [34]. This association appeared to be attributable to an increase in breathlessness—i.e., patients with a low mean body mass having worse health because of higher levels of dyspnea. However, in another study, impaired health status in patients with low free fat mass could not be explained just in terms of breathlessness [35]. In patients with chronic hypoxia, arterial oxygen tension is correlated with health status [30,36].

There is a degree of intercorrelation between factors that determine health status impairment. Within the limits of what is measurable in the same population of patients, multivariate analysis has shown that 50% of the SGRQ Total score could be attributed to a combination of cough, wheeze, MRC Dyspnoea Grade, 6-min walking distance, and anxiety score (each as statistically significant covariates) [18]. Thus it appears that health status questionnaires can bring together a range of effects of COPD into one summary measure of the overall impact of the disease—which is their primary purpose.

B. Mortality and Health Status

Two recent studies in male COPD patients, one in Spain [37], the other in Japan [38], have shown that health status measured using the SGRQ was a predictor of mortality. This was not observed with the CRQ, however [38]. The association between SGRQ score and mortality was independent of the effect of age, FEV_1, and BMI on mortality [37].

C. FEV_1 and Health Status

FEV_1 and health status scores are correlated, but only weakly [13,18,30,31, 36,39,40]. A typical example is shown in Fig. 2. There is a significant cor-

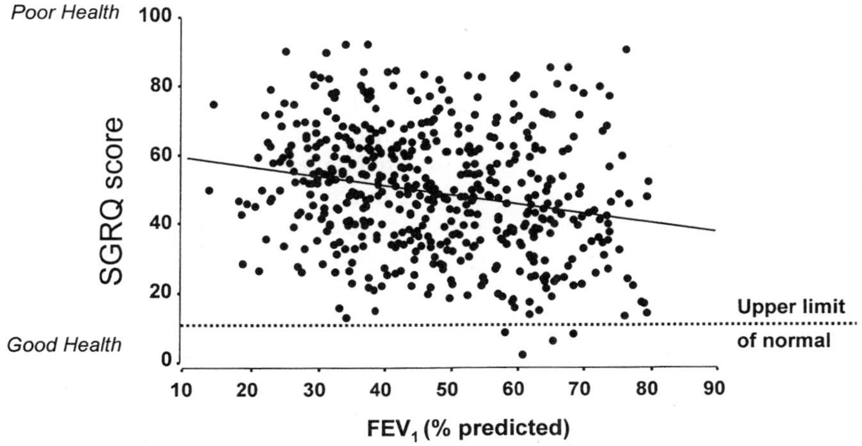

Figure 2 Correlation between SGRQ score and postbronchodilator FEV_1, $r = 0.23$, $p < 0.0001$. Note: A high SGRQ score indicates poor health. Many patients with relatively mild airflow limitation may have very poor health. Most of those patients will report breathlessness on walking up a slight hill or on stairs.

relation between lower FEV_1 and worse health, but the regression line is rather flat. Many patients may have impaired health despite having only moderate airway obstruction, although there are also some with severe obstruction who appear to have little disturbance to their daily lives. The weak correlation between FEV_1 and level of symptoms and their effect on patients' daily life and health has important implications for clinical practice, since assessments based solely on lung spirometry will be inadequate, even in routine practice.

D. Assessment of Patients with COPD

Questionnaires such as the CRQ and SGRQ are too long and complex to be used in routine practice, and an alternative would be to use one of the shorter questionnaires such as the BPQ or AQ20. The five-point MRC Dyspnoea scale is even easier to use and provides a reliable and simple method of assessing disability due to breathlessness [33]. In practice it is very easy to identify COPD patients with poor health, since most of them who have an SGRQ score > 40 will report breathlessness on walking up one flight of stairs or on slight hills. This simple assessment, coupled with FEV_1 measurement and a record of the frequency of exacerbations, will provide a very good and comprehensive assessment of a patient with COPD.

IV. Thresholds for Clinical Significance

One of the most useful aspects of health status measurement is the identification of a score that is described variously as a "threshold for clinical significance," "minimum important difference," "minimum clinically important difference," etc. These terms are used to convey the concept that there is a particular health status score or change in score that indicates a clinically significant boundary. Methods of assessing these thresholds are complex and are discussed in depth elsewhere [41]. For any given questionnaire, the threshold value appears to be consistent across the different methods of estimation. With the CRQ, the minimum clinically important difference appears to be 0.5, for all four components of that instrument [42]. The corresponding value for the SGRQ is 4 units for both the Total and Impacts scores [43]. No estimate has been calculated for the Symptoms and Activity components. In a recent study, a 4-unit difference in SGRQ score was associated with a 5.1% increased risk of all-cause mortality and a 12.9% increase in risk of respiratory-related mortality after 3 years [37].

These thresholds are average values that have been estimated in populations of patients. As a result, they can be applied only to groups of patients, because health status questionnaires treat each patient as if he or she were an average patient. As a result, the clinically significant threshold or minimum important difference applies only to the "average" or "typical" patient. For this reason it is inappropriate to use a 4-point change in SGRQ score or a 0.5-unit change in CRQ score to indicate whether an individual patient had a worthwhile response to therapy. One final point to bear in mind is the fact that any estimate of one of these thresholds is an average calculated from measurements made in many patients. Thus there is both sampling and measurement error. It is a mistake to think of these estimates as being absolutely precise. Rather, they should be considered as indicative values. This issue is discussed in greater depth elsewhere [41].

V. Health Status Changes Following Treatment

Following treatment for COPD, both FEV_1 and health status scores improve, but the correlation is weak [44]. Furthermore FEV_1 data may be misleading in terms of the health gain associated with treatment. In a 16-week study that compared two doses of salmeterol with placebo in COPD, the improvement in FEV_1 was similar with both doses of the drug ($\approx$110 mL) [44]. In the patients given salmeterol 50 μg twice daily (i.e., the standard dose), the SGRQ total score improved by a clinically and statistically significant amount. Clearly, in those patients, the improvement in FEV_1 was associated with a worthwhile symptomatic improvement. By contrast, patients given salmeterol 100 μg twice daily experienced neither a clinically nor a statistically significant improvement in SGRQ, despite having an improvement in FEV_1 of the same size as that obtained with the lower dose. This lack of symptomatic benefit appears to have been due to side effects [1]. A similar finding has now been made with formoterol in COPD [44]. This is an important observation, since physicians are often tempted to increase drug doses in the face of a poor response or to get an even better effect. The use of direct measurements of health status has shown that such an approach with long-acting β-blockers may lead to a loss of any benefit, rather than additional gain.

Another example of the value of health status measurement is the ability to compare the overall efficacy of two drugs of the same class, but with different durations of action. The long-acting bronchodilator tiotropium produces a similar peak daytime effect on FEV_1 its older short-acting analog ipratropium given 4 times daily, although with less variation during the day. However, the biggest benefit was seen in the trough measurement of FEV_1 made in the morning [46]. This effect appears to be fully established over the first week of treatment and then changes very little over 1 year of follow-up. By contrast, the pattern of changes in health status over a 1-year period are very interesting (Fig. 3). Both the short- and long-acting treatments produced similar small improvements by 1 week, but thereafter they diverged. There was only a very modest further improvement in ipratropium-treated patients, but the patients who received tiotropium continued to improve for up to 6

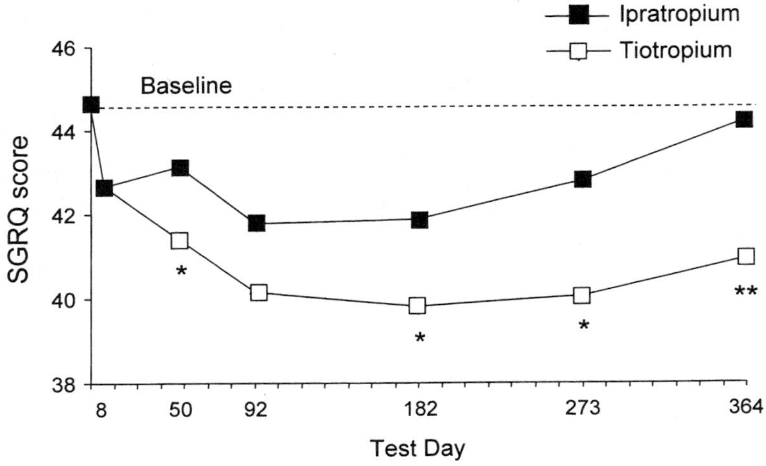

Figure 3 Changes in health status over 1 year following treatment with ipratropium, 40 μg qds, or tiotropium, 12 μg od. Note: $*p < 0.05$; $**p < 0.01$ for difference between ipratropium and tiotropium.

months. After 6 months the two treatments group diverged progressively, so that after 1 year the effect of ipratropium was almost lost. A similar pattern was seen in a separate study that compared tiotropium with placebo [47]. When comparing these studies, it appears that regular ipratropium is little better than placebo, at least in terms of health status gain. This conclusion is supported by another study in which there was a direct comparison of ipratropium and placebo [45].

VI. Longitudinal Trends in Health Status

The anticholinergic studies just described show a pattern of worsening health after the initial small improvement with both ipratropium and placebo [46,47]. A measurable decline in FEV_1 is a feature of COPD, but only recently has the accompanying decline in health status been documented [40,48]. In patients with a mean postbronchodilator FEV_1 of 50% predicted and treated with bronchodilators alone, the SGRQ score declines at 3.2 units per year. On average, the patients reach a clinically significant level of deterioration of 4 units every 15 months. This is much faster than the age-associated worsening of SGRQ score reported in a cross-sectional study in subjects without COPD [37]. The mechanisms of this decline have yet to be fully established, although the rate of decline FEV_1 and exacerbations are both factors [40]. Quite clearly there will be "fast" and "slow" health status decliners, and the challenge will be to identify "fast decliners" early on and develop appropriate interventions.

The demonstration of a measurable decline in health status has important implications for the design and interpretation of long-term clinical trials in COPD, and for the management of patients in routine practice. Progressive worsening of the patients' health over time will appear to erode earlier therapeutic gains. This may not mean that the treatment effect has worn off, however, it may just be a reflection of the fact that COPD is a relentlessly progressive disease. The most encouraging finding in the ISOLDE study was that fluticasone reduced the rate of decline in SGRQ score by nearly 40% and that the difference between steroid- and placebo-treated groups widened progressively over the 3-year study period [48].

VII. Implications for Practice

Health status questionnaires are developed and validated in populations of patients as research tools that allow standardised assessments. Each is made up of a set of items that are applicable to most patients with COPD. In clinical trials they provide a measure of the average response in a group of patients whose disease and its effects have been measured in a standardized way. In routine practice clinicians treat individuals, not standardized patients. This presents a challenge in terms of how we can assess whether an individual patient has had a worthwhile improvement.

Physiological changes do not provide an adequate surrogate for symptomatic or health status improvement. For example, the correlation between changes in FEV_1 and health status is weak [44]. There is statistically significant correlation, but the degree of shared variance is low ($\approx$12%), so it is not possible to predict whether an individual patient has had a significant improvement in health status score. Furthermore, the typical improvement in FEV_1 with a bronchodilator in COPD lies within the limits of day-to-day repeatability of the measurement. Use of spirometry as the sole method of assessing benefit would deny many patients a worthwhile treatment. Long-acting bronchodilators may produce symptomatic benefit by improving inspiratory flow rates [2], minimizing the effects of dynamic hyperinflation [4,5] and by improving sleep. The absence of a strong correlation between symptomatic and spirometric gain is not surprising, but does form a challenge for assessment of benefit in routine practice.

To identify patients who have had a worthwhile symptomatic improvement, assessment by spirometry must be supplemented by other methodologies. Use of standardized questionnaires will not be the answer, for a number of reasons. First, long questionnaires are too complex and time-consuming. Second, questionnaires short enough for routine use can contain only a small number of selected items that are common to all patients with COPD. That gives very little opportunity for individual patients to indicate how they personally experience benefit from treatment. The third issue is statistical. In a population of stable COPD patients, the short-term repeatability of these questionnaires is good. For example, the correlation between SGRQ measurements made 2 weeks apart is 0.92 [18]. Unfortunately, this still means that about half of the patients will show a change in SGRQ score that is greater than the 4-unit threshold for a clinically significant change, whether or not there has been a real change in their state. This problem is not unique to health status measurement, it also arises when assessing an individual patient's spirometric response to long-acting bronchodilator.

VIII. Assessment of Individual Patient Benefit

Most treatments for COPD are for symptomatic benefit, so it is only worth continuing to prescribe the treatment if the patient can report benefit. This leads naturally to concerns about placebo effects, but these may be overstated. It is possible to "back-calculate" a 4-unit change in SGRQ score into clinical treatment scenarios. For example, a 4-unit change corresponds to a patient who returns after a period of treatment with a new therapy to report that he or she no longer takes so long to wash or dress, can now walk up stairs without stopping, and is now able to leave the house for shopping or entertainment [41]. (Note: A 4-unit improvement would occur with the SGRQ only if the patient reported all three improvements). A smaller improvement, for example, 2.7 units on the SGRQ, would occur if the patient reported that treatment allowed him to get washed or dressed more quickly and to walk up stairs without stopping. Even these criteria for improvement appear to be quite strict when compared with the first attempt at a definition of a minimum clinically significant improvement: "The smallest difference in score which patients perceive as beneficial and would mandate, in the absence of troublesome side effects and excessive cost, a change in the patient's management" [42]. Such improvements can be identified quite readily in the course of a consultation. Indeed, the patient's simple retrospective assessment of the treatment's effect correlates well with the improvement in SGRQ score [44]. Recent studies have shown that health status benefits can be detectable after 2 weeks and are quite clearly apparent at 4–6 weeks [49], thus it is reasonable to carry out an assessment of benefit after 1 month of treatment.

IX. Summary

Health status measurements provide a valid standardized estimate of the overall effect of COPD on a patient's daily life and well-being. In routine practice they can usefully complement spirometric measurements when making baseline assessments. In a clinical trial they provide a measure of the average level of symptomatic benefit to be obtained with that therapy. In the individual patient seen in routine practice, assessment of symptomatic benefit and quality-of-life improvement requires that a careful clinical history be taken.

References

1. Killian KJ, Jones NL. Respiratory muscles and dyspnea. Clin Chest Med 1988; 9:237–248.
2. Taube C, Burghart L, Paasch K, Kirsten DK, Jörres RA, Magnussen H. Factor analysis of changes in dyspnea and lung function parameters after bronchodilation in chronic obstructive pulmonary disease. Am J Respir Crit Care Med 2000; 162:216–220.

3. Begin A, Grassino A. Role of inspiratory muscle function in chronic hypercapnia. Am Rev Respir Dis 1991; 143:905–912.
4. Belman MJ, Botnick WC, Shin JW. Inhaled bronchodilators reduce dynamic hyperinflation during exercise in patients with chronic obstructive pulmonary disease. Am J Respir Crit Care Med 1996; 153:967–975.
5. O'Donnell DE, Lam M, Webb KA. Spirometric correlates of improvement in exercise performance after anticholinergic therapy in chronic obsructuve pulmonary disease. Am J Respir Crit Care Med 1999; 160:542–549.
6. Killian KJ, Summers E, Jones NL, Campbell EJM. Dyspnea and leg effort during incremental cycle ergometry. Am Rev Respir Dis 1992; 145:1339–1345.
7. Guyatt GH, Townsend M, Berman LB, Pugsley SO. Quality of life in patients with chronic airflow limitation. Br J Dis Chest 1987; 81:45–54.
8. Gosselink R, Troosters T, DeCramer M. Peripheral muscle weakness contributes to exercise limitation in COPD. Am J Respir Crit Care Med 1996; 153:976–980.
9. Bernard S, Whittom F, Leblanc P, et al. Aerobic and strength training in patients with chronic obstructive pulmonary disease. Am J Respir Crit Care Med 1999; 159:896–901.
10. Engelen MPKJ, Schols AMWJ, Baken WC, Wesseling GJ, Wouters EFM. Nutritional depletion in relation to respiratory and peripheral skeletal muscle function in out-patients with COPD. Eur Respir J 1994; 7:1793–1797.
11. Schols AMWJ, Buurman WA, Staal-van den Brekel AJ, Dentener MA, Wouters EFM. Evidece for a relation between metabolic derangements and increased levels of inflammatory mediators in a subgroup of patients with chronic obstructive pulmonary disease. Thorax 1996; 51:819–824.
12. Janssens JP, Rochat T, Frey JG, Dousse N, Pichard C, Tschopp JM. Health-related quality of life in patients under long-term oxygen therapy: a home-based descriptive study. Respir Med 1997; 91:592–602.
13. Engstrom CP, Persson LO, Larsson S, Ryden A, Sullivan M. Functional status and well being in chronic obstructive pulmonary disease with regard to clinical parameters and smoking: a descriptive and comparative study. Thorax 1996; 51: 825–830.
14. Jones PW, Willits LR, Burge PS, Calverley PMA. Disease severity and the effect of fluticasone proprionate on chronic obstructive pulmonary disease exacerbations. Eur Respir J 2003; 21:1–6.
15. Seemungal TAR, Donaldson GC, Paul EA, Bestall JC, Jefferies DJ, Wedzicha JA. Effect of exacerbation on quality of life in patients with chronic obstructive pulmonary disease. Am J Respir Crit Care Med 1998; 157:1418–1422.
16. Seemungal TA, Donaldson GC, Bhowmik A, Jeffries DJ, Wedzicha JA. Time course and recovery of exacerbations in patients with chronic obstructive pulmonary disease. Am J Respir Crit Care Med 2000; 161:1608–1613.
17. Guyatt GH, Berman LB, Townsend M, Pugsley SO, Chambers LW. A measure of quality of life for clinical trials in chronic lung disease. Thorax 1987; 42:773–778.
18. Jones PW, Quirk FH, Baveystock CM, Littlejohns P. A self-complete measure

for chronic airflow limitation—the St George's Respiratory Questionnaire. Am Rev Respir Dis 1992; 145:1321–1327.

19. Maille AR, Koning CJ, Zwinderman AH, Willems LN, Dijkman JH, Kaptein AA. The development of the 'Quality-of-Life for Respiratory Illness Questionnaire (QOL-RIQ)': a disease-specific quality-of-life questionnaire for patients with mild to moderate chronic non-specific lung disease. Respir Med 1997; 91:297–309.
20. Lareau SC, Breslin EH, Meek PM. Functional status instruments: outcome measure in the evaluation of patients with chronic obstructive pulmonary disease. Heart & Lung 1996; 25:212–224.
21. Weaver TE, Narsavage GL, Guilfoyle MJ. The development and psychometric evaluation of the Pulmonary Functional Status Scale: an instrument to assess functional status in pulmonary disease. J Cardiopulm Rehab 1998; 18:105–111.
22. Hyland ME, Bott J, Singh S, Kenyon CA. Domains, constructs and the development of the breathing problems questionnaire. Quality of Life Res 1994; 3: 245–256.
23. Hyland ME, Singh SJ, Sodergren SC, Morgan MP. Development of a shortened version of the Breathing Problems Questionnaire suitable for use in a pulmonary rehabilitation clinic: a purpose-specific, disease-specific questionnaire. Quality of Life Res 1998; 7:227–233.
24. Barley EA, Quirk FH, Jones PW. Asthma health status in clinical practice: validity of a new short and simple instrument. Respir Med 1998; 92:1207–1214.
25. Hajiro T, Nishimura K, Jones PW, et al. A novel, short and simple questionnaire to measure health-related quality of life in patients with chronic obstructive pulmonary disease. Am J Respir Crit Care Med 1999; 159:1874–1878.
26. Alemayehu B, Aubert RE, Feifer RA, Paul LD. Comparative analysis of two quality-of-life instruments for patients with chronic obstructive pulmonary disease. Value in Health 2002; 5:436–441.
27. Yohannes AM, Roomi J, Waters K, Connolly MJ. Quality of life in elderly patients with COPD: measurement and predictive factors. Respir Med 1998; 92: 1231–1236.
28. Hajiro T, Nishimura K, Tsukino M, Ikeda A, Koyama H, Izumi T. Comparison of discriminative properties among disease-specific questionnaires for measuring health-related quality of life in patients with chronic obstructive pulmonary disease. Am J Respir Crit Care Med 1998; 157:785–790.
29. Singh SJ, Smith DL, Hyland ME, Morgan MD. A short outpatient pulmonary rehabilitation programme: immediate and longer-term effects on exercise performance and quality of life. Respir Med 1998; 92:1146–1154.
30. Carone M, Bertolotti G, Anchisi F, Zotti AM, Donner CF, Jones PW. Analysis of factors that chraracterize health impairment in patients with chronic respiratory failure. Eur Respir J 1999; 13:1293–1300.
31. Hajiro T, Nishimura K, Tsukino M, Ikeda A, Koyama H, Izumi T. Analysis of clinical methods used to evaluate dyspnea in patients with chronic obstructive pulmonary disease. Am J Respir Crit Care Med 1998; 158:1185–1189.
32. Hajiro T, Nishimura K, Tsukino M, Ikeda A, Oga T, Izumi T. A comparison of

the level of dyspnea vs disease severity in indicating the health-related quality of life of patients with COPD. Chest 1999; 116:1632–1637.
33. Bestall JC, Paul EA, Garrod R, Garnham R, Jones PW, Wedzicha JA. Usefulness of the Medical Research Council (MRC) dyspnoea scale as a measure of disability in patients with chronic obstructive pulmonary disease. Thorax 1999; 54:581–586.
34. Shoup R, Dalsky G, Warner S, et al. Body composition and health-related quality of life in patients with obstructive airways disease. Eur Respir J 1997; 10:1576–1580.
35. Mostert R, Goris A, Weling-Scheepers C, Wouters EFM, Schols AMWJ. Tissue depletion and health related quality of life in patients with chronic obstructive pulmonary disease. Respir Med 2000; 94:859–867.
36. Okubadejo AA, Jones PW, Wedzicha JA. Quality of life in patients with chronic obstructive pulmonary disease and severe hypoxaemia. Thorax 1996; 51:44–47.
37. Domingo-Salvany A, Lamarca R, Ferrer M, et al. Health-related quality of life and mortality in male patients with chronic obstructive pulmonary disease. Am J Respir Crit Care Med 2002; 166:680–685.
38. Oga T, Nishimura K, Tsukino M, Sato S, Hajiro T. Analysis of the factors related to mortality in chronic obstructive pulmonary disease. Am J Respir Crit Care Med 2003; 167:544–549.
39. Rutten-van Molken M, Roos B, Van Noord JA. An empirical comparison of the St George's Respiratory Questionnaire (SGRQ) and the Chronic Respiratory Disease Questionnaire (CRQ) in a clinical trial setting. Thorax 1999; 54:995–1003.
40. Spencer S, Calverley PMA, Burge PS, Jones PW. Health status deterioration in COPD. Am J Respir Crit Care Med 2001; 163:122–128.
41. Jones PW. Interpreting thresholds for a clinically significant change in health status ('quality of life') with treatment for asthma and COPD. Eur Respir J 2002; 19:398–404.
42. Jaeschke R, Singer J, Guyatt GH. Measurement of health status: ascertaining the minimal clinically important difference. Controlled Clin Trials 1989; 10:407–415.
43. Jones PW, Quirk FH, Baveystock CM. The St George's Respiratory Questionnaire. Respir Med 1991; 85(suppl B):25–31.
44. Jones PW, Bosh TK. Quality of life changes in COPD patients treated with salmeterol. Am J Respir Crit Care Med 1997; 155:1283–1289.
45. Dahl R, Greefhorst LAPM, Nowak D, Nonikov V, Byrne AM, Thomson MH, et al. Inhaled formoterol dry powder versus ipratropium bromide in chronic obstructive pulmonary disease. Am J Respir Crit Care Med 2001; 164:778–784.
46. Vincken W, van Noord JA, Greefhorst AP. Improved health outcomes in patients with COPD during 1 yr's treatment with tiotropium. Eur Respir J 2002; 19:209–216.
47. Casaburi R, Mahler DA, Jones PW, et al. A long-term evaluation of once daily inhaled tiotropium in chronic obstructive pulmonary disease. Eur Respir J 2002; 19:209–216.

48. Burge PS, Calverley PM, Jones PW, Spencer S, Anderson JA, Maslen TK. Randomised, double blind, placebo controlled study of fluticasone propionate in patients with moderate to severe chronic obstructive pulmonary disease: the ISOLDE trial. Br Med J 2000; 320:1297–1303.
49. Calverley PMA, Pauwels R, Vestbo J, Jones PW, Pride NAG. Combined salmeterol and fluticasone in the treatment of chronic obstructive pulmonary disease. Lancet 2003; 361:449.

11

Health Resource Utilization

MITCHELL FRIEDMAN[†]

Tulane University Health Sciences Center
New Orleans, Louisiana, U.S.A.

I. COPD—The Challenge

Chronic respiratory diseases represent a challenge in both industrialized and developing countries because of their frequency and economic impact [1]. Understanding the burden of health care utilization and costs is important in developing strategies for prevention and management of chronic obstructive pulmonary disease (COPD), due to the fact that health planners in these countries have limited resources. COPD is a disease state characterized by chronic, progressive airflow limitation that is not fully reversible, with a precise definition varying from different management guidelines [2]. COPD refers to disorders including chronic bronchitis, emphysema, and a combination of the two disorders [3].

In the Global Burden of Disease Study conducted under the auspices of the World Health Organization (WHO) and the World Bank, the worldwide prevalence of COPD in 1990 was estimated to be 9.34/1000 men and 7.33/1000 in women [4–6]. The prevalence of COPD varies among countries,

[†]Deceased.

due most likely primarily to tobacco consumption habits [2]. It has been estimated that over 15 million individuals are affected with COPD in the United States, with a majority of them having either chronic bronchitis or a combination of chronic bronchitis and emphysema. [3]. There are an estimated 450,000 new cases per year [27]. A recent surveillance study showed that between the period 1988–1994 compared to the period 1971–1975, the number of persons with mild COPD ($FEV_1 \geq 80\%$ predicted values and FEV_1/FVC of $< 70\%$) increased from 6.5 million to 12.1 million persons. Over the same time periods, persons with worse COPD ($FEV_1 < 80\%$ predicted values) rose from 6.8 million to 12.1 million [8]. As reviewed by Vermiere [2], a study of 625 primary-care physicians and 280 respiratory specialists across eight countries reported that the prevalence of COPD had increased over the past 10 years. It is presently the fourth leading cause of death in the United States, with an increase in mortality of over 160% over the past 30 years [7]. A recent report by the Centers for Disease Control continues to report increased mortality from COPD, and in 2000, more women than men died of COPD (59,936 versus 59,118) [8]. The increase in mortality is not limited to the United States, since increased mortality has been found in other countries, e.g., Sweden [9]. This increase in mortality in COPD is especially remarkable since the rates for the other top three causes of mortality (coronary heart disease, stroke, other cardiovascular disease) have remained flat or actually decreased over the same period of time [7].

As pointed out by Sin et al. [10], COPD has traditionally been thought of as a disease of the elderly, but data from the National Ambulatory Medical Care Survey [11] demonstrated that approximately 70% of COPD patients were under the age of 65 and they consumed 67% of total COPD office visits and 43% of all hospitalizations. Thus COPD significantly affects the working-age population. Using population-based data from the Third National Health and Nutrition Examination Survey [10,12], the relationship between COPD and labor force participation in the United States was determined. The participants with COPD in the NHANES III survey were 3.9% less likely to be in the labor force compared to those without COPD. Mild, moderate, and severe COPD was associated with a 3.4%, 3.9%, and 14.4% reduction in the labor-force participation rate relative to those without COPD [10]. Others have shown similar data, with one study demonstrating that patients with COPD lost, on average, 3.6 work days per year because of their COPD [10,13].

Sin et al. [10] also computed an estimate of the economic impact of this reduction of employment. They estimated an excess unemployment of 366,600 persons in 1994 due to their COPD. This would result in a loss of productivity of approximately $9.9 billion [10].

II. Health Care Utilization in COPD

COPD, besides resulting in loss of productivity and causing increasing morbidity and mortality, also affects medical resource use, daily life, self-reported health status, and other activities for persons with this disease [14]. Furthermore, due to the increasing rates for disease incidence, its related use of health care resources (i.e., outpatient visits, hospital days, tests, and pharmaceutical interventions) are also continuing to increase. Strassels et al. recently reported a description of medical resource use in the United States [11]. Data for this study were derived from the 1987 National Medical Expenditure Survey. On a per-person basis, individuals with COPD spent nearly 5 days in the hospital during 1987. In this study, COPD accounted for approximately 28% of all hospitalizations among persons with COPD. On average, persons with COPD visited outpatient clinics twice, generalists more than four times, and specialists almost five times during that year. With regard to indirect resource use, persons with COPD reported 24.4 bed days, 27.5 restricted-activity days, and 3.6 lost work days over that year. The data from this study are self-reported. The recent surveillance report from the Centers for Disease Control [8] demonstrated that between 1980 and 2000, the annual number of physician office visits and hospital outpatient visits increased from 5.5 million to 8 million visits. Over the same period of time, the annual number of emergency department visits increased from 1.1 million to 1.5 million and the annual number of hospitalizations increased from 652,000 to 726,000 [8]. Studies from several countries, including the Netherlands, Sweden, and the United States, have all demonstrated increasing hospital and outpatient days from COPD.

Similar data have been recently reported using a large observational database of 1522 patients with a diagnosis of COPD enrolled in a health maintenance organization [15]. Medical charts for the whole of 1997 were reviewed from 200 COPD cases and also from 200 control patients obtained from a matched group of 4566 control patients of similar age and gender. Patients with COPD were more likely than the control group to smoke during the study period (46% versus 13.5%). Of those who had ever smoked, COPD patients had significantly greater smoking exposure than those without COPD (49.5 versus 34.9 pack-years). On average, patients with COPD had 3.7 chronic medical conditions (including lung disease), compared with 1.8 for the control group, particularly for heart disease, cancer, neurological injuries, and gastritis. Patients with COPD had significantly greater use of outpatient services than controls, with an average of 27.9 outpatient encounters per person compared to 16.2 for the control group. The services utilized included increased utilization of all services (including respiratory care services), particularly cardiology and emergency services. Compared with the control group, patients with COPD were 2–3 times more likely to be admitted to the hospital during the study year (1.8 versus 1.4), and those admitted had longer average duration of stays (4.7 versus 3.9 days).

Health care resources would be predicted to increase with increasing severity of COPD. Several organizations have proposed management of patients with COPD based on a staging system for the severity of the disease. This staging system has several potential applications, including clinical recommendations, prognostication, and health care resource planning [4,16]. It is unknown, however, if the severity of the disease based on these staging systems correlates with health care resource utilization and/or cost of treating the disease. In order to determine the exact health care resource utilization in COPD, based on a staging system a more recent study has been published [17]. This study was a retrospective evaluation of patients with a diagnosis of COPD identified between January 1993 and December 1994. Patients aged 35 to 80 years without restriction to gender or race were included. Patients with a diagnosis of COPD, emphysema, and/or chronic bronchitis as defined by the American Thoracic Society (ATS) were eligible to be included [16]. Patients were included regardless of whether COPD was the primary, secondary, most responsible, or a complicating diagnosis. Eligible patients had a maximum ratio of $FEV_1/FVC < 0.7$; a maximal $FEV_1 \leq 65\%$ of predicted, and a smoking history of at least 20 pack-years. All patients who could be identified with a diagnosis of COPD treated at a university medical center hospital and/or outpatient clinics were eligible to be included in this analysis, regardless of the severity of the disease. The majority of patients (n = 351; 85%) were followed by a primary-care physician (family medicine or internal medicine), while a smaller percentage (n = 62; 15%) were followed by a pulmonologist. Of the 351 patients followed by primary-care physicians, 209 were Stage I, 82 were Stage II, and 60 were Stage III. Of the 62 patients followed by pulmonologists, none were Stage I, 32 were Stage II, and 30 were Stage III. Patients were identified through a review of hospital and clinic billing records, hospital admission records, clinic visit logs, and pharmacy records. Patients were stratified according to the ATS statement on interpretation of lung function: Stage I included patients with an $FEV_1 \geq 50\%$ to $\leq 65\%$ predicted; Stage II included patients with an $FEV_1 \geq 35\%$ to 49% predicted; and Stage III included patients with an $FEV_1 < 35\%$ predicted. Eligible patients had to have filled ≥70% of their prescriptions (based on pharmacy refill records) for their pulmonary drugs in the year prior to study entry. Exclusion criteria were as follows: a history primarily consistent with asthma characterized by paroxysmal wheezing or dyspnea; allergic rhinitis or atopy; a total blood eosinophil count greater than $500/mm^3$; end-stage renal disease requiring dialysis; active tuberculosis or lung cancer; or fulminant hepatic failure.

A total of 413 patients were initially identified and included in the analysis. Patients were stratified by the severity of COPD based on $FEV_1\%$ predicted criteria. There were 209 patients with Stage I COPD, 114 patients with Stage II COPD, and 90 patients with Stage III COPD. Patients were followed for a maximum of 60 months. The average duration of follow-up was 47 ± 10 months. The percentages of Stage I patients completing 1, 2, 3, 4, and 5 years of follow-up were 100%, 98%, 96%, 94%, and 91%, respectively. No deaths were recorded among Stage I patients, with all 19 dropouts lost to follow-up. The percentages of Stage II patients completing 1, 2, 3, 4, and 5 years of follow-up were 97%, 90%, 88%, 83%, and 74%, respectively. Of the 30 dropouts, 10 were lost to follow-up and 20 expired (8 secondary to COPD and 12 due to non-COPD-related causes). The percentages of Stage III patients completing 1, 2, 3, 4, and 5 years of follow-up were 94%, 91%, 78%, 77%, and 58%, respectively. Of the 38 dropouts, 8 were lost to follow-up, and 30 expired (24 due to COPD and 6 due to non-COPD-related causes). The percentage of patients lost to follow-up was identical (9%) in each of these disease severities. The percentage of patients who expired was significantly different between the three severity groups ($p < 0.01$). Mortality over the 5-year follow-up in Stage I, II, and III COPD was 0%, 17%, and 33%, respectively.

The frequency of clinic, emergency department, and hospital visits in the study patients is summarized in Fig. 1. The frequency of each type of visit was significantly correlated with disease severity ($p < 0.001$). Stage III

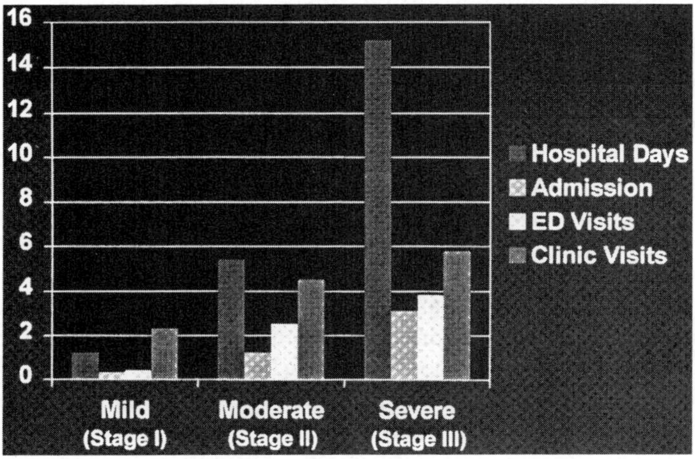

Figure 1 Health care resource utilization in patients with COPD (episodes/year).

patients had significantly greater utilization than Stage I or II patients, while Stage II patients had significantly greater utilization than Stage I patients. The mean lengths of hospitalization for Stage I, II, and III patients were 3.4 ± 4.2 days, 4.2 ± 5.0 days, and 4.9 ± 3.9 days, respectively. As a result, the mean number of days of hospitalization increased from just over 1 day per patient per year in Stage I patients to 5.5 days for Stage II and 15 days for Stage III patients. Oxygen therapy was not used by any patient with Stage I COPD. Oxygen therapy was used initially in 5% of Stage II patients and in 43% of Stage III patients. Oxygen therapy was subsequently added to 29% of Stage II patients and to 33% of Stage III patients. The final percentages of Stage II and Stage III patients using oxygen were 34% and 76%, respectively. The final distributions of patients receiving nocturnal and continuous oxygen were 37% and 63%, respectively. This study has some limitations. It is retrospective and there is always some risk of bias. Another limitation of the analysis was the inability to confirm that patients did not receive additional health care services provided elsewhere. Despite these limitations, this study provides one of the first comprehensive health care resource evaluations of a large cohort of patients with COPD.

III. Economic Burden of COPD

The increased health care resources utilized by persons with COPD obviously result in an increased economic burden to all countries. Estimating the economic and medical costs of COPD, is difficult, however, due to the lack of large prospective studies. However, there are several studies (including modeling) that can be used to determine the economic burden accrued to society due to COPD.

The total costs associated with illnesses comprise directs costs, indirect costs, and intangibles [9]. Directs costs are those associated with the prevention, diagnosis, and treatment of the disease. Indirect costs are those arising from a reduced working capacity among the patients. Intangible costs arise from a patient's pain, suffering, and decreased quality of life. As pointed out by Jacobson et al. [9] these costs are seldom reported, partly due to difficulty to measure and partly because there are different opinions regarding how to value reductions in quality of life. Thus, direct and indirect costs are reasonable estimates of the economic burden of COPD [9]. In data from the National Heart, Lung and Blood Institute, (NHLBI), the direct and indirect costs from COPD for the United States, compared to other common respiratory illnesses, are shown in Figure 2.

There are several reports, utilizing various national surveys, that have estimated the medical costs of COPD. As reviewed [11], an early study used

Condition	Total Costs	Direct Medical Costs	Mortality	Morbidity	Total
COPD	23.9	14.7	4.5	4.7	9.2
Asthma	12.6	9.8	0.9	0.9	2.8
Influenza	14.6	1.4	0.1	13.1	13.2
Pneumonia	7.8	1.7	4.6	1.5	6.1
Tuberculosis	1.1	0.7	-	-	0.4
Respiratory cancer	25.1	5.1	17.1	2.9	20.0

Figure 2 Estimates of direct and indirect costs of lung disease, 1993 (in billions of U.S. dollars).

the 1970 Health Interview Survey to estimate the costs of emphysema [18]. The authors estimated the total costs due to emphysema in 1970 to be greater than $15 billion. Ward et al. used a public payor prospective to estimate the direct costs of COPD from various surveys [3]. They estimated the total annual payment for COPD in the United States to be $6.6 billion for these surveys conducted in 1985–1992. Intangible and indirect costs for COPD were not valued in this study. Medicare and Medicaid reimbursement rates were applied as fee structures for valuing the services studied (except pharmaceuticals).

About one-third of the cost of hospitalizations for persons with COPD used the billing codes for "medical management of COPD." More than half the costs for hospitalizations of COPD patients was for other respiratory conditions. The analysis of COPD on length of stay for hospitalizations suggested a slightly longer length of stay for those with COPD versus those without. The annual cost was $628 million, with an average cost for these services of $2361. The annual payment for emergency room visits for COPD was $148 million. On a per-visit basis, the cost was $237. The annual outpatient visit cost for COPD was $156 million. The average per-visit cost was $25 excluding physician fees. The annual payments for diagnostic/screening procedures was $55 million. Eighty-four percent of the costs were for chest radiographs, 15% for electrocardiograms, and only 1% for spirometry. The average per-visit cost was $8.43. The annual payments for nursing home care were $942 million, with an average yearly cost of $17,868 for nursing home care. The costs for COPD-related hospice care were estimated to be $28 million with an annual cost of $17,274. The estimated total cost for home health care for COPD was $309 million, with an average annual cost of $5386.

The costs of pharmaceutical agents used in COPD (predominantly bronchodilators and corticosteroids) were estimated to be $462 million. The annual expenditure for oxygen expenses was $2.3 billion.

Strassels et al., using data derived from the 1987 Medical Expenditure Survey, estimated the mean per-person direct medical expenditures among persons with COPD were $6469 (1987 U.S. dollars), about 25% of which was COPD-related [11]. The authors made two main observations. The first was that individuals with COPD incurred significant amounts of per-person resource use expenditures. The second observation was that COPD- related resource use and expenditures represented a relatively small proportion of costs and resource use among persons with COPD. For example, they demonstrated that inpatient admissions accounted for 68.5% of total mean COPD admission expenditures ($4430), but only 27.8% of admissions in this group was related to COPD. For prescribed drugs, the mean COPD expenditure was $509 and represented 7.9% of COPD total expenditures, but only 34.6% of the expenditures in this group were COPD-related. Outpatient visit costs were $782 and were 12.1% of COPD total expenditures but only 14.2% of total expenditures. Similar relationships were seen for office and emergency department visits. However, the majority of patients were older than 65 years of age, and no determination of the severity of COPD was made. These data suggest that persons with COPD experience a substantial burden of health care resources and costs due to co-morbid conditions besides the COPD.

Further evidence is the 1982 data demonstrating that persons with COPD who are enrolled in Medicare spent $8850, 2.5 times the amount for persons without COPD who were enrolled in Medicare [19]. Likewise, Ruchlin et al. found that Medicare expenditures were $11,841 (year 2000 dollars) for individuals with COPD, compared to $4901 for all covered patients [20]. In 1996, persons with chronic bronchitis spent $770, and those with emphysema spent $1285 [21]. Similar to other studies [21], a majority of the costs were related to hospital care. According to estimates from the National Heart, Lung and Blood Institute in 1993, the annual cost of COPD was $23.9 billion. The largest contribution to the cost of COPD was hospitalization [22].

In the study reviewed previously [17], the investigators also evaluated costs in a cohort of patients who were stratified with regard to severity of illness. Costs in this analysis were identified for drugs, oxygen therapy, laboratory tests, diagnostic tests, procedures, clinic visits, emergency department visits, and hospitalizations. Acquisition costs of pulmonary drug therapy was based on 1999 PC-Price Check data. Average wholesale prices (AWP) prices were based on the actual product (generic or brand) and dose regimen used. Pulmonary drugs included β-agonists, ipratropium, theophylline, steroids, and antibiotics. Initial drug treatment was defined as pulmonary drugs used in the first 30 days after patients were identified in 1993 or 1994. Add-on drug therapy was defined as pulmonary drug therapy added during disease exacerbations or for persistent symptoms of COPD 30 days after study entry. Oxygen therapy was classified as nocturnal or continuous. Continuous oxygen therapy cost was estimated to be $232 per month, while nocturnal oxygen therapy cost was estimated to be $149 per month. Laboratory tests and other diagnostic procedures obtained during a clinic visit, emergency room visit, or hospitalization for COPD were included in the analysis. These typically included pulmonary function tests, chest X-rays, arterial blood gases, theophylline levels, blood glucose, hepatic function tests, complete blood counts, and sputum Gram stains. The costs of laboratory tests, procedures, and other monitoring tests were estimates of institutional costs provided by the individual departments conducting each test. These estimates were based on reagents consumed, disposable supplies, equipment maintenance, personnel salaries, and overhead, where appropriate. Inclusion of cost for clinic visits, emergency room visits, and hospitalization were restricted to those identified specifically for COPD, including initial diagnosis and work-up, routine follow-up, disease progression or exacerbation, and drug toxicity. Cost per clinic visit was estimated on the basis of personnel salaries and overhead. This estimate was $28 per visit and was used for all clinic visits regardless of the actual time of the individual visit. Emergency room visit costs were fixed at $125 per visit, and hospitalization at $650 per day in the intensive care unit and $375 per day in a non-intensive care unit. Clinic visit, emergency room, and hospital costs represent estimates of institutional cost, not charges. In addition, these costs were on a "per-diem" basis. Tests, procedures, or treatments occurring during these visits were reported separately.

The resultant annual median health care costs are summarized in Figure 3. The median total treatment costs were significantly greater for Stage III patients compared to Stage II or Stage I patients ($p < 0.01$). The median total treatment costs for Stage II patients were also significantly greater compared to Stage I patients ($p < 0.01$). Total treatment costs increased over the 5 years of follow-up for all stage of COPD. The increases in total cost for Stage I, II, and III over the 5 years of follow-up were 9%, 14%, and 11%, respectively. The magnitude of the increase was not significantly different across the three disease severities. Hospitalization represented the greatest percentage of total cost regardless of the severity of disease ($p < 0.01$). In Stage I COPD, drug acquisition costs accounted for 31% of the total cost. In comparison, drug acquisition cost accounted for only 14% and 7% of total cost in Stage II and

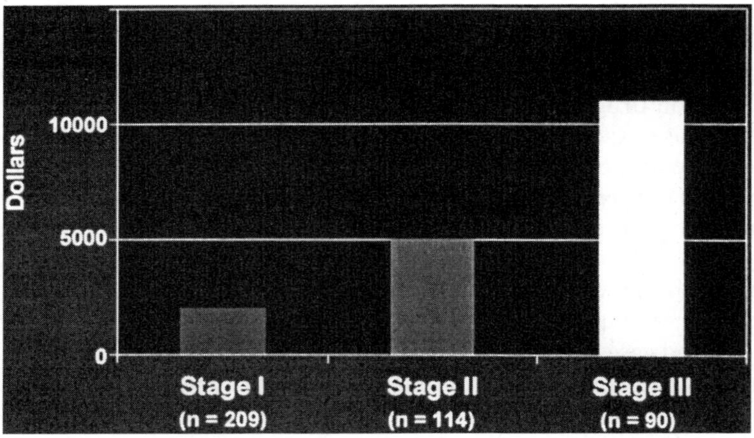

Figure 3 Annual median treatment costs stratified by severity of COPD.

III patients, respectively. Laboratory and diagnostic test costs accounted for 20% of total cost in Stage I patients, but only 10% and 6% of total cost in Stage II and Stage III patients, respectively. Emergency room and clinic visit costs each contributed 6% or less to the total treatment cost, regardless of the severity of the disease. Our data are also important because they underscore the relative importance of the different cost variables contributions to the total cost of COPD. In Stage I COPD, hospitalization, drugs, and laboratory/diagnostic tests were the most important cost variables. In Stage II and III COPD, hospitalization and oxygen therapy were the most important cost variables.

These data are also similar for other countries. In Sweden, by 1991, the direct costs for all respiratory disease were 8% of the cost of all diseases. The total costs related to COPD increased from 699 SEK in 1989 to 1085 SEK in 1991. Total costs increased from 2021 to 2784. For COPD, the costs related to inpatient care increased more than drug costs. The number of life-years lost as a result of COPD increased from 1960–1062 to 1990–1992. In contrast, the number of life-years lost decreased for asthma over the same time period [9]. Similar data for Sweden has been shown by Lofdahl [23]. As indicative of the increasing economic burden of COPD, Feenstra et al. have projected a 90% increase in health care costs in the Netherlands related to COPD [24]. The projected costs are greatly influenced by the impact of hospital costs and medication costs. These data clearly demonstrate that hospitalizations are the largest cost factor in COPD. As reviewed, persons with COPD who are hospitalized for co-morbidities unrelated to COPD have longer length of stays, thus incurring additional costs due to COPD. Attempts to decrease the prevalence of cigarette smoking will clearly have an impact on the incidence of COPD and its progression and thus is the major factor to decrease costs of COPD. Other strategies designed to decrease exacerbations and hospitalizations in COPD will also have a significant impact on the economic burden of COPD [25,26].

References

1. Ait-Khaled N, Enarson D, Bousquet J. Chronic respiratory diseases in developing countries: the burden and strategies for prevention and management. Bull WHO 2001; 79:971–979.
2. Vermiere P. The burden of chronic obstructive pulmonary disease. Respir Med 2002; 96(suppl C):S3–S10.
3. Ward M, Mavitz HS, Smith WW, Baskt A. Direct medical cost of chronic obstructive pulmonary disease in the U.S.A. Respir Med 2000; 94:1123–1129.
4. Pauwels RA, Buist AS, Calverley PMA, Jenkins C, Hurd SS. Global strategy for the diagnosis, management, and prevention of chronic obstructive pulmonary disease. Am J Respir Crit Care Med 2001; 163:1256–1276.
5. Murray C, Lopez AD. Evidence-based health policy—lessons from the Global Burden of Disease Study. Science 1996; 274:740–743.
6. Murray C, Lopez AD, eds. The Global Burden of Disease: A Comprehensive Assessment of Mortality and Disability from Diseases, Injuries and Risk Factors in 1990 and Projected to 2020. Cambridge, MA: Harvard University Press, 1996.
7. Pauwels R, Buist SA, Calverley PMA, Jenkins CR, Hurd SS. Global strategy for the diagnosis, management, and prevention of chronic obstructive pulmonary disease. Am Rev Respir Dis 2001; 163:1256–1276.
8. Mannino D, Homa DM, Akinbami LJ, et al. Chronic obstructive pulmonary disease surveilance—United States, 1971-200. MMWR 2002; 51:1–34.
9. Jacobson L, Hertzman P, Lofdahl CG, Skoogh BE, Lindgren B. The economic impact of asthma and chronic obstructive pulmonary disease (COPD) in Sweden in 1980 and 1992. Respir Med 1999; 94:247–255.
10. Sin D, Stafinski T, Ying CN, Bell NR, Jacobs P. The impact of chronic obstructive pulmonary disease on work loss in the United States. Am J Respir Crit Care Med 2002; 165:704–707.
11. Strassels SA, Smith DH, Sullivan SD, Mahajan PS. The costs of treating COPD in the United States. Chest 2001; 110:334–352.
12. National Center for Health Statistics. Plan and Operation of the Third National Health and Nutrition Examination Survey, 1988–1994, PHS 94-1308. Hyattsville, MD: U.S. Department of Health and Human Services, 1994.
13. Strassels SA, Sullivan S, Smith D. Characteristics of the costs of chronic obstructive pulmonary disease (COPD). Eur Respir J 1996; 9(suppl 23):421S.

14. Stewart A, Greenfield S, Hays RD, et al. Functional status of patients with chronic conditions: results from the Medical Outcomes Study. JAMA 1989; 262:907–913.
15. Mapel D, Pearson M. Obtaining evidence for use by healthcare payers on the success of chronic obstructive pulmonary disease management. Respir Med 2002; 96(suppl C):S23–S30.
16. American Thoracic SocietyStandards for the diagnosis and care of patients with chronic obstructive pulmonary disease (COPD). Am J Respir Crit Care Med 1995; 152:77–120.
17. Hilleman DE, Dewan N, Maleskar M, Friedman M. Pharmacoeconomic evaluation of COPD: stratification of costs according to severity of the disease and initial drug therapy. Chest 2000; 118:1278–1285.
18. Freeman R, Rowland CR, Smith EC, et al. Economic cost of pulmonary emphysema: implications for policy making on smoking. Inquiry 1976; 13:15–22.
19. Grasso ME, Wellerm WE, Shaffer TJ, et al. Capitation, managed care, and chronic obstructive pulmonary disease. Am J Respir Crit Care Med 1998; 158: 133–138.
20. Ruchlin HS, Dasbach EJ. An economic obverview of chronic obstructive pulmonary disease. Pharmacoeconomics 2001; 19:623–642.
21. Wilson L, Devine EB, So K. Direct medical costs of chronic obstructive pulmonary disease: chronic bronchitis and emphysema. Respir Med 2000; 94:204–213.
22. Sullivan SD, Ramsey SD, Lee TA. The economic burden of COPD. Chest 2000; 117:5S–9S.
23. Lofdahl C-G. Cost development of obstructive airway disease in Sweden. Eur Respir J 1996; 6:113–115.
24. Feenstra T, van Genugten MLL, Hoogenveen RT, Wouters EF, Rutten-van Molken MPMH. The impact of aging and smoking on the future burden of chronic obstructive pulmonary disease. Am J Respir Crit Care Med 2001; 164: 590–595.
25. Friedman M, Witek TJ Jr, Serby CW, Menjoge SS, Wilson JD, Hilleman DE. Pharmacoeconomic evaluation of a combination of ipratropium plus albuterol compared to ipratropium alone and albuterol alone in chronic obsctructive pulmonary disease. Chest 1999; 115:635–641.
26. Friedman M, Hilleman DE. Economic burden of chronic obstructive disease: impact of new treatment options. Pharmacoeconomics 2001; 19:245–254.
27. Ward M, Mavitz HS, Smith WW, Baskt A. Direct medical cost of chronic obstructive pulmonary disease in the U.S.A. Respir Med 2000; 94:1123–1129.

12

Anticholinergics

PETER J. BARNES

Imperial College
London, England

I. Introduction

Bronchodilators are the mainstay of current therapy in chronic obstructive pulmonary disease (COPD), and while they provide relatively little improvement in spirometric lung function compared to asthma, they may significantly reduce symptoms of dyspnea by reducing the increased lung volumes, and may also improve exercise tolerance [1]. Anticholinergics are the most effective class of brochodilators in the management of COPD [2,3]. Currently available anticholinergic drugs include ipratropium bromide, oxitropium bromide, and, more recently, tiotropium bromide, which work by blocking the receptors (muscarinic receptors) for the neurotransmitter acetylcholine, which is released from cholinergic nerve endings in the airways. Recently there have been important advances in this field, with the discovery of several distinct types of muscarinic receptor, raising the possibility that more selective drugs may be developed. Existing anticholinergic drugs have to be delivered several times a day so, as with β_2-agonists, once-daily preparations would be of great advantage in the long-term management of patients with chronic airway diseases. Important advances have been made in both areas of drug development, leading to the first of a new generation of anticholinergics.

II. Rationale for Anticholinergic Therapy in COPD

Anticholinergics are antagonists of muscarinic receptors and, in therapeutic use, have no other significant pharmacological effects. In animals and humans there is a small degree of resting bronchomotor tone due to tonic vagal nerve impulses, which release acetylcholine in the vicinity of airway smooth muscle. This can be blocked by section of the vagal nerve in animals and also by anticholinergic drugs in humans. Recent evidence suggests that acetylcholine may also be released from cells in the airways other than nerves, including epithelial cells, but the role of extraneuronal acetylcholine un human airways is currently uncertain [4]. The synthesis of acetylcholine in epithelial cells is increased by inflammatory stimuli which increase the expression of choline acetyltransferase, and this could therefore contribute to cholinergic effects in airway diseases. Since muscarinic receptors are expressed in airway smooth muscle of small airways which do not appear to be innervated by cholinergic nerves [5], this might be an important mechanism of cholinergic narrowing in peripheral airways that could be relevant in COPD (Fig. 1).

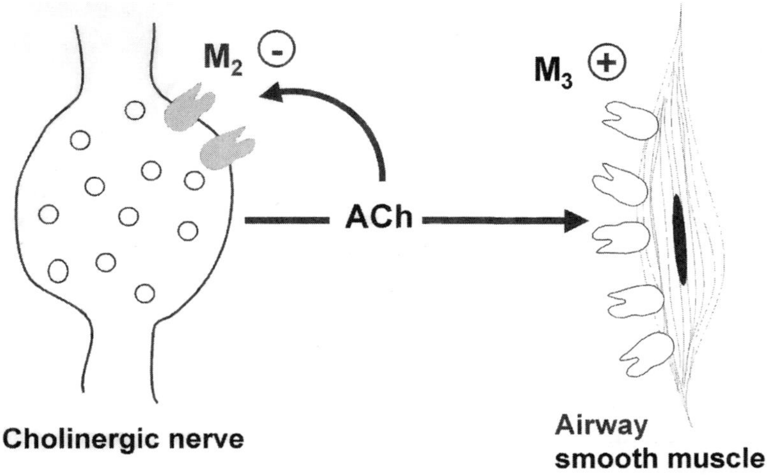

Figure 1 In proximal airways acetylcholine (ACh) is released from vagal parasympathetic nerves to activate M_3 receptors on airway smooth muscle cells. In peripheral airways M_3 receptors are expressed but there is no cholinergic innervation; however, these may be activated by ACh released from epithelial cells, which may express choline acetyltransferase (ChAT) in response to inflammatory stimuli, such as tumor necrosis factor-α (TNF-α).

There is considerable evidence that cholinergic pathways may play an important role in regulating acute bronchomotor responses in animals, and there are a wide variety of mechanical, chemical, and immunological stimuli that are capable of eliciting reflex bronchoconstriction via vagal pathways. Anticholinergic drugs afford some protection against acute challenge by sulfur dioxide, inert dusts, cold air, and emotional factors, but are less effective against antigen challenge, exercise, and fog. This is not surprising, as anticholinergic drugs will only inhibit reflex cholinergic bronchoconstriction and have no significant blocking effect on the *direct* effects of inflammatory mediators such as histamine and leukotrienes on bronchial smooth muscle. This is the reason that anticholinergics are less effective as bronchodilators than β_2-agonists, which act as antagonists of all bronchoconstrictor mediators that are released from inflammatory cells in asthma. Furthermore, cholinergic antagonists probably have little or no effect on mast cells, microvascular leak, or the chronic inflammatory response.

Anticholinergics are the most effective bronchodilators in COPD [6]. Vagal cholinergic tone appears to be the only reversible element of airway obstruction in COPD, and its effects are exaggerated by geometric factors due to narrowed airways, since airway resistance is inversely proportional to the fourth power of the airway radius (Fig. 2). Since cholinergic nerves cause mucus secretion in addition to bronchoconstriction, anticholinergics may reduce airway mucus secretion and clearance, but this does not appear to happen in most clinical studies. However, oxitropium bromide has been shown to reduce mucus hypersecretion in patients with COPD, and this could be an added advantage [7] which may account for the superiority of anticholinergics compared to β_2-agonists as bronchodilators in COPD. This is in marked contrast to asthma, in which β-agonists are much more effective bronchodilators than anticholinergics, and act as functional antagonists to inhibit the bronchoconstrictor effect of multiple mediators, including histamine, leukotrienes, and kinins. This also implies that these bronchoconstrictor mediators, derived largely from mast cells and eosinophils, cannot play a key role in COPD, in which other inflammatory mediators are more important.

III. Muscarinic Receptor Subtypes in the Airways

Pharmacological studies have revealed the presence of several subtypes of muscarinic receptor, and this has been confirmed by the cloning of five distinct muscarinic receptor genes [8]. Three muscarinic receptor subtypes have been found in human airways, and they have different functional effects [9]. Autoradiographic mapping of muscarinic receptors in human airways has

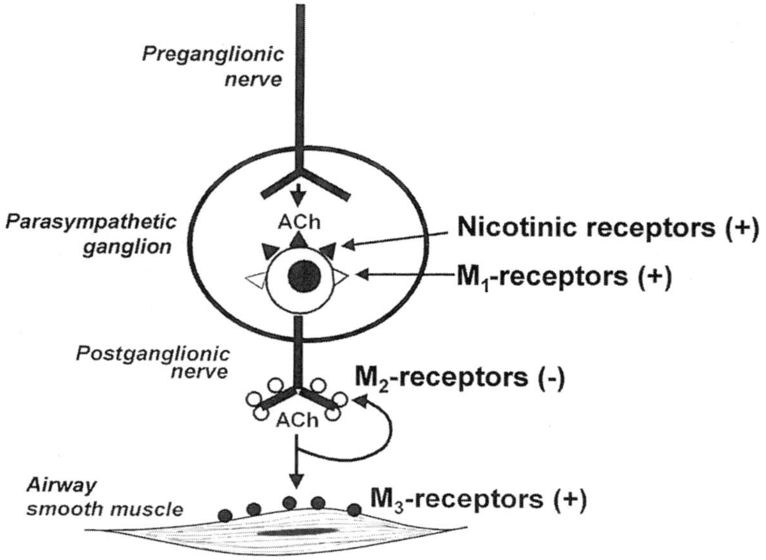

Figure 2 Anticholinergic drugs inhibit vagally mediated airway tone, leading to bronchodilatation. This effect is small in normal airways but is greater in airways of patients with chronic obstructive COPD, which are structurally narrowed.

demonstrated predominant localization to airway smooth muscle of all airways, although there is a higher density of receptors in proximal airways [5]. Muscarinic receptors are also localized in high density to submucosal glands.

A. M_1 Receptors

M_1 receptors are localized to parasympathetic ganglia in the airways, where they appear to function as regulators of ganglionic transmission (Fig. 3). Normally, preganglionic nerves release acetylcholine, which acts on nicotinic receptors on ganglionic cells to activate postganglionic nerves, but normally there is a high level of filtering, so that only a proportion of preganglionic signals are translated into postganglionic impulses. M_1 receptors facilitate neurotransmission through these ganglia and therefore enhance cholinergic reflex bronchoconstriction. This implies that blocking M_1 receptors would be beneficial in treating COPD. The M_1-selective antagonist pirenzepine is more effective at blocking reflex bronchoconstriction than the direct contractile effect of a cholinergic agonist [10]. However, another M_1-selective agonist telenzepine was not effective as a bronchodilator in COPD

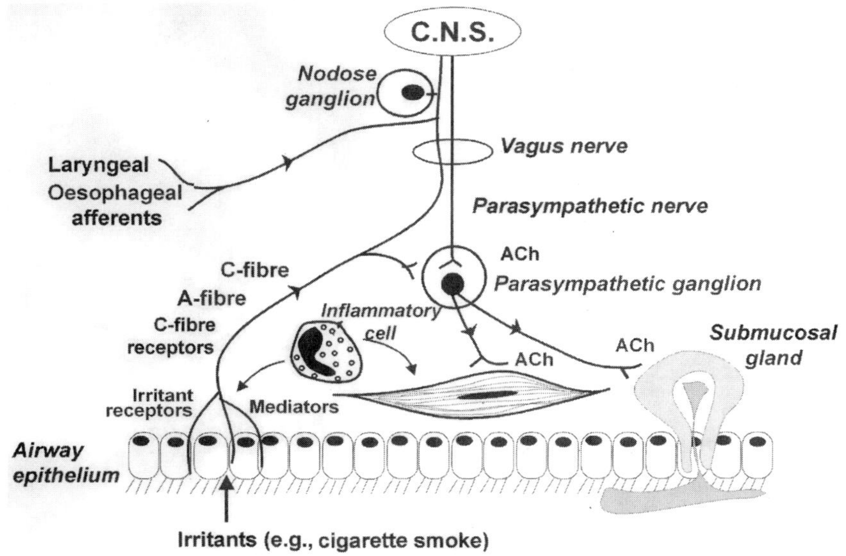

Figure 3 Muscarinic receptor subtypes in airways. Ganglionic neurotransmission is mediated via nicotinic receptors (ion channels), but M_1 receptors may facilitate this transmission. M_2 receptors on postganglionic cholinergic nerve terminals inhibit the release of acetylcholine (ACh), thus reducing the stimulation of postjunctional M_3 receptors which constrict airway smooth muscle.

when given orally [11]. M_1 receptors are also weakly expressed on submucosal glands in human airways, but do not appear to have any functional role [12], although in human nasal mucosa there is a weak stimulatory effect [13].

B. M_2 Receptors

M_2 receptors are located on the ends of cholinergic nerve endings and act as feedback inhibitors of acetylcholine release from the nerve (autoreceptors) (Fig. 4). Muscarinic autoreceptors have been demonstrated functionally in human airways in vitro [14] and in vivo [15]. These autoreceptors have been shown to be of the M_2-receptor subtype in human airways, and blockade of these receptors results in increased release of acetylcholine and therefore increased bronchoconstrictor responses to cholinergic nerve stimulation [16]. It is possible that this may explain some of the cases of paradoxical bronchoconstriction reported after use of ipratropium bromide. More selective anticholinergics that avoid blockade of M_2 receptors would therefore be

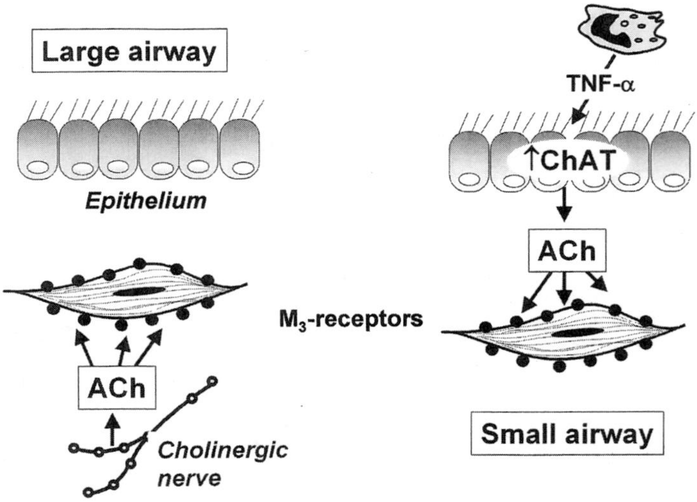

Figure 4 Muscarinic autoreceptors. Acetylcholine (ACh) released from cholinergic nerves activates M_3 receptors on airway smooth muscle, causing bronchoconstriction. At the same time, M_2 receptors on cholinergic nerve endings are activated and inhibit further acetylcholine release. A nonselective inhibitor such as ipratropium bromide inhibits M_3 receptors, thus giving bronchodilatation, but also blocks M_2 receptors, thereby increasing acetylcholine release and counteracting its bronchodilator action.

desirable. M_2 receptors are also found in airway smooth muscle, but do not appear to play a role in bronchoconstrictor responses to cholinergic agonists [17].

C. M_3 Receptors

The bronchoconstrictor response to cholinergic nerve stimulation and cholinergic agonists is mediated via M_3 receptors on airway smooth muscle [18], and M_3 receptors are expressed in airway smooth muscle of all airways, including peripheral airways [12]. M_3 receptors also mediate mucus secretion in response to cholinergic agonists [19,20]. Thus, blockade of M_3 receptors is the main therapeutic objective of anticholinergic therapy in COPD.

D. M_4 and M_5 Receptors

Although both M_4 and M_5 receptors are expressed in human tissues, these subtypes have not been detected in human airways [12]. M4 receptors have been detected in rabbit lung and appear to function like M_2 receptors, emphasizing the differences in muscarinic regulation between species [21].

IV. The Search for Selective Anticholinergics

Ipratropium and oxitropium bromide are nonselective blockers and therefore block M_2 receptors, which increases acetylcholine release, and this could then reduce the degree of blockade or reduce the duration of action on the drug M_3 receptors [16]. This has suggested that development of selective anticholinergics that block M_1 and M_3 receptors, but avoid blocking M_2 receptors, may have advantages. It was also hoped that more selective drugs might have fewer side effects, if some of these were mediated by receptor subtypes other than M_3 receptors. In practice, the major side effects of anticholinergics, including dry mouth, glaucoma, and urinary retention, are all mediated by M_3 receptors, so it is not possible to reduce these adverse effects. In practice these side effects are a minimal problem with currently available anticholinergics, as they are not absorbed.

As discussed above, selective inhibitors of M_1 receptors have been tested in clinical studies but do have any clinically useful effect in COPD or asthma. Selective inhibitors of M_3 receptors have also been developed, but existing drugs, such as darifenacin and YM905, are only weakly selective and are short-acting, so are unlikely to be of any clinical advantage [22]. Some drugs appear to have selectivity for M_1 and M_3 receptors compared to M_2 receptors. Both tiotropium bromide and glycopyrrolate dissociate more slowly from M_1 and M_3 receptors than from M_2 receptors and therefore have a kinetic selectivity [23,24].

V. Tiotropium Bromide

A major development in this area has been the discovery of tiotropium bromide, a quaternary ammonium compound similar to ipratropium, which has kinetic selectivity and dissociates very slowly from M_1 and M_3 receptors, but rapidly from M_2 receptors [3,25–28]. However, even more important than its selectivity is its very long duration of action.

A. In Vitro Pharmacology

Tiotropium bromide binds to muscarinic receptors with high affinity and is approximately 10-fold more potent than ipratropium bromide in binding to human lung muscarinic receptors [29]. Tiotropium bromide has a long-lasting protective effect against the binding of a radiolabeled cholinergic antagonist compared to atropine and ipratropium bromide. Similarly, [^{3}H]-labeled tiotropium bromide dissociates extremely slowly from human lung membranes, predicting a very long duration of action.

The pharmacological mechanism for the slow dissociation from M_1 and M_3 receptors is currently unknown. It cannot be accounted for by the high affinity of binding, since the drug dissociates much more rapidly from M_2 receptors, for which there is an equally high affinity of binding. It is possible that the fit of the molecule in the binding cleft of M_1 and M_3 receptors is such that it causes a change in receptor shape that prevents the drug leaving the ligand-binding cleft.

Tiotropium is a potent muscarinic receptor antagonist, with a prolonged duration of blockade in guinea pig trachea in vitro [25]. The long duration of action of tiotropium bromide in binding studies has been confirmed in functional studies with cholinergic neural responses in guinea pig and human airways in vitro [30]. Tiotropium bromide potently inhibits cholinergic nerve-induced contraction of guinea pig trachea and is approximately fivefold more potent than ipratropium bromide or atropine. The onset of action of tiotropium bromide is somewhat slower than is seen with atropine or ipratropium bromide but, after washout, its duration of action in blocking cholinergic neural responses is greatly prolonged, with a $t_{1/2}$ of over 6 hr, compared with just over 1 hr for ipratropium bromide. In human bronchi, tiotropium bromide has a similar inhibitory effect and is 10 times more potent than atropine, in agreement with the receptor-binding studies.

Tiotropium bromide, ipratropium bromide, and atropine all increase acetylcholine release to a similar extent (30–40%), but this is lost 2 hr after washout of all the antagonists [30]. Thus, although tiotropium bromide causes very prolonged blockage of airway smooth muscle M_3 receptors after washout, this does not apply to prejunctional M_2 autoreceptors. This demonstrates that the kinetic selectivity of tiotropium bromide, first demonstrated in binding studies to transfected cells, also applies to in-vitro functional studies.

B. Animal Studies in Vivo

Inhaled tiotropium bromide gives long-lasting protection against methacholine-induced bronchoconstriction in dogs and guinea pigs, with a protective effect of over 12 hr [25].

C. Clinical Pharmacology Studies

Several clinical studies have now demonstrated that tiotropium bromide is a very long-lasting bronchodilator [27]. Single doses of inhaled tiotropium bromide have been investigated in clinical studies in patients with COPD and asthma. In asthmatic patients, there is a prolonged bronchodilator effect after a single dose, lasting for up to 36 hr. There is also a prolonged dose-dependent protection against inhaled methacholine challenge [31]. At an inhaled dose of 40 μg there is a protection of over 7 doubling dilutions against methacholine, and the protection lasts for >48 hr. This should be compared with a protective effect of oxitropium bromide of less than 6 hr [32]. There is no adverse effects of inhaled tiotropium bromide and no effects on heart rate or blood pressure. In patients with COPD, tiotropium bromide gives a dose-related bronchodilatation which persists for over 24 hr [33,34].

These studies demonstrated that tiotropium is suitable for once-daily dosing and that at the lower doses where most improvement is seen there are unlikely to be significant side effects. This has subsequently been borne out by long-term clinical studies in patients with COPD [35–37]. More recent studies over 12 months have demonstrated not only improvement in spirometry that is sustained over this periods, but also significant improvement in health status [38,39]. There is also a surprising reduction in exacerbations, which may reflect a "stabilization" of the airways by an effective long-lasting bronchodilator.

Once-daily tiotropium is significantly more effective than four-times-daily ipratropium bromide at recommended doses. There may be several reasons for this. First, the increased potency of tiotropium bromide may mean that there is more effective blockade of muscarinic receptors. Dose-ranging studies have demonstrated a maximal effect at relatively low doses, whereas this may not be achieved at the recommended doses of ipratropium or oxitropium [35]. Second, the kinetic selectivity for M_3 and M_1 receptors over M_2 receptors may result in less increase in acetylcholine release, and this would make blockade of M_3 receptors on airway smooth muscle more efficient. Third, the prolonged duration of action may have a better long-term bronchodilator effect than repeated doses of short-acting drugs. Long-acting bronchodilators appear to have a much better controlling effect than short-acting drugs, and this has been well illustrated by the superiority of long-acting inhaled β_2-agonists (salmeterol, formoterol), compared to short-acting β_2-agonists (albuterol, terbutaline) [40,41]. It is possible that, by maintaining a prolonged bronchodilator effect in airway smooth muscle cells, they behave in a different way to recurrent bronchodilatation with constant forming and reforming of latch-bridges [42].

VI. Pharmacokinetics

Although inhaled anticholinergics have a long history in the treatment of airway disease, drugs such as atropine and strammonium fell out of favor because of the problem with anticholinergic side effects, and particularly central nervous system effects that included hallucinations. Anticholinergics came back into fashion only when quaternary ammonium derivatives, such as ipratropium bromide, were found to have none of these side effects. Quaternary ammonium compounds are electrically charged and thus are not absorbed from the gastrointestinal tract and do not pass the blood–brain barrier. They largely avoid anticholinergic side effects. Oral anticholinergics are not a possibility for the treatment of airway diseases because of unacceptable anticholinergic side effects.

Similarly, tiotropium bromide, another quaternary ammonium compound, is not absorbed from the gastrointestinal tract. After inhalation of a 10-μg dose there is rapid absorption into the circulation, with a peak plasma concentration within 5 min of 6 pg/mL, followed by a rapid fall within 1 hr to the stead-state level of 2 pg/mL and a terminal half-life of 5–6 days that is independent of the dose [23]. It has been calculated that this concentration would occupy $<5\%$ of muscarinic receptors and this may account for the relatively low incidence of systemic side effects. There is no evidence for drug accumulation after repeated administration.

VII. Side Effects

Inhaled anticholinergic drugs are usually well tolerated, and there are almost no side effects with either ipratropium or oxitropium bromide because there is virtually no systemic absorption of these positively charged quaternary ammonium compounds [43]. The expected side effects of anticholinergic drugs are dryness of the mouth, urinary retention, and glaucoma (secondary to mydriasis). However, these have not proved to be a problem in clinical practice, even in an elderly population. These side effects are all mediated via blockade of M_3 receptors, and therefore development of more selective drugs is unlikely to provide any clinical advantage.

Reports of paradoxical bronchoconstriction with ipratropium bromide, particularly when given by nebulizer, were largely explained by the hypotonicity of the nebulizer solution and by antibacterial additives, such as benzalkonium chloride. Nebulizer solutions free of these problems are less likely to cause bronchoconstriction. Occasionally, bronchoconstriction may occur with ipratropium bromide given by metered-dose inhaler. One theoretical concern with anticholinergics has been that inhibition of mucus secretion might slow mucus clearance or may make the mucus more viscous and difficult to expectorate. In clinical practice this does not appear to be a problem, perhaps indicating that cholinergic mechanisms are not important for basal mucus secretion, but only in the mucus hypersecretion that occurs in COPD.

Tiotropium bromide is well tolerated. There are no local side effects reported and no effects have been reported on sputum production, consistent with previous experience with regular doses of inhaled ipratropium bromide, even when high doses are used. There is a potential danger of induction of glaucoma in susceptible patients after accidental topical administration, but this is not a possibility with the dry powder inhaler formulation that will be marketed. In trials that have involved chronic treatment with inhaled tiotropium bromide in patients with COPD there is a low incidence of anticholinergic side effects. Approximately 10% of patients experience dryness of the mouth, but this is not of sufficient magnitude to cause withdrawal from the trial [37]. There are no other consistent side effects that can be attributed to systemic effects of anticholinergics. In the study that compared tiotropium once daily with ipratropium four times daily, there was a 15% incidence of dry mouth compared to a 10% incidence with ipratropium [36].

VIII. Future Prospects

Inhaled anticholinergics are the bronchodilators of choice in COPD, and at the moment bronchodilators are the only effective drug therapy available for COPD. As the worldwide prevalence of COPD is increasing, it is likely that the use of anticholinergic drugs will increase, particularly as the diagnosis and treatment become more widely disseminated through international treament guidelines [44]. Long-acting inhaled β_2-agonists are also effective in controlling symptoms in COPD [45], and there is a useful additive bronchodilator effect of ipratropium bromide with salmeterol [46]. Anticholinergics are much less effective than β_2-agonists in patients with asthma and therefore have only a minor role as an additional bronchodilator. However, elderly asthmatics and patients with a degree of fixed airflow obstruction appear to respond better.

Tiotropium bromide is likely to be an important advance in the management of COPD, as once-daily medication is effective and this will improve compliance with long-term therapy. Indeed, the long duration of action of tiotropium bromide means that even if occasional daily doses are missed this will not affect symptom control, as it takes 2 weeks for the effects of the drug to disappear [35]. Tiotropium bromide may also have additive effects with long-acting β_2-agonists, but such studies have not yet been reported. Whether tiotropium bromide will have a role in asthma remains to be determined, but it may be useful as an additional bronchodilator in patients with fixed airflow obstruction and patients with severe disease. It may also be useful for treating exacerbations.

It has proved difficult to develop M_3-selective antagonists, but it is possible that such drugs will be discovered in the future. However, the long duration of action is likely to be a more important property of tiotropium bromide than its kinetic selectivity. It is likely that other long-acting anticholinergics will be discovered, as there is a large therapeutic market.

References

1. Barnes PJ. Chronic obstructive pulmonary disease. New Engl J Med 2000; 343: 269–280.
2. Barnes PJ, Buist AS. The Role of Anticholinergics in COPD and Chronic Asthma. Macclesfield: Gardner Caldwell, 1997.
3. Disse B. Antimuscarinic treatment for lung diseases from research to clinical practice. Life Sci 2001; 68:2557–2564.
4. Wessler I, Kirkpatrick CJ, Racke K. Non-neuronal acetylcholine, a locally acting molecule, widely distributed in biological systems: expression and function in humans. Pharmacol Ther 1998; 77:59–79.
5. Mak JCW, Barnes PJ. Autoradiographic visualization of muscarinic receptor subtypes in human and guinea pig lung. Am Rev Respir Dis 1990; 141:1559–1568.
6. Rennard SI, Serby CW, Ghafouri M, Johnson PA, Friedman M. Extended therapy with ipratropium is associated with improved lung function in patients with COPD. A retrospective analysis of data from seven clinical trials. Chest 1996; 110:62–70.
7. Tamaoki J, Chiyotani A, Tagaya E, Sakai N, Konno K. Effect of long term treatment with oxitropium bromide on airway secretion in chronic bronchitis and diffuse panbronchiolitis. Thorax 1994; 49:545–548.
8. Eglen RM, Hegde SS, Watson N. Muscarinic receptor subtypes and smooth muscle function. Pharmacol Rev 1996; 48:531–565.
9. Barnes PJ. Muscarinic receptor subtypes in airways. Life Sci 1993; 52:521–528.
10. Lammers J-WJ, Minette P, McCusker M, Barnes PJ. The role of pirenzepine-sensitive (M_1) muscarinic receptors in vagally mediated bronchoconstriction in humans. Am Rev Respir Dis 1989; 139:446–449.
11. Ukena D, Wehinger C, Engelstatter R, Steinijans V, Sybrecht GW. The muscarinic M_1-receptor selective antagonist telenzepine has no bronchodilator effects in patients with chronic obstructive airways disease. Eur Respir J 1993; 6: 378–382.
12. Mak JCW, Baraniuk JN, Barnes PJ. Localization of muscarinic receptor subtype mRNAs in human lung. Am J Respir Cell Mol Biol 1992; 7:344–348.
13. Mullol J, Baraniuk JN, Logun C, Merida M, Hausfeld J, Shelhamer JH, Kaliner MA. M_1 and M_3 muscarinic antagonists inhibit human nasal glandular secretion in vitro. J Appl Physiol 1992; 73:2069–2073.

14.
15. Minette PA, Barnes PJ. Prejunctional inhibitory muscarinic receptors on cholinergic nerves in human and guinea-pig airways. J Appl Physiol 1988; 64: 2532–2537.
16. Minette PAH, Lammers J, Dixon CMS, McCusker MT, Barnes PJ. A muscarinic agonist inhibits reflex bronchoconstriction in normal but not in asthmatic subjects. J Appl Physiol 1989; 67:2461–2465.
17. Patel HJ, Barnes PJ, Takahashi T, Tadjkarimi S, Yacoub MH, Belvisi MG. Characterization of prejunctional muscarinic autoreceptors in human and guinea-pig trachea *in vitro*. Am J Respir Crit Care Med 1995; 152:872–878.
18. Watson N, Magnussen H, Rabe KF. Antagonism of b-adrenoceptor-mediated relaxations of human bronchial smooth muscle by carbachol. Eur J Pharmacol 1995; 275:307–310.
19. Roffel AF, Elzinga CRS, Zaagsma J. Muscarinic M_3-receptors mediate contraction of human central and peripheral airway smooth muscle. Pulm Pharmacol 1990; 3:47–51.
20. Ramnarine SI, Haddad EB, Khawaja AM, Mak JC, Rogers DF. On muscarinic control of neurogenic mucus secretion in ferret trachea. J Physiol (Lond) 1996; 494:577–586.
21. Rogers DF. Motor control of airway goblet cells and glands. Respir Physiol 2001; 125:129–144.
22. Mak JCW, Haddad E-B, Buckley NJ, Barnes PJ. Visualization of muscarinic m_4 mRNA and M_4-receptor subtypes in rabbit lung. Life Sci 1993; 53:1501–1508.
23. Alabaster VA. Discovery and development of selective M_3 antagonists for clinical use. Life Sci 1997; 60:1053–1060.
24. Disse B, Speck GA, Rominger KL, Witek TJ, Hammer R. Tiotropium (Spiriva): mechanistical considerations and clinical profile in obstructive lung disease. Life Sci 1999; 64:457–464.
25. Haddad E-B, Patel H, Keeling JE, Yacoub MH, Barnes PJ, Belvisi MG. Pharmacological characterization of the muscarinic receptor antagonist, glycopyrrolate, in human and guinea-pig airways. Br J Pharmacol 1999; 127:413–420.
26. Disse B, Reichal R, Speck G, Travnecker W, Rominger KL, Hammer R. Ba679BR, a novel anticholinergic bronchodilator: preclinical and clinical aspects. Life Sci 1993; 52:537–544.
27. Barnes PJ, Belvisi MG, Mak JCW, Haddad EB, O'Connor B. Tiotropium bromide (Ba 679 BR), a novel long-acting muscarinic antagonist for the treatment of obstructive airways disease. Life Sci 1995; 56:853–859.
28. Hansel TT, Barnes PJ. Tiotropium bromide: a novel once-daily anticholinergic bronchodilator for the treatment of COPD. Drugs Today 2002; 38:585–600.
29. Barnes PJ. Tiotropium bromide. Expert Opin Investig Drugs 2001; 10:733–740.
30. Hvizdos KM, Goa KL. Tiotropium bromide. Drugs 2002; 62:1195–1203.
31. Haddad E-B, Mak JCW, Barnes PJ. Characterization of [^{3}H]Ba 679, a slow-dissociating muscarinic receptor antagonist in human lung: radioligand binding and autoradiographic mapping. Mol Pharmacol 1994; 45:899–907.
32. Takahashi T, Belvisi MG, Patel H, Ward JK, Tadjkarimi S, Yacoub MH,

Barnes PJ. Effect of Ba 679 BR, a novel long-acting anticholinergic agent, on cholinergic neurotransmission in guinea-pig and human airways. Am J Respir Crit Care Med 1994; 150:1640–1645.
33. O'Connor BJ, Towse LJ, Barnes PJ. Prolonged effect of tiotropium bromide on methacholine-induced bronchoconstriction in asthma. Am J Respir Crit Care Med 1996; 154:876–880.
34. Wilson NM, Green S, Coe C, Barnes PJ. Duration of protection by oxitropium bromide against cholinergic challenge. Eur J Respir Dis 1987; 71:455–458.
35. Maesen FPV, Smeets JJ, Costongs MAL, Wald FDM, Cornelissen PJG. BA 1993; 6:1031–1036.
36. Maesen FPV, Smeets JJ, Sledsens TJM, Wald FDM, Cornelissen JPG. Tiotropium bromide, a new long-acting antimuscarinic bronchodilator: a pharmacodynamic study in patients with chronic obstructive pulmonary disease (COPD). Eur Respir J 1995; 8:1506–1513.
37. Littner MR, Ilowite JS, Tashkin DP, Friedman M, Serby CW, Menjoge SS, Witek TJ. Long-acting bronchodilation with once-daily dosing of tiotropium (Spiriva) in stable chronic obstructive pulmonary disease. Am J Respir Crit Care Med 2000; 161:1136–1142.
38. van Noord JA, Bantje TA, Eland ME, Korducki L, Cornelissen PJ. A randomised controlled comparison of tiotropium nd ipratropium in the treatment of chronic obstructive pulmonary disease. The Dutch Tiotropium Study Group. Thorax 2000; 55:289–294.
39. Casaburi R, Briggs DDJ, Donohue JF, Serby CW, Menjoge SS, Witek TJJ. The spirometric efficacy of once-daily dosing with tiotropium in stable COPD: a 13-week multicenter trial. Chest 2000; 118:1294–1302.
40. Casaburi R, Mahler DA, Jones PW, Wanner A, San PG, ZuWallack RL, Menjoge SS, Serby CW, Witek T. A long-term evaluation of once-daily inhaled tiotropium in chronic obstructive pulmonary disease. Eur Respir J 2002; 19: 217–224.
41.
42. Vincken W, van Noord JA, Greefhorst AP, Bantje TA, Kesten S, Korducki L, Cornelissen PJ. Improved health outcomes in patients with COPD during 1 years treatment with tiotropium. Eur Respir J 2002; 19:209–216.
43. Pearlman DS, Chervinksy P, Laforce C, Seltzer JM, Southern DL, Kemp JP, Dockhord RJ, Grossman J, Liddle RF, Yancey SW, Cocchetto DM, Alexander WJ, van As A. A comparison of salmeterol with albuterol in the treatment of mild-to-moderate asthma. New Engl J Med 1992; 327:1420–1425.
44. Kesten S, Chapman KR, Broder I, Cartier A, Hyland RH, Knight A, Malo J-L, Mazza JA, Moote DW, Small P, Tarlo S, Gontovnick L, Rebuck AS. A 3 month comparison of twice daily inhaled formoterol versus four times daily inhaled albuterol in the management of stable asthma. Am Rev Respir Dis 1991; 144:622–625.
45. Fredberg JJ, Inouye DS, Mijailovich SM, Butler JP. Perturbed equilibrium of myosin binding in airway smooth muscle and its implications in bronchospasm. Am J Respir Crit Care Med 1999; 159:959–967.

46. Gross NJ. Ipratropium bromide. New Engl J Med 1988; 319:486–494.
47. Pauwels RA, Buist AS, Calverley PM, Jenkins CR, Hurd SS. Global strategy for the diagnosis, management, and prevention of chronic obstructive pulmonary disease. NHLBI/WHO Global Initiative for Chronic Obstructive Lung Disease (GOLD) Workshop summary. Am J Respir Crit Care Med 2001; 163: 1256–1276.
48. Appleton S, Smith B, Veale A, Bara A. Long-acting b2-agonists for chronic obstructive pulmonary disease. Cochrane Database Syst Rev 2000; 2: CD001104.
49. van Noord JA, de Munck DR, Bantje TA, Hop WC, Akveld ML, Bommer AM. Long-term treatment of chronic obstructive pulmonary disease with salmeterol and the additive effect of ipratropium. Eur Respir J 2000; 15:878–885.

13

β-Adrenergic Receptor Agonist Bronchodilators in the Treatment of COPD

STEPHEN I. RENNARD

University of Nebraska Medical Center
Omaha, Nebraska, U.S.A.

I. Introduction

After smoking cessation, bronchodilators are first-line therapy in the treatment of chronic obstructive pulmonary disease (COPD) [1]. Among the bronchodilators currently available, selective β-adrenergic receptor agonists have been extensively used over the last 30 years. An interesting paradox is that lack of response to β-agonists has often been used to define patients with COPD, particularly in clinical trials. This has often led to a general impression that treatment of COPD offers little benefit. Available data, however, clearly demonstrate that the majority of COPD patients respond to bronchodilators, including β-agonists [2,3]. Moreover, evidence is accumulating that β-agonists may benefit patients by mechanisms different from simple bronchodilatation. This chapter will review the current understanding of β-agonist bronchodilators and their role in the treatment of COPD.

II. Mechanism of Action

Adrenergic receptors mediate a myriad of physiological effects in response to agonists released by adrenergic nerves, the adrenal gland, and other cellular sources [4]. They are classified into two major categories, α and β, based on pharmacological properties. The β-receptors located in airway smooth muscle cause bronchodilatation. As a result, adrenergic agents have been used over the centuries for the treatment of acute bronchospasm. Epinephrine, with effects on both α- and β-receptors, has largely been replaced for this purpose by more selective agents with a higher therapeutic index.

Several classes of β-receptors have been described [4]. β_2-receptors are primarily responsible for airway smooth muscle relaxation. In contrast, β_1-receptors are largely responsible for the tachycardia observed with nonselective β-agonists. The β_3-receptors, located on brown fat, have a thermogenic effect, which is believed to be important in hibernating animals but also contributes to smooth muscle relaxation, particularly in the gastrointestinal tract [5]. β-Receptors have also been described on skeletal muscle, where they may have an anabolic effect [6]. Whether this is mediated by β_2- or by a novel class of β-receptors (β_4) remains controversial. Agents that are selectively active on the β_2-receptor have proven useful, as they bronchodilate airway smooth muscle with less adverse effects than the nonselective β-agonists. New advances in the understanding of the β-receptor and its signaling mechanisms suggest that further generations of β-agonists will have added clinical benefits.

The β_2-adrenergic receptor is a seven-membrane-spanning receptor [7]. Receptors of this class are barrel-shaped, the membrane-spanning units forming a cylinder. The active binding site for β-agonists is in the center of the barrel. In the "classical" model for β-receptor activation (Fig. 1), ligand binding causes a conformational change in the receptor, which then binds and activates the G protein, G_s. The α unit of G_s then dissociates from the β–γ subunits and activates adenyl cyclase, leading to the production of cAMP which in turn activates protein kinase A. This substance phosphorylates a number of substrates, leading to calcium sequestration and bronchodilatation.

Protein kinase A, however, can phosphorylate and regulate the activity of a large number of substrates, creating the possibility for β-adrenergic agonists to exert other effects and to interact with other signaling pathways. Several of these interactions may have clinical significance for the patient with COPD. In this context, β-adrenergic agonists are often used together with glucocorticoids. Glucocorticoids can increase β-adrenergic receptor expression [8], and this may account for some of the benefits when these agents are used in combination. β-Agonists, however, can also lead to phosphorylation of the glucocorticoid receptor. This facilitates receptor activation, and thus β-agonists may potentiate the action of glucocorticoids [9,10].

Several mechanisms help terminate signaling [11]. First, the receptor can be desensitized by phosphorylation, leading to uncoupling from G_s. The receptor can also be internalized, where it can be degraded or recycled, and finally, receptor numbers can be downregulated by alterations in receptor gene expression. Second, cAMP, can be degradated by phosphodiesterases [12]. More than 50 phosphodiesterases have been described, many of which degrade cAMP. Their expression and activity varies among types of cells. This provides another level at which β-agonist actions can be modulated therapeutically. Because of its rapid production and subsequent degradation, β-adrenergic agonists generally result in a transient increase in cAMP and a transient initiation of signaling cascades. Activated proteins can be dephosphylated by specific phosphatases, thus resetting the system. Some agonists, such as PGE_2 that acts on a separate set of G-protein-coupled receptors, can cause a more sustained increase in cAMP. As might be expected from the complex signaling pathways initiated by cAMP, the biological consequences of these two signaling paradigms are not identical. The β-agonists of prolonged duration of action and the combination of β-agonists together with inhibitors of phosphodiesterase have the capability of altering the cAMP kinetics. These agents, therefore, have the potential for biological effects that differ from those of shorter-acting β-adrenergic agonists.

Activity of the β-receptor can be modulated by a number of other signaling pathways, a number of which are likely to be of importance in COPD. Cholinergic stimulation can modulate β-adrenergic responsiveness. The M_1 and M_3 receptors, by activation of protein kinase C, can lead to phosphorylation of the β-receptor and thereby decrease its activity [13,14]. In addition, activation of the M_2 muscarinic receptor can lead to activation of G_i. In contrast to G_s, G_i inhibits adenylyl cyclase and can therefore antagonize the ability of β-agonists to increase the levels of cAMP [15].

Other interactions are also likely important. The pro-inflammatory cytokines IL-1 and TNF-α decrease β-agonist responsiveness [16]. Similar effects were observed with the Th2 cytokines IL-5, IL-10, and IL-13. In addition, TGF-β, a multifunctional cytokine believed to play an important role in tissue repair and remodeling, can downregulate β-receptors on airway smooth muscle [17].

Interestingly, while knowledge about the β-receptor and its signaling mechanisms have increased, uncertainty remains about the exact mechanisms that lead to smooth muscle relaxation. Through protein kinase A-mediated phosphorylation, increases in cAMP have been believed to activate the BK_{Ca} channel, leading to a decrease in intracellular calcium and smooth muscle relaxation [18]. Other mechanisms may also play a role. cAMP can also activate protein kinase G, which can active BK_{Ca}. Recently, mitochondrial uncoupling protein 1 has also been suggested to play a role in cAMP-mediated Ca sequestration and smooth muscle relaxation [5]. In

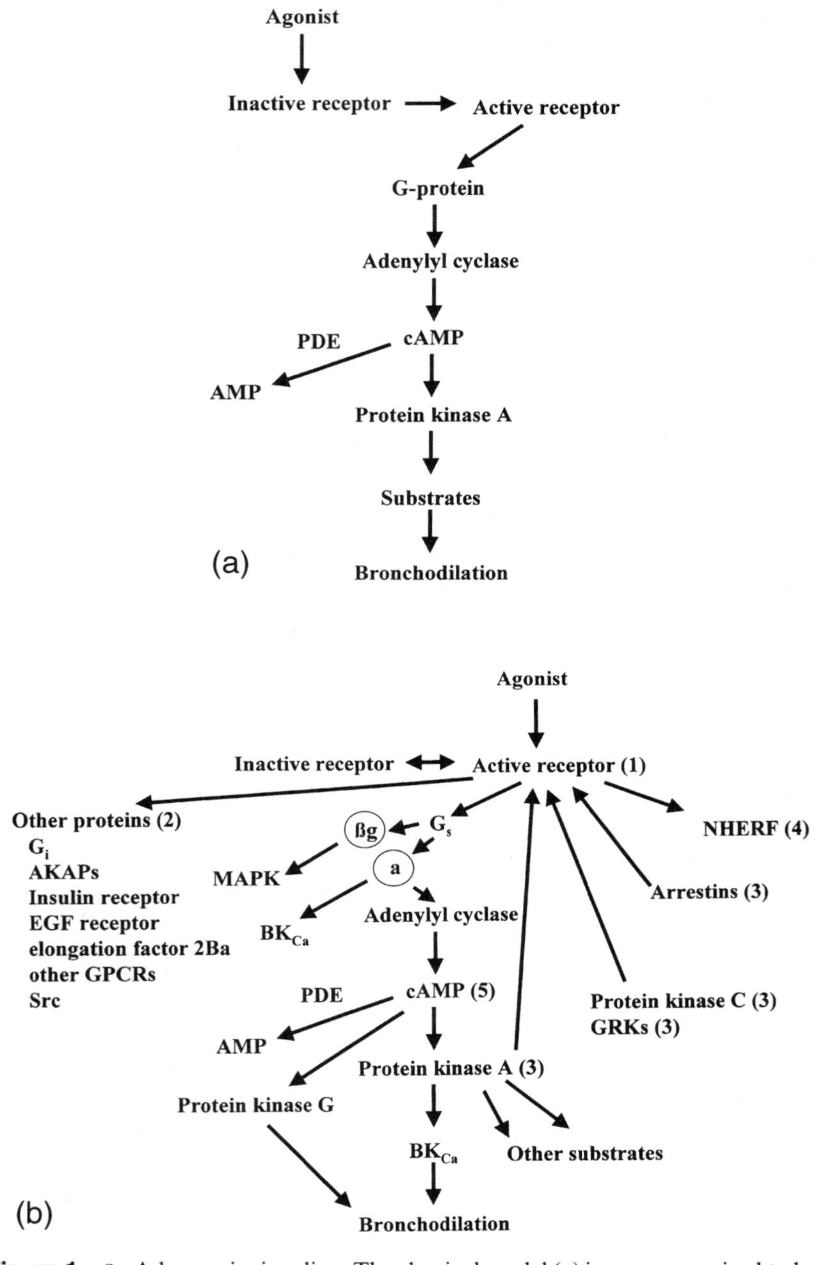

Figure 1 β_2-Adrenergic signaling. The classical model (a) is now recognized to be an oversimplification at every step. The complexity of β-receptor signaling can both lead to subtle biological effects and create interesting opportunities for therapeutic intervention (b). Some of the key differences from the classical pathway are specified below and discussed in the text. (Also see Refs. 4, 7, 11, 18, and 96 for reviews.)

(1) Receptor activation is no longer thought to be a simple agonist-induced switch from inactive to active. Rather, the receptor is believed to exist in an equilibrium between inactive and active states that are stabilized by agonist. There are, moreover, likely multiple active states that permit the receptor to interact with multiple signaling pathways. There are several clinical implications of this model. First, not all ligands will necessarily have the same effects, as they may stabilize different conformations of the receptor. This may account for the clinical observation that some patients seem to respond better to one β-agonist than to others. Second, a certain fraction of the receptors can be spontaneously active. This may account for the biological changes that are observed with a small reduction in receptor number even though only a very small number of receptors are needed for maximal agonist-induced signaling.

(2) The β-receptor not only can couple to G_s, but also can interact with several other proteins. These can have a variety of signaling functions and provide cross-talk with other pathways. This can lead to agonist-induced transactivation of the EGF receptor and can potentiate the actions of the insulin receptor, interactions which may depend on receptor phosphorylation at specific sites on the β-receptor. It is possible that different activated states of the receptor have different signaling functions.

(3) Several proteins can regulate β-receptor activity. In the activated state, the β-receptor becomes a substrate for G-protein receptor kinases (GRKs). GRK-2 phosphorylates specific receptors on the β-receptor, which then permit the binding of arrestins 2 and 3. Both arrestins equally desensitize the receptor, that is, prevent activation of G_s. Arrestin 3 is much more active in promoting internalization of the receptor, where it may be degraded or recycled. Arrestin binding can, moreover, stabilize the receptor in an active conformation and can lead to binding to tyrosine kinases including Src family members. Consistent with the model of multiple receptor conformations, agonists may differ in their ability to induce activation of G_s and to permit GRK phosphorylation. This creates a possibility for development of therapeutic compounds with further degrees of selectivity.

Protein kinase A can also phosphorylate the β-receptor. This has several important effects. First, it decreases the ability of the β-receptor to activate G_s, and thus desenstitizes the receptor. Second, it allows the β-receptor to activate G_i, a G protein which inhibits adenylyl cyclase, an effect which could further limit cAMP-mediated signaling. G_i, moreover, can also initiate signaling through other pathways, including the MAPK pathways. Protein kinase C can also phosphorylate the β-receptor, leading to desensitization. Protein phosphotase 2B can dephosphorylate the receptor, restoring activity. Finally, the β-receptor can bind to A kinase-anchoring proteins (AKAPs), structural proteins which can assemble complexes of kinases and their substrates, thus facilitating their interactions.

(4) Agonist binding also allows the β-receptor to interact with Na/H exchanger regulatory factor (NHERF), a regulatory molecule which inhibits Na/H exchange mediated by Na/H exchanger 3. By virtue of this action, intracellular calcium levels may be reduced and smooth muscle relaxation can be induced.

(5) Once formed, cAMP can activate several signaling mechanisms. In addition to protein kinase A, of which there are two forms, cAMP can activate ePAC. cAMP can, moreover, also activate protein kinase G, an action which can also lead to relaxation of smooth muscle.

addition, $G_s\alpha$ can also bind and activate BK_{Ca} [11]. Finally, the β-receptor can alter Na/H exchange directly, and, by this action, can alter intracellular calcium. A major role for cAMP-independent relaxation of airway smooth muscle in response to β-agonists has been suggested by in-vitro studies [19]. It is likely that more than one pathway contributes to the clinically effective smooth muscle relaxation observed in response to the administration of β-agonists.

These advances in the understanding of the mechanisms of action of β-agonists have several implications for the clinician. The development of β-agonists with long duration of action (see below) permit dosing on a less frequent basis. It is likely, however, that the clinical effects of these agents, which have the potential to cause sustained increases in cAMP, may differ in important ways from the shorter-acting agents. It should not be assumed, therefore, that more frequent dosing with shorter-acting agents is "equivalent" to use of longer-acting agents.

The number of potential mechanisms by which β-agonists can interact with other therapeutic agents in COPD, including phosphodiesterase inhibitors and anticholinergics, make synergistic, or at least "collaborative" interactions likely. Again, the clinical effects of such combination therapy will need to be assessed empirically. Finally, while currently used primarily as bronchodilators, β-agonists have considerable potential to exert additional effects of potential benefit to the COPD patient, either alone or in combination with other therapeutic agents. It seems plausible that the popularity of β-agonists among patients derives, at least in part, from such nonbronchodilator effects.

The β-adrenergic receptors are present not only on airway smooth muscle cells but on most cells. A series of in-vitro and in-vivo studies have demonstrated several biological effects which may be relevant to patients with COPD (Table 1) [20,21]. Among these, β-agonists inhibit several aspects of inflammatory cell recruitment and activation, which could have an anti-inflammatory effect. In this context, cAMP can decrease neutrophil expression of the adhesion molecule Mac1 [22]. Both salmeterol and formoterol inhibit adhesion of neutrophils to endothelial cells [23,24]. Expression of this receptor is required for interaction between neutrophils and endothelial cells and for subsequent neutrophil migration into tissue. Formoterol has been reported to inhibit neutrophil chemotaxis directly [25]. Consistent with these observations, β-adrenergic agonists have been reported to decrease neutrophil accumulation in subjects with asthma [26]. Salmeterol, but not short-acting β-adrenergic agonists, also appears to reduce neutrophil activation, as evidenced by reduced oxidant production [27] and release of IL-8 [28]. Interestingly, these effects of salmeterol were not blocked by the β-blocker propranolol. Moreover, while cAMP can have similar effects on neutrophil

Table 1 Non-bronchodilator Effects of β-Agonists of Potential Benefit in COPD

Anti-inflammatory
Neutrophil
Monocyte
Lymphocyte
Mast cell
Eosinophil
Inhibition of mediator release
Edema resolution
Airway epithelial
Cilia beating
Mucociliary clearance
Secretions
Cytoprotective
Augmented repair
Augmented skeletal muscle function
Inhibited remodeling
Smooth muscle hyperthrophy
Fibrosis
Contraction

activation, the activity of salmeterol did not parallel its cAMP-stimulating activity and was not blocked by the β-blocker propanolol [29]. This suggests that the antineutrophil actions of salmeterol may be mediated through a different receptor or through the β-receptor via one of the novel mechanisms discussed above (see Fig. 1). Finally, cAMP promotes neutrophil apoptosis, as does salmeterol [30], and thus β-agonists have the potential for accelerating neutrophil clearance. To what degree β-agonists affect neutrophil recruitment and activation in COPD patients is unknown.

The β-agonists have been evaluated on other cell types [21]. They seem to have an inhibitory action on both eosinophil and mast cell activation and mediator release. Lymphocytes and monocytes contain β-receptors, and β-agonists have been reported to have inhibitory actions on both cell types. Thus, β-agonists decrease monocyte release of TNF-α, IL-8, GMCSF, IL-1β, and Il-2 [21,31]. Similarly, reductions in lymphocyte release of TNF-α, IL-2, GMCSF, IL-3, IL-4, and IL-5 have also been reported [21,32]. In contrast to monocytes, macrophages express fewer β-receptors and are less sensitive to β-agonists. The effect of β-agonists on these functions in vivo has been evaluated in several relatively small studies in asthmatics. While some reduction in lymphocyte activation markers has been reported, these results have not been uniformly observed [33–35]. Evaluations of potential anti-inflammatory effects of β-agonists have not been reported in vivo in patients with COPD.

Airway epithelial cells express β-adrenergic receptors, and the demonstrable effects of β-agonists on epithelial cells may have clinical relevance. Ciliary beating frequency [36] and mucociliary clearance [37] are increased by β-agonists. They may also modify the damage resulting from bacterial products. In this context, salmeterol attenuated the bacterial damage induced both by *Haemophilus influenzae* [38] and the *Pseudomonas aeruginosa* toxins pyocyanin and elastase [39] in in-vitro models. β-Agonists can also accelerate the ability of epithelial cells to repair a defect in vitro [40]. Whether similar actions occur in vivo is unknown. However, such actions may protect the airway in the presence of bacterial colonization as well as accelerate restoration of epithelial integrity and function following cell damage. Such effects may be important in COPD patients, who often are chronically colonized with bacteria. Interestingly, β-agonist actions on epithelial cells may also be pro-inflammatory. Formoterol, for example, has been demonstrated to increase IL-8 secretion of cultures of human airway epithelial cells [41]. The clinical relevance of these observations remains unknown.

The β-agonists can also affect edema. In a nasal allergen challenge model, salmeterol reduced vascular leak [42]. Similarly, salmeterol accelerated the clearance of albumin from the lower respiratory tract in a sheep model of pulmonary edema [43], and terbutaline accelerated fluid resorption from human airways in vitro [44]. Finally, salmeterol reduced the severity of high-altitude pulmonary edema in a group of susceptible individuals who ascended rapidly to altitude [45]. Edema is believed to play an important role in the inflamed airway in COPD. To what degree β-agonist-induced resolution of edema contributes to therapeutic benefit has not been directly assessed.

The β-agonists can also affect the structural elements in the lung. In this context, both smooth muscle cells and fibroblasts are potential sources of inflammatory mediators, the production of which can be inhibited by β-agonists [46]. Airway structure may also be affected by β-agonist action on mesenchymal cells. In addition, cAMP has an inhibitory effect on both smooth muscle and fibroblast proliferation and on fibroblast recruitment and matrix production [47]. Isoproterenol can inhibit fibroblast collagen production [48], and salmeterol can attenuate thrombin-induced smooth muscle proliferation [49], although the latter may be independent of the β-receptor. In addition, β-agonists can inhibit the ability of fibroblasts to contract extracellular collagenous matrices [50].

The small airways are a major site of airflow limitation in COPD, particularly in patients with moderately severe disease. The pathology of airways is characterized by the accumulation of fibroblasts and myofibroblasts together with the collagenous extracellular matrix produced by these cells. These fibrotic airways are contracted and narrowed. By inhibiting these detrimental remodeling processes, β-agonists have the potential to alter the architectural changes that contribute to progressive airflow limitation in COPD and perhaps alter the natural history of the disorder.

Taken together, the large and growing body of literature demonstrates that β-agonists have a number of actions that may benefit patients with COPD. Of these, improvement in airflow over the short time frame is most likely due to acute relaxation of airway smooth muscle. Other effects, however, are entirely plausible. Their effective evaluation is likely to require new paradigms for the assessment of the COPD patient. Despite the lack of consensus on how best to make such assessments, clinical evidence supports the concept that such beneficial effects actually may occur.

III. Clinical Response

A large number of β-agonist bronchodilators have been developed (Table 2). Two major classes of β-agonists are currently available, which differ in their duration of action. The short-acting β-agonists, when administered by inhalation, generally have an onset of action of 5 min, reaching a peak in 30 min. Their activity has largely waned by 2–4 hr. Long-acting β-agonists (LABAs), in contrast, have duration of action of at least 12 hr. Two agents are currently available. Formoterol is believed to achieve its long duration of action by its lipophilic property [51]. As a result, it binds into the cell membrane and resides there as a depot. The drug can then diffuse from the cell membrane into the aqueous environment and interact with the receptor in a manner similar to that of the short-acting β-agonists. Its onset of action is similar to that of albuterol, beginning within 5 min [52]. In contrast, salmeterol achieves its long duration of action by a different mechanism. It is also lipophilic but, after binding into the membrane, the tail of the salmeterol molecule interacts with a specific site on the receptor, amino acids 149–158 [53]. Binding at this site is not believed to activate the receptor, but it allows salmeterol to serve as a tethered ligand. The saligenin head of the molecule can then interact repeatedly with the agonist-binding site, resulting in receptor activation. Salmeterol has an onset of action distinctly slower than that of short-acting β-agonists, commencing after 30 min and achieving a peak at 2 hr. Like formoterol, its duration of action is at least 12 hr, making both of the LABAs appropriate for twice-daily dosing.

The short-acting β-agonists that have been evaluated do show reduced effectiveness with continued use [54]. This is particularly true in asthma, where an increase in bronchial responsiveness has been associated with

Table 2 Selected Formulations of β-Agonist Bronchodilators

Agonist	Selectivity	Formulations	Comment
Epinephrine	α and all β's	IV, nebulized,[a] MDI	
Isoproterenol	all β's		Not currently available in USA
Albuterol	β_2	Nebulizer solution, MDI, oral[b]	Also available in an MDI in combination with ipratropium
Levalbuterol	β_2	Nebulizer solution	
Metaproterenol	β_2	MDI, nebulizer solution, oral	
Pirbuterol	β_2	MDI[c]	
Salmeterol	β_2	MDI, DPI	Long-acting; also available in a DPI in combination with fluticasone
Formoterol	β_2	DPI	Long-acting; also available in some countries in combination with budesonide

MDI = metered-dose inhaler; DPI = dry-powder inhaler.
[a] The IV formulation has been administered via nebulizer following dilution.
[b] Delayed-release oral formulations provide a "long-acting" preparation.
[c] Available in a self-actuated MDI.

continued use of the compounds. For albuterol, which, like most β-agonists, is chiral, the bronchodilator effect is due to the levo-isomer [55]. The s-isomer, in contrast, has been suggested to contribute to toxicity, induce airway inflammation, and contribute to reduced effectiveness with time [56]. A new preparation containing only the d-isomer is an effective bronchodilator [55] in asthmatics but has not been evaluated in COPD. Short-acting β-agonists retain effectiveness with regular chronic use in COPD patients, but there is a slight but demonstrable decrease in bronchodilator effect [3]. This has not been reported for either of the long-acting β-agonists [52,57]. The reasons why LABAs should not demonstrate tachyphyllaxis are unclear. One possibility for salmeterol is that it is only a partial agonist. Other possibilities include differences in the time course of cAMP activation or other biological effects initiated by LABAs.

As noted above, the β-adrenergic agonists are clinically effective bronchodilators in the majority of COPD patients [2,3]. In this context, the "resting" smooth muscle tone likely contributes to improved airflow. The response in COPD patients is similar to that of normal individuals, namely, a somewhat modest bronchodilator response after the admistration of the β-adrenergic agonists. This contrasts markedly with the response in asthma, where airway tone may be markedly increased and β-agonists can have very large effects on airflow.

There are several reasons why COPD patients may benefit by the modest improvement in airflow that results from β-agonists. First, while a normal individual experiencing a 200-mL improvement in FEV_1 on top of a normal lung function of several liters may have no noticeable effect, a similar improvement in a COPD patient with a baseline FEV_1 of 1 L would represent a large improvement over baseline. Such an effect may be readily noticeable and of clinical significance for a patient with clinically important airflow limitation. Bronchodilators may also improve lung emptying, resulting in reduced lung volumes [58]. Reductions in residual volume generally exceed the reduction in total lung capacity, thus vital capacity increases. Reduction in end expiratory lung volume decreases inspiratory work and is associated with reduced dyspnea. In this context, reduction in end expiratory lung volume following β-agonist bronchodilators is better correlated with improved dyspnea than is improved airflow measured as FEV_1 [59]. Finally, dyspnea for the COPD patient is most severe with exertion. The increased respiratory rate associated with exertion results in dynamic hyperinflation, and it is this process which is believed to be the main cause of dyspnea in COPD patients [60]. Even modest improvements in airflow can have important effects on dynamic hyperinflation and hence on dyspnea and exercise tolerance [59,61].

When compared to the anticholinergic ipratropium, β-agonists, in general, have an equal or superior effect on the FEV_1. Ipratropium, however, has a relatively greater effect on the vital capacity [3,57]. The similarity of response to both β-agonists and anticholinergics has raised the question of whether maximal bronchodilatation can be achieved with a single bronchodilator or whether combinations can achieve more than individual components [62]. Several studies have used a sequential design in which β-agonist and anticholinergic bronchodilators, with or without dose escalation, were given [63]. These studies have reported that maximal bronchodilatation can be achieved with a single agent. However, these studies have been limited by small size and, in some cases, by the evaluation of patients during acute exacerbations, when the maximal bronchodilatation is reduced by the acute effect of the episode.

Studies using drugs in combination have demonstrated superior bronchodilatation with both short- [64] and long-acting [65,66] β-agonist bronchodilators. Most of the available studies, however, have used the

FDA-indicated dose of ipratropium, 2 puffs (36 μg), which is likely to be suboptimal in some subjects [63,67]. While some controversy exists about the benefit of β-agonists in combination with anticholinergics, their combined use is common clinical practice and is recommended by current guidelines. A study by Van Noord and co-workers compared salmeterol administered together with either a placebo or with ipratropium. Interestingly, even after 10 hr following the administration of drug, the combination was superior to salmeterol alone [65]. At this time point, no residual bronchodilator effect of the ipratropium would be expected. Persistent superiority of the combination is consistent with the concept of a synergistic action. The additive effect of the long-acting β-agonists and the long-acting anticholinergic tiotropium remain to be assessed.

The β-agonist bronchodilators can also be combined with theophylline. As β-agonists increase cAMP, and theophylline, among its other effects, may prevent its breakdown, a synergistic effect is likely. Indeed, both SABAs [68] and salmeterol [69] induce more effective broncodilatation when combined with theophylline. Data on formoterol are not available. One study has evaluated albuterol and ipratropium together in combination with theophylline or placebo and has demonstrated benefit from the triple combination [70]. Studies such as these have not yet been performed with the selective phosphodiesterase inhibitors currently under clinical development.

The role of glucocorticosteroids in COPD has been a controversial issue [71,72]. Several recent reports indicate that glucocorticosteroids can result in modest increases in airflow and may also reduce exacerbation frequency [73,74], thus accounting for a beneficial effect on health status [75]. Inhaled glucocorticoids have also been assessed in combination with long-acting β-agonist bronchodilators. Both budesonide combined with formoterol [76] and fluticasone in combination with salmeterol [77] have been assessed. Both have demonstrated greater clinical benefits than the individual components used alone. Because of the possibility for synergistic interactions between β-agonists and glucocorticoids, these combinations have attracted considerable attention. Because combined formulations are currently marketed, these agents have proved very popular in clinical practice.

IV. Adverse Effects of β-Agonists

Pharmacologically based adverse effects of β-agonists include palpitations, tachycardia, tremor, hypokalemia, and worsening ventilation-perfusion (V/Q) matching [54]. The cardiac effects are partially due to β_2-receptors located in the heart, and cannot be completely prevented by selective agonists. By relaxing vascular smooth muscle, V/Q matching may actually worsen. This has been associated with worsened oxygenation in acutely ill COPD patients [78]. This is not regarded as a major clinical problem because the small effect can be compensated with the administration of supplemental oxygen. Compared to clinically indicated doses, increasing the dose of LABAs has been associated with a reduction in exercise performance in a study with formoterol [79] and with a reduction in health status in a study with salmeterol [80]. The mechanisms for these effects are undefined.

V. Clinical Assessment of the COPD Patient

The most common measure of disease severity in COPD has been airflow assessed by FEV_1 [1]. This measure has been the primary endpoint for all clinical trials evaluating bronchodilator therapy in COPD. However, it has become clear in recent years that the FEV_1 correlates relatively poorly with other clinical features of COPD [81]. Indeed, symptomatic response may occur when improvement in FEV_1 is very modest. For these reasons, more recent clinical trials have begun to assess a number of additional clinical outcomes of importance to patients with COPD. Prominent among these are symptoms, especially dyspnea, exercise performance, health status (sometimes termed "quality of life" when referring to an individual subject), exacerbations, and health care resource utilization. Because of their relatively recent routine use in clinical trials, more data are available assessing these parameters for the recently introduced LABAs. However, there is no established consensus on the best methods to assess these parameters. Nevertheless, while the clinical studies available vary somewhat in their results, a general pattern is emerging.

VI. Effect on Dyspnea

Both SABAs [82] and LABAs [52,57,83] are associated with improved symptoms, particularly dyspnea. As noted above, the "responsiveness" of COPD patients has generated considerable controversy. Exclusion of patients who responded to β-agonists was felt by some investigators and regulatory agencies to be important to exclude asthmatics. Using an approach consistent with the recent GOLD definition of COPD, in which some degree of reversibility is expected [1], several clinical trials have evaluated subjects as a function of reversibility [57,83]. The population of COPD patients is unimodally distributed, suggesting that the classification of "reversible" and "irreversible" is arbitrary. Those individuals who reversed more generally show greater improvement with treatment. However, those who reverse less also show clinical benefit. As noted above, these benefits may be due to reduced hyperinflation not clearly reflected by the FEV_1 improvement. Reversibility testing, therefore, should not be used to determine who should receive β-agonist treatment, though it may guide the clinician by helping to define the expected clinical response.

VII. Effect on Exercise

Improvement in exercise endurance following β-agonist bronchodilator treatment has been reported in several trials [59,79,84]. However, while acute treadmill tests using constant workload in laboratories have shown improvement in small numbers of subjects, larger studies evaluating walking distance have failed to do the same [57,83,85,86]. This raises the interesting possibility that bronchodilators can improve the functional capacity of the lungs, but that performance may depend on other factors as well. Some of these include peripheral muscle and cardiovascular function. More information is needed before the final mechanism underlying this discrepancy can be elucidated.

VIII. Quality of Life

Health status assessed using disease specific questionnaires such as the St. George's Respiratory Questionnaire or the Chronic Respiratory Disease Questonnaire improves following treatment with both SABAs [82] and LABAs [57,80,83,85,86]. This important outcome is of great value to assess in large populations the true significance of the physiological changes that may be modest in absolute terms.

IX. Exacerbations

Exacerbations have recently received considerable attention. They are a major source of health care expenditures and have a major adverse effect on health status [87]. While one study has demonstrated a reduced time to first exacerbation following salmeterol, another did not [57,83]. Again, while statistically significant results were not observed in most trials, the trend has been for treatment with LABAs to reduce exacerbations [86]. Interestingly, this does not appear to be an effect associated with SABAs [88].

The magnitude of the effects noted above varies among studies. The trends, however, are generally in favor of a benefit in favor of β-agonist treatment. Meta-analyses assessing these parameters pose some problems, as the measures and definitions used vary among studies. Nevertheless, the pattern emerges that the COPD patient can derive considerable clinical benefit from β-agonist bronchodilator therapy, and that these benefits may take multiple forms.

X. Use of β-Agonist Bronchodilators in Clinical Practice

As noted above, the majority of patients with COPD demonstrate a response to β-agonist bronchodilators. Simple prescription of β-agonist bronchodilators, however, is unlikely to result in optimal clinical benefit. In this regard, it is essential to understand how the COPD patient adjusts to physiological limitation and disability.

Airflow limitation in COPD patients develops insidiously over many years [89]. Dyspnea is generally worse with increasing respiratory rate, particularly with exertion. As a result, most COPD patients decrease their level of activity [90]. This can result in an extraordinarily sedentary existence. During early stages of the illness, COPD patients may attribute their developing dyspnea to their smoking or to aging. Even when severely disabled, COPD patients have often reset their expectations so that there is little anticipation of improvement with treatment [90]. This makes clinical assessment of the individual COPD patient difficult. Simply asking "How are you doing?" is unlikely to provide much insight.

Similarly, administering a medication that results in significant physiological improvement may be of no perceptible benefit for an individual who has a completely sedentary existence. Thus, integration of bronchodilator therapy into a complete management program, including rehabilitation, is essential. A rehabilitation program can have dramatic effects on performance and on health status without having any effect on physiological functioning [91,92]. The β-agonist bronchodilators, which have little effect on walking distance by themselves, by improving the sensation of dyspnea following exercise could improve adherence to a rehabiliation program. Evidence suggests that a combined approach, which includes optimizing physiological functioning and then implementing the most aggressive rehabilitation program possible, can achieve optimum clinical results [93]. Such an approach may be appropriate even in milder stages of the disease [1].

According to most guidelines, as needed (prn) short-acting bronchodilators are recommended for the "rescue" of patients with COPD [1]. However, acute episodes of dyspnea result not from changes in lung function, but rather from changes in respiratory rate. For this reason, and in marked contrast to the strategy used in asthma, regular bronchodilator therapy to optimize physiological functioning should be the hallmark of symptomatic management of COPD patients [1]. Such a strategy is appropriate not only for patients with severe end-stage disease, but also for patients with milder disease who are only symptomatic with exercise.

For patients taking regular bronchodilators, long-acting formulations have the obvious advantage of convenience. Twice-daily dosing is considerably more acceptable to patients than dosing four to six times daily. In addition, the long-acting β-agonist bronchodilators provide steady bronchodilatation throughout the day, avoiding the peaks and troughs associated with shorter-acting agents. Several of the short-acting β-agonist bronchodilators are available in oral, slow-release formulations. Such preparations are also "long-acting," but this is a function of the formulation rather than of the pharmacology of the agent.

Oral formulations may be useful in selected patients who have difficulty with inhaled medications, but they have much greater systemic effects. In general, this is associated with adverse effects of β-agonists, particularly tremor and palpitations. As a result, the inhaled route is preferred [1]. On the other hand, the possibility of beneficial systemic effects, for example, on skeletal muscle, suggests a theoretical advantage for systemic administration.

Several formulations for inhaled use are available. Self-contained devices, including both pressurized metered-dose inhalers and dry-powder inhalers, are most widely used. The general consensus is that dry-powder inhalers are easier to use since the current generation of metered-dose inhalers delivers the drug in a high-velocity jet, requiring considerable patient coordination for effective administration [94,95]. Preparations of short-acting β-agonist bronchodilators are also available for administration as nebulized solutions. This route of administration may be beneficial for individuals with very low inhaled airflows. Many patients seem to prefer the slow administration of a bronchodilator using a face mask. In addition, in the United States, nebulized solutions are often fully covered by insurance, while other forms of inhaled medications are not. Thus, despite the fact that the nebulizer equipment requires cleaning and maintenance, some patients prefer nebulizers over the metered-dose inhalers.

XI. Summary

The β-agonist bronchodilators have been among the mainstays in the treatment of the COPD patient for decades. Recent understanding of the β-receptor and its signaling mechanisms suggest that newer generations of drugs will be available with improved clinical utility. Moreover, recent understanding of the multiple effects of β-agonists suggest that clinical benefits go well beyond simple bronchodilatation. Effective treatment of the COPD patient requires a comprehensive approach with both pharmacological and nonpharmacological interventions. However, β-agonist bronchodilators remain key components in this comprehensive management program.

References

1. Pauwels RA, et al. Global strategy for the diagnosis, management, and prevention of chronic obstructive pulmonary disease. NHLBI/WHO Global Initiative for Chronic Obstructive Lung Disease (GOLD) Workshop summary. Am J Respir Crit Care Med 2001; 163(5):1256–1276.
2. Anthonisen NR, Wright E. Bronchodilator response in chronic obstructive pulmonary disease. Am Rev Respir Dis 1986; 133:814–819.
3. Rennard SI, et al. Extended therapy with ipratropium is associated with improved lung function in COPD: a retrospective analysis of data from seven clinical trials. Chest 1996; 110:62–70.
4. Hoffman BB. Catecholamines, sympathomimetic drugs, and adrenergic receptor antagonists. In: Hardman JG, Limbird LE, eds. Goodman and Gilman's The Pharmacologic Basis of Therapeutics. New York: McGraw-Hill, 1996:215–268.
5. Shabalina I, et al. Uncoupling protein-1: involvement in a novel pathway for beta-adrenergic, cAMP-mediated intestinal relaxation. Am J Physiol Gastrointest Liver Physiol 2002; 283(5):G1107–G1116.
6. Ricart-Firinga C, et al. Effects of beta(2)-agonist clenbuterol on biochemical and contractile properties of unloaded soleus fibers of rat. Am J Physiol Cell Physiol 2000; 278(3):C582–C588.
7. Liggett SB. Update on current concepts of the molecular basis of beta2-adrenergic receptor signaling. J Allergy Clin Immunol 2002; 110(suppl 6):S223–S228.
8. Davies AO, Lefkowitz RJ. Regulation of beta-adrenergic receptors by steroid hormones. Annu Rev Physiol 1984; 46:119–130.
9. Adcock IM, Maneechotesuwan K, Usmani O. Molecular interactions between glucocorticoids and long-acting beta2-agonists. J Allergy Clin Immunol 2002; 110(suppl 6):S261–S268.
10. Tseng YT, et al. Molecular interactions between glucocorticoid and catecholamine signaling pathways. J Allergy Clin Immunol 2002; 110(suppl 6):S247–S254.
11. Benovic JL. Novel beta2-adrenergic receptor signaling pathways. J Allergy Clin Immunol 2002; 110(6 suppl):S229–S235.
12. Essayan DM. Cyclic nucleotide phosphodiesterases. J Allergy Clin Immunol 2001; 108:671–680.
13. Houslay MD. Crosstalk: a pivotal role for protein kinase C in modulating relationships between signal transduction pathways. Eur J Biochem 1991; 195(1):9–27.
14. Abdel-Latif AA. Cross talk between cyclic AMP and the polyphosphoinositide signaling cascade in iris sphincter and other nonvascular smooth muscle. Proc Soc Exp Biol Med 1996; 211(2):163–177.

15. Roffel AF, Meurs H, Zaagsma J. Muscarinic receptors and the lung: relevance to chronic obstructive pulmonary disease and asthma. In: Barnes PJ, Buist AS, eds.The Role of Anticholinergics in Chronic Obstructive Pulmonary Disease and Chronic Asthma. Cheshire, UK: Gardiner-Caldwell, 1997:92–125.
16. Shore SA. Cytokine regulation of beta-adrenergic responses in airway smooth muscle. J Allergy Clin Immunol 2002; 110(suppl 6):S255–S260.
17. Nogami M, et al. TGF-beta modulates beta-adrenergic receptor number and function in cultured human tracheal smooth muscle cells. Am J Physiol 1994; 266:L187–L191.
18. Torphy TJ. Beta-adrenoceptors, cAMP and airway smooth muscle relaxation: challenges to the dogma. Trends Pharmacol Sci 1994; 15(10):370–374.
19. Spicuzza L, et al. Evidence that the anti-spasmogenic effect of the beta-adrenoceptor agonist, isoprenaline, on guinea-pig trachealis is not mediated by cyclic AMP-dependent protein kinase. Br J Pharmacol 2001; 133(8):1201–1212.
20. Johnson M, Rennard S. Alternative mechanisms for long-acting beta(2)-adrenergic agonists in COPD. Chest 2001; 120(1):258–270.
21. Johnson M. Effects of beta2-agonists on resident and infiltrating inflammatory cells. J Allergy Clin Immunol 2002; 110(suppl 6):S282–S290.
22. Bloemen PGM, et al. Increased cAMP levels in stimulated neutrophils inhibit their adhesion to human bronchial epithelial cells. Am Physiol Soc 1997; 272: 580–587.
23. Bolton PB, Lefevre P, McDonald DM. Salmeterol reduces early- and late-phase plasma leakage and leukocyte adhesion in rat airways. Am J Respir Crit Care Med 1997; 155(4):1428–1435.
24. Bowden JJ, Sulakvelidze I, McDonald DM. Inhibition of neutrophil and eosinophil adhesion to venules of rat trachea by beta 2-adrenergic agonist formoterol. J Appl Physiol 1994; 77(1):397–405.
25. Eda R, Townley RG, Hopp RJ. Effect of terfenadine on human eosinophil and neutrophil chemotactic response and generation of superoxide. Ann Allergy 1994; 73(2):154–160.
26. Ii D, Wang D, Venge P. Comparison of the anti-inflammatory effects of inhaled fluticasone propionate and salmeterol in asthma: a placebo-controlled cross-over study of bronchial biopsies. Eur Respir J 1997; 25:444S.
27. Ottonello L, et al. Inhibitory effect of salmeterol on the respiratory burst of adherent human neutrophils. Clin Exp Immunol 1996; 106:97–102.
28. Ward C, et al. Salmeterol reduces BAL IL-8 levels in asthmatics on low dose inhaled corticosteroids. Eur Respir J 1998; 12:380S.
29. Nials AT, et al. The duration of action of non-beta 2-adrenoceptor mediated responses to salmeterol. Br J Pharmacol 1997; 120(5):961–967.
30. Lee E, Smith J, Robertson T. Salmeterol and inhibitors of phosphodiesterase 4 (PDE-4) induce apoptosis in neutrophils from asthmatics: beta-adrenergic receptor-mediated salmeterol activity and additive effects with PDE4 inhibitors. Am J Respir Cell Mol Biol 1999; 159:A329.
31. Pennings HJ, et al. Salbutamol and salmeterol moedulate cytokine production by peripheral blood monocytes. Eur Respir J 1995; 19:1871.

32. Sekut L, et al. Anti-inflammatory activity of salmeterol: down-regulation of cytokine production. Clin Exp Immunol 1995; 99(3):461–466.
33. Li X, et al. An antiinflammatory effect of salmeterol, a long-acting beta(2) agonist, assessed in airway biopsies and bronchoalveolar lavage in asthma. Am J Respir Crit Care Med 1999; 160(5 pt 1):1493–1499.
34. Orsida BE, et al. Effect of a long-acting beta2-agonist over three months on airway wall vascular remodeling in asthma. Am J Respir Crit Care Med 2001; 164(1):117–121.
35. Sue-Chu M, et al. Bronchial biopsy study in asthmatics treated with low and high dose fluticasone propionate (FP) compared to low dose FP combined with salmeterol. Eur Respir J 1999; 14:1245.
36. Salathe M. Effects of beta-agonists on airway epithelial cells. J Allergy Clin Immunol 2002; 110(suppl 6):S275–S281.
37. Bennett WD. Effect of beta-adrenergic agonists on mucociliary clearance. J Allergy Clin Immunol 2002; 110(suppl 6):S291–S297.
38. Dowling RB, et al. Effect of salmeterol on *Haemophilus influenzae* infection of respiratory mucosa *in vitro*. Eur Respir J 1998; 11(1):86–90.
39. Dowling RB, et al. Effect of salmeterol on *Pseudomonas aeruginosa* infection of respiratory mucosa. Am J Respir Crit Care Med 1997; 155(1):327–336.
40. Puchelle E, Peault B. Human airway xenograft models of epithelial cell regeneration. Respir Res 2000; 1(3):125–128.
41. Korn SH, Jerre A, Brattsand R. Effects of formoterol and budesonide on GM-CSF and IL-8 secretion by triggered human bronchial epithelial cells. Eur Respir J 2001; 17(6):1070–1077.
42. Proud D, et al. Intransal salmeterol inhibits allergen-induced vascular permeability but not mast cell activation or cellular infiltration. Clin Exp Allergy 1998; 28:868–875.
43. Frank JA, et al. Beta-adrenergic agonist therapy accelerates the resolution of hydrostatic pulmonary edema in sheep and rats. J Appl Physiol 2000; 89(4): 1255–1265.
44. Sakuma T, et al. Alveolar fluid clearance in the resected human lung. Am J Respir Crit Care Med 1994; 150(2):305–310.
45. Sartori C, et al. Salmeterol for the prevention of high-altitude pulmonary edema. N Engl J Med 2002; 346(21):1631–1636.
46. Panettieri RA Jr. Airway smooth muscle: an immunomodulatory cell. J Allergy Clin Immunol 2002; 110(suppl 6):S269–S274.
47. Rennard SI. Inflammation and repair processes in chronic obstructive pulmonary disease. Am J Respir Crit Care Med 1999; 160(5 pt 2):S12–S16.
48. Rennard SI, et al. Modulation of fibroblast production of collagen types I and III: effects of PGE1 and isoproterenol. Fed Proc 1981; 40:1813.
49. Harris T, et al. Salmeterol modulates cell proliferation and cyclin D1 protein levels in thrombin-stimulated humn cultured airway smooth muscle cells via an action independent of the β2 adrenoreceptor. Am J Respir Crit Care Med 1999; 159:A530.
50. Mio T, et al. Beta-adrenergic agonists attenuate fibroblast-mediated contraction of released collagen gels. Am J Physiol 1996; 270(5 pt 1):L829–L835.

51. Anderson GP, Linden A, Rabe KF. Why are long-acting beta-adrenoceptor agonists long-acting? Eur Respir J 1994; 7(3):569–578.
52. Friedman M, Della Cioppa G, Kottakis J. Formoterol therapy for chronic obstructive pulmonary disease: a review of the literature. Pharmacotherapy 2002; 22(9):1129–1139.
53. Green SS, et al. Sustained activation of a G protein-coupled receptor bia "anchored" agonist binding. Molecular localization of the salmeterol exosite within the 2-adrenergic receptor. J Biol Chem 1996; 271:24029–24035.
54. Sears MR. Adverse effects of beta-agonists. J Allergy Clin Immunol 2002; 110(6 suppl):S322–S328.
55. Nelson HS. Clinical experience with levalbuterol. J Allergy Clin Immunol 1999; 104(2 pt 2):S77–S84.
56. Cockcroft DW, Swystun VA. Effect of single doses of S-salbutamol, R-salbutamol, racemic salbutamol, and placebo on the airway response to methacholine. Thorax 1997; 52(10):845–848.
57. Rennard SI, et al. Use of a long-acting inhaled beta(2)-adrenergic agonist, salmeterol xinafoate, in patients with chronic obstructive pulmonary disease. Am J Respir Crit Care Med 2001; 163(5):1087–1092.
58. Mahler DA. The effect of inhaled beta2-agonists on clinical outcomes in chronic obstructive pulmonary disease. J Allergy Clin Immunol 2002; 110(6 suppl):S298–S303.
59. Belman MJ, Botnick WC, Shin JW. Inhaled bronchodilators reduce dynamic hyperinflation during exercise in patients with chronic obstructive pulmonary disease. Am J Respir Crit Care Med 1996; 153:967–975.
60. Manning HL, Mahler DA. Pathophysiology of dyspnea. Monaldi Arch Chest Dis 2001; 56(4):325–330.
61. O'Donnell DE, Lam M, Webb KA. Measurement of symptoms, lung hyperinflation, and endurance during exercise in chronic obstructive pulmonary disease. Am J Respir Crit Care Med 1998; 158(5 pt 1):1557–1565.
62. Levy SF. Bronchodilators in COPD. Chest 1991; 99:793–794.
63. Rennard SI. Anticholinergics in combination bronchodilator therapy in COPD. In: Spector SL, ed. Anticholinergic Agents in the Upper and Lower Airways. New York: Marcel Dekker, 1999:119–136.
64. Group, CIAS. In chronic obstructive pulmonary disease, a combination of ipratropium and albuterol is more effective than either agent alone. Chest 1994; 105:1411–1419.
65. van Noord JA, et al. Long-term treatment of chronic obstructive pulmonary disease with salmeterol and the additive effect of ipratropium. Eur Respir J 2000; 15(5):878–885.
66. D'Urzo AD, et al. In patients with COPD, treatment with a combination of formoterol and ipratropium is more effective than a combination of salbutamol and ipratropium: a 3-week, randomized, double-blind, within-patient, multicenter study. Chest 2001; 119(5):1347–1356.
67. Gross NJ, et al. Dose response to ipratropium as a nebulized solution in patients with chronic obstructive pulmonary disease. Am Rev Respir Dis 1989; 139:1188–1191.

68. Taylor DR, et al. The efficacy of orally administered theophylline, inhaled salbutamol, and a combination of the two as chronic therapy in the management of chronic bronchitis with reversible air-flow obstruction. Am Rev Respir Dis 1985; 131:747–751.
69. ZuWallach RL, et al. Salmeterol plus theophylline combination therapy in the treatment of COPD. Chest 2001; 119(6):1661–1670.
70. Nishimura K, et al. The additive effect of theophylline on a high-dose combination of inhaled salbutamol and ipratropium bromide in stable COPD. Chest 1995; 107:718–723.
71. Barnes PJ. Inhaled corticosteroids are not beneficial in chronic obstructive pulmonary disease. Am J Respir Crit Care Med 2000; 161(2 pt 1):342–344. (Discussion 344).
72. Calverley PM. Inhaled corticosteroids are beneficial in chronic obstructive pulmonary disease. Am J Respir Crit Care Med 2000; 161(2 pt 1):341–342. (Discussion 344).
73. Thompson WH, et al. Controlled trial of inhaled fluticasone propionate in moderate to severe COPD. Lung 2002; 180(4):191–201.
74. Paggiaro PL, et al. Multicentre randomised placebo-controlled trial of inhaled fluticasone propionate in patients with chronic obstructive pulmonary disease. Lancet 1998; 351:773–780.
75. Spencer S, et al. Health status deterioration in patients with chronic obstructive pulmonary disease. Am J Respir Crit Care Med 2001; 163(1):122–128.
76. Milanowski J, Nahavedian S, Larus E. Budesonide/formoterol in a single inhaler acts rapidly to improve lung function and relieve symptoms in patients with moderate to severe COPD. Eur Respir J 2002; 20:P1576.
77. Mahler DA, et al. Improvemetns in FEV1 and symptoms in COPD patients following 24 weeks of twice daily treatment with salmeterol 50/fluticasone propionate 50 combination. Am J Respir Crit Care Med 2001; 163:A279.
78. Gross NJ, Bankwala Z. Effects of an anticholinergic bronchodilator on arterial blood gases of hypoxemic patients with chronic obstructive pulmonary disease. Comparison with a beta-adrenergic agent. Am Rev Respir Dis 1987; 136(5): 1091–1094.
79. Liesker JJ, et al. Effects of formoterol (Oxis Turbuhaler) and ipratropium on exercise capacity in patients with COPD. Respir Med 2002; 96(8):559–566.
80. Jones PW, Bosh TK. Quality of life changes in COPD patients treated with salmeterol. Am J Respir Crit Care Med 1997; 155:1283–1289.
81. Jones PW. Issues concerning health-related quality of life in COPD. Chest 1995; 107(suppl 5):187S–193S.
82. Guyatt GH, Townsend M, Pugsley SO, et al. Bronchodilators in chronic air-flow limitation. Am Rev Respir Dis 1987; 135:1069–1074.
83. Mahler DA, et al. Efficacy of salmeterol xinafoate in the treatment of COPD. Chest 1999; 115(4):957–965.
84. Patakas D, et al. Comparison of the effects of salmeterol and ipratropium bromide on exercise performance and breathlessness in patients with stable chronic obstructive pulmonary disease [see comments]. Respir Med 1998; 92(9): 1116–1121.

85. Dahl R, et al. Inhaled formoterol dry powder versus ipratropium bromide in chronic obstructive pulmonary disease. Am J Respir Crit Care Med 2001; 164(5): 778–784.
86. Aalbers R, et al. Formoterol in patients with chronic obstructive pulmonary disease: a randomized, controlled, 3-month trial. Eur Respir J 2002; 19(5):936–943.
87. Seemungal TA, et al. Effect of exacerbation on quality of life in patients with chronic obstructive pulmonary disease. Am J Respir Crit Care Med 1998; 157(5 pt 1):1418–1422.
88. Friedman M, et al. Pharmacoeconomic evaluation of a combination of ipratropium plus albuterol compared with ipratropium alone and albuterol alone in COPD. Chest 1999; 115(3):635–641.
89. Fletcher C, et al. The Natural History of Chronic Bronchitis and Emphysema. New York: Oxford University Press, 1976:1–272.
90. Rennard S, et al. Impact of COPD in North America and Europe in 2000: subjects' perspective of Confronting COPD International Survey. Eur Respir J 2002; 20(4):799–805.
91. Ries AL, et al. Effects of pulmonary rehabilitation of physiologic and psychosocial outcomes in patients with chronic obstructive pulmonary disease. Ann Intern Med 1995; 122:823–832.
92. Lacasse Y, et al. Pulmonary rehabilitation for chronic obstructive pulmonary disease. Cochrane Database Syst Rev 2002(3), CD003793.
93. Weiner P, et al. The cumulative effect of long-acting bronchodilators, exercise, and inspiratory muscle training on the perception of dyspnea in patients with advanced COPD. Chest 2000; 118(3):672–678.
94. van der Palen J, et al. Evaluation of the effectiveness of four different inhalers in patients with chronic obstructive pulmonary disease. Thorax 1995; 50(11): 1183–1187.
95. van Beerendonk I, et al. Assessment of the inhalation technique in outpatients with asthma or chronic obstructive pulmonary disease using a metered-dose inhaler or dry powder device. J Asthma 1998; 35(3):273–279.
96. Hurley JH. Structure, mechanism, and regulation of mammalian adenylyl cyclase. J Biol Chem 1999; 274:7599–7602.

14

Theophylline and Phosphodiesterase Inhibitors in COPD

ALICIA R. ZuWALLACK

Kent County Memorial Hospital
Warwick, and College of Pharmacy
University of Rhode Island
Kingston, Rhode Island, U.S.A.

RICHARD L. ZuWALLACK

St. Francis Hospital and Medical Center
Hartford, and University of Connecticut
School of Medicine
Farmington, Connecticut, U.S.A.

I. Introduction

Naturally occurring plant alkaloids such as theophylline, caffeine, and theobromine, a constituent of chocolate, have been used to treat airway obstruction since the middle of the nineteenth century. Caffeine in the form of strong coffee or tea was used as a remedy for asthma until the early 1900s, when theophylline was first used. Widespread use of theophylline did not occur until the mid-1930s, but it soon became and remained a cornerstone in the treatment of asthma and chronic obstructive pulmonary disease (COPD) until only recently. With the increasing use of inhaled steroids and long-acting β-agonists in asthma, and anticholinergics and long-acting β-agonists in COPD, the use of theophylline is decreasing in industrialized countries. However, this drug remains one of the most frequently prescribed asthma medications in the world [1,2].

Theophylline can be classified by its chemical structure or by one of its known modes of action. The chemical structure of theophylline is 1,3-dimethylxanthine, and it is similar in structure to other naturally occurring methylxanthines such as caffeine and theobromine. As a nonselective inhibitor of the ubiquitous phosphodiesterase enzyme (PDE), theophylline is also classified as a phosphodiesterase inhibitor. However, as the following discussion will point out, it is far from clear how much of the drug's beneficial and detrimental actions are mediated by this pharmacological action.

II. Molecular Mechanisms of Action of Theophylline and Other PDE Inhibitors

Although several mechanisms for the pharmacological effects of theophylline have been proposed, only two occur at therapeutic drug concentrations: nonselective inhibition of phosphodiesterase isoenzymes and nonselective antagonism of adenosine receptors [3]. Other proposed mechanisms of less clear clinical significance include increasing the levels of circulating catecholamines, direct and indirect actions on intracellular calcium concentration, and antagonism of inflammatory mediators such as prostaglandins and tumor necrosis factor-α.

A. Phosphodiesterase Inhibition

The phosphodiesterase enzymes (PDEs) are a family of enzymes that are widely distributed in a variety of tissues. Individual members of this family, or isoenzymes, have unique biological activities. At least 10 genetically distinct isoenzymes have been identified [4,5]. The PDEs all hydrolytically cleave the 3′-phosphoester bond to form inactive 5′-nucleotide products, thus inactivating cyclic AMP and GMP, second messengers that play an important role in the physiological response of certain hormones, neurotransmitters, autacoids, and drugs. This action is depicted in Fig. 1. The main differences among members of this enzyme family are their relative affinities for cyclic AMP and cyclic GMP [4]. Evidence strongly suggests that cyclic AMP and GMP mediate the relaxation of airway smooth muscle through the activation of protein kinase A and protein kinase B. Cyclic AMP also decreases inflammation by inhibiting mast cells, eosinophils, neutrophils, monocytes, and lymphocytes, increasing ciliary beat frequency to improve pulmonary toilet, and decreasing airway smooth muscle mitogenesis [4]. Cyclic GMP has not been shown to have these effects. PDE3, PDE4, PDE7, and PDE5 are the isoenzymes that co-regulate cyclic AMP and cyclic GMP in airway smooth muscle [1,4]. The amount of inhibition of the PDE enzyme system at therapeutic concentrations of theophylline does not appear to explain the extent of the pharmacological effects of the drug [1,6,16,17]. Therefore, the action of theophylline is likely more complex than PDE inhibition alone.

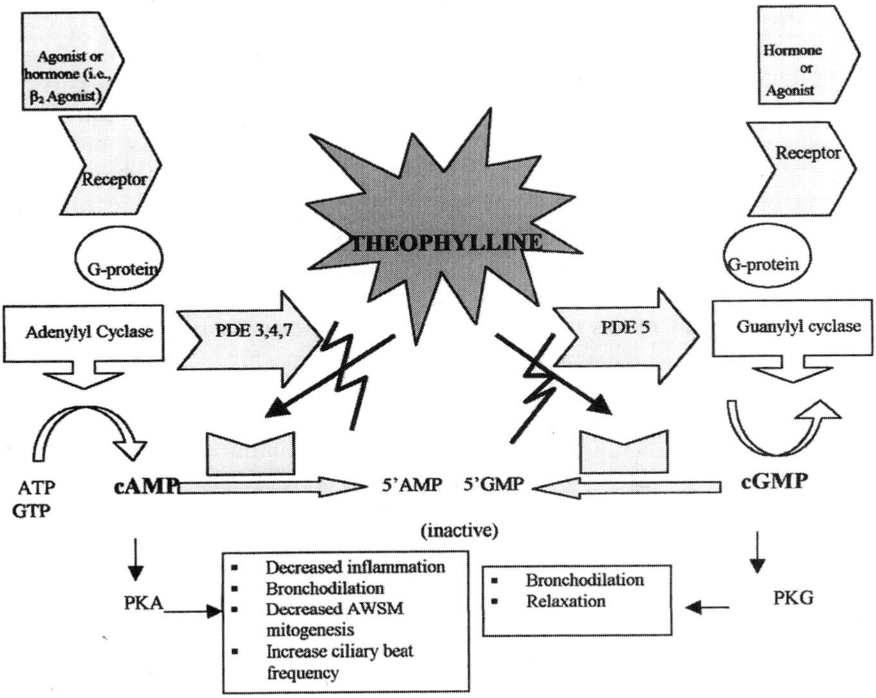

Figure 1 Proposed mechanism of action of theophylline as a nonselective phosphodiesterase inhibitor. PDE, phosphodiesterase; cAMP, cyclic AMP; cGMP, cyclic GTP; PKA, protein kinase; PKG, protein kinase G; AWSM, airway smooth muscle.

B. Adenosine Receptor Antagonism

Adenosine has been shown to cause bronchoconstriction in asthmatic patients when given by inhalation, and theophylline is a potent inhibitor of adenosine receptors at therapeutic concentrations [7,8]. The mechanism of bronchoconstriction is via the release of histamine and leukotrienes from mast cells in the airway. It is unclear if this effect is significant because enprofylline, a methylxanthine that does not antagonize adenosine receptors, is a more potent bronchodilator than theophylline [3,6]. Adenosine antagonism may, however, be responsible for some of the toxicity associated with theophylline, such as arrhythmia, central nervous system stimulation, gastric acid hypersecretion, and diuresis. Caffeine, which may also antagonize adenosine receptors, has a similar side-effect profile.

III. Pharmacological Effects of Theophylline

Although its mechanism of action cannot be fully described by any current theory, it remains that theophylline has many pharmacological effects, both therapeutic and detrimental. A list of some of the respiratory and nonrespiratory potential beneficial effects is given in Table 1. Theophylline is a proven bronchodilator, an effect which may mediate the reduction in trapped-gas volume in COPD. Its beneficial effect on gas exchange, which is modest, is probably due to in large part to bronchodilation and respiratory stimulation [9]. Theophylline reduces pulmonary artery pressure and pulmonary vascular resistance, and increases right and left ventricular systolic function [10].

Although controversy exists [11], it appears that a plasma level of theophylline in the therapeutic range can increase diaphragm muscle contractility following phrenic nerve stimulation in normal subjects [12]. A positive effect of therapeutic levels of this drug on diaphragmatic fatigue in COPD patients is also controversial [11,13,14], and possibly confounded by alterations in blood flow to the respiratory muscles or the recruitment of respiratory muscles with this drug [11]. Theophylline may also improve respiratory muscle efficiency, although the clinical significance of this is uncertain [15].

Table 1 Examples of Beneficial Positive Respiratory and Nonrespiratory Effects of Theophylline and PDE Inhibitors

Respiratory
Bronchodilation [29,31,32,39,42,58–63]
Decrease in static lung volumes [58,62]
Improved gas exchange [28,64,65]
Respiratory stimulation [9]
Increased diaphragm muscle strength and reduced diaphragm fatigue [13]
Improved respiratory muscle efficiency [66]
Increased mucociliary clearance [67,68]
Decreased dyspnea [28,31,38,58,62]
Improved exercise ability [32,58,62,65]
Improved health status [31,32,39]
Reduction in airway inflammation [42]
Nonrespiratory
Improved cardiovascular performance [10]
Decreased pulmonary artery pressure [10]
Diuresis
Caffeine-like central nervous stimulation
Protection from renal insufficiency following intravenous contrast medium [69]

The above-described beneficial effects may explain the modest, dose-dependent improvements in exercise performance and dyspnea. Other potential favorable effects of theophylline are an enhanced mucociliary clearance and an immunomodulator effect, through inhibiting the movement of T-cells from the circulation into the airways, and reduced microvascular leak of plasma into the airways [1,3,16,17]. The anti-inflammatory effect of theophylline in COPD is underscored by a recent study which showed substantial reductions in sputum neutrophils, interleukin-8 concentrations, and neutrophil chemotaxis in patients treated with this drug [18].

The effects of theophylline on sleep are complex. In normal subjects, a 6-mg/kg dose of non-sustained-release theophylline given at nighttime had a clear disruptive effect on sleep, characterized by a delayed sleep onset and increased awakenings [19]. These detrimental effects were not present at night with lower doses. When given during the daytime, the alerting effect of this drug was present even at lower doses. In a double-blind, crossover study of 20 patients with COPD [20], sustained-release theophylline dosed in the evening to a target serum concentration of between 6.7 and 12.0 mg/L was compared to inhaled albuterol given four times daily. There was less of an overnight drop in FEV_1 with theophylline than with albuterol. Of note, the overnight sleep parameters were similar with the two treatments, including total sleep time, time in bed, sleep efficiency, sleep latency, awake time after sleep onset, and the proportion of time spent in each sleep stage. Theophylline use was associated with less time with oxygen saturation levels less than 90%. Thus, although this drug can clearly have negative effects on sleep, sustained-release theophylline dosed conservatively and at night to COPD patients may lead to beneficial effects on nocturnal pulmonary function and oxygen saturation, without significant detrimental effects on sleep quality.

Untoward pharmacological effects of theophylline include nausea, vomiting, irritability, heartburn, tremor, diarrhea, headache, seizures, toxic encephalopathy, hyperthermia, hyperglycemia, hypokalemia, hypotension, and cardiac arrhythmias [1,3,6,16]. Toxicity will be discussed in more depth later in this chapter.

IV. Pharmacokinetics

A basic understanding of the pharmacokinetics of theophylline is important in the clinical application of the drug. Multiple factors can influence the absorption, distribution, metabolism, and elimination of theophylline, including age, hepatic function, diet, concomitant drug use, and disease state itself. Because of the narrow therapeutic range and low toxic index, consideration of pharmacokinetic parameters regarding an individual patient and a specific dosage form of theophylline is crucial.

A. Absorption

Non-sustained-release theophylline is 100% bioavailable after oral administration, and serum concentrations peak at 1–2 hr after a dose [21]. This type of formulation has to be dosed multiple times daily. Now that sustained-release dosage forms are available from generic manufacturers at a low cost, the only rationale for using non-sustained-release theophylline is for patients who cannot swallow tablets or capsules and require a liquid dose form. The mechanism of sustained-release theophylline is a decreased rate of absorption. A variety of products, listed in Table 2, are currently available that increase the absorption time from 6 to 12 hr. Most products also have complete bioavailability as they are absorbed, however as absorption rate increases, it may exceed gastrointestinal transit time, reducing bioavailability [21].

B. Distribution

The apparent volume of distribution (which is the ratio of total amount of drug in the body to the plasma concentration of the drug) is 0.5 L [3,6]. This suggests that the drug is not extensively present in tissues outside the plasma compartment, therefore dose increases are not needed in obese patients, and doses are best calculated using ideal body weight. Distribution follows a two-compartment model, where theophylline initially distributes to the plasma compartment, and then distributes to the second compartment, the airways.

Table 2 Available Dosage Forms of Oral Theophylline

Dosage form	Manufacturer	Time to peak absorption (hr)	Dosing frequency	Notes
Theo-24®	UCB	13	Q 24 H	Contains coated beads of drug designed to dissolve at different times over 24 hr
Uniphyl®	Purdue	7–10	Q 24 H	Tablets may be split at the score, but not crushed or chewed
T-Phyl®	Purdue	6	Q 12 H	
Theolair®	3M	5	Q 8–12 H	Should be taken consistently with regard to meals
Theophylline ER capsules	Inwood	7–10	Q 8–12 H	AB-rated generic of SloBid® (no longer manufactured)
Theophylline ER tablets	Sidmark	8	Q 12–24 H	AB-rated generic of TheoDur® (no longer manufactured)

The toxicities of theophylline occur from concentrations that are too high in the plasma, which result from too high a dose or too rapid administration.

C. Metabolism and Elimination

Theophylline does not undergo first-pass metabolism. Approximately 90% of a dose is metabolized hepatically into several compounds via cytochrome P450 isoenzymes 1A2, 3A3, and 2E1 [3]. Only two metabolites are pharmacologically active: 3-methylxanthine, with approximately 10% of the bronchodilator activity of the parent compound; and caffeine. However, the amount of caffeine found in adults treated with theophylline is negligible.

Cigarette smoking increases theophylline metabolism by 1.5 to 2 times, and dosage may have to be adjusted accordingly. Other conditions that increase metabolism include cystic fibrosis and hyperthyroidism. Congestive heart failure, hypothyroidism, acute febrile illness, hepatic impairment, and severe COPD decrease metabolism. Elimination of the metabolites occurs by urinary excretion. Because only 10% of the dose of theophylline is excreted unchanged, there is no need to adjust the dose in patients with renal impairment. In addition to associated clinical conditions, drugs can also effect the metabolism of theophylline by either inhibiting or inducing its metabolism. A summary of pertinent drug interactions involving theophylline can be found in Table 3.

V. Dosing and Monitoring of Theophylline

When considering an initial dose regimen of theophylline, the clinician must first review the factors that may alter distribution and elimination. Factors that require special consideration include advanced age, concurrent medications, smoking status, concomitant disease states, and weight. Ideally, initial theophylline doses should be dosed based on ideal body weight and rounded to the nearest available strength of theophylline. The initial daily dose should be low, thereby allowing for the patient to develop tolerance to the minor caffeine-like side effects that are common when commencing therapy. The dose can then be carefully titrated to clinical response while monitoring serum concentrations of the drug. Practically, since more rapidly acting inhaled bronchodilators with excellent safety profiles are available as maintenance therapy, there is rarely a need for rapid increments or aggressive dosing of this drug. The theophylline package inserts recommend dosing to serum levels of 10–20 μg/mL. However, it is more reasonable to aim for levels between 10–15 μg/mL. Indeed, some clinical responses may occur at lower, so-called subtherapeutic levels. Dosing for elderly patients, who are at higher risk for toxicity, should be very conservative.

Table 3 Drugs Affecting Theophylline Level

Drugs that increase theophylline levels by inhibiting metabolism	
Ethanol	Interferon
Allopurinol (>600 mg/day)	Isoniazid
β-Blockers	Loop diuretics
Calcium channel blockers	Methotrexate
Carbamazepine	Mexiletine
Cimetidine	Pentoxiphylline
Ciprofloxacin	Propafenone
Corticosteroids	Propranolol
Clarithromycin	Tacrine
Disulfiram	Thiabendazole
Erythromycin	Thyroid hormones
Estrogen & oral contraceptives	Ticlodipine
Fluvoxamine	Troleandomycin
Influenza vaccine	Zileuton
Drugs that decrease theophylline levels by inducing metabolism	
Aminoglutethimide	
Barbiturates	
Carbamazepine	
Isoniazid	
Isoproterenol IV	
Ketoconazole	
Loop diuretics	
Moricizine	
Phenytoin	
Rifampin	
Sulfinpyrazone	
Sympathomimetics	

The clinician initiating theophylline therapy for an adult may consider starting at 300 mg/day of a sustained-release theophylline product given either once daily or divided into two doses. Doses may be adjusted in 150-mg intervals following periods of at least 3 days, based on serum concentration monitoring. Alternately, theophylline may be dosed at 10 mg/kg ideal body weight per day, rounded to the nearest practical dose availability but not to exceed 900 mg daily. For patients who smoke and are less than 50 years old, initial doses may be started higher, at approximately 16 mg/kg per day, whereas patients with cardiac decompensation or liver dysfunction should be started at 5 mg/kg per day (Table 4).

Table 4 Theophylline Dosing for Adults with COPD

	Dose	Comments and dose adjustments
Initial dose[a]	300 mg/day	Increase dose in 3 days if initial dose is tolerated
First increment = 150 mg	450 mg/day	Increase dose in 3 days if initial dose is tolerated and clinical response is not sufficient
Second increment = 150 mg	600 mg/day	Measure level at peak concentration, after at least 3 days
Theophylline level <10 μg/mL		May increase dose by 25%; recheck level in 3 days
Theophylline 10–15 μg/mL		Maintain dose if tolerated; recheck level in 6–12 months[b]
Theophylline 15.1–19.9 μg/mL		Consider reducing dose by 10% after withholding one dose; recheck level in 3 days
Theophylline 20–25 μg/mL		Withhold one dose, resume dose with next lower increment; recheck level in 3 days
Theophylline >25 μg/mL		Withhold next two doses, then resume treatment with initial dose or lower dose; recheck level in 3 days

[a] Single dose or divided into a twice-daily dose of sustained-release theophylline preparation.
[b] Recheck levels sooner if toxicity or inefficacy is suspected, or a change in clearance is anticipated.
Source: Adapted from Weinberger M, Hendeles L. Theophylline in asthma. N Engl J Med 1996; 334:1380–1388.

Monitoring levels is crucial to avoid potentially fatal toxicities. As mentioned above, when initiating therapy or making any changes in therapy, a theophylline serum concentration should be measured after 3 days. Once the dose is adjusted that both manages the patient's symptoms while remaining in the therapeutic range, serum levels need only be monitored every 6–12 months unless toxicity or inefficacy are suspected. Peak levels should generally be obtained for monitoring purposes. A peak level should be drawn approximately 2 hr after an oral dose. If a low level is suspected, a trough level may be drawn immediately prior to the next scheduled dose. Patients should be counseled to alert the health care provider of changes in smoking status, new medications, or changes in health status that might alter theophylline clearance. Patients should ideally use only one pharmacy for medications, due to the high propensity for drug interactions with theophylline. This ensures that screening is occurring for drug interactions, which is especially important for patients with multiple health care providers.

VI. Toxicity

Theophylline has a low toxicity index, meaning the difference between the effective dose and the lethal dose is relatively small. The range of toxicity symptoms is wide and includes everything from mild symptoms of nausea, headache, and nervousness to life-threatening seizures and cardiac arrhythmia. Unfortunately, mild symptoms of toxicity are not a reliable precursor of more serious toxicity, and may not precede seizures or arrhythmia [22]. Theophylline-induced seizures, which often begin as focal in onset and then become generalized, are associated with high mortality [23]. Overdosage of theophylline is often accidental rather than intentional. Patients may increase their dose or wrongly take "as needed" doses for increasing symptoms. Of clinical importance, toxicity associated with chronic ingestion may be more serious and occur at lower serum levels than with intentional acute ingestion. Elderly patients are at especially high risk of serious toxicity, with nearly a 17-fold increase risk of developing life-threatening seizures or arrhythmia than younger individuals, despite similar theophylline levels [24].

The best treatment of theophylline toxicity is prevention. This includes regular serum concentration monitoring, recognition and prevention of drug interactions, and patient education not to self-escalate dosing. Management of patients with acute toxicity includes charcoal administration as well as supportive care. Hemoperfusion or hemodialysis may be considered for levels greater than 100 μg/mL in the acute overdose setting, and for all patients over 60 years of age in the chronic overdose setting [25].

VII. The Effectiveness of Theophylline on Important Outcomes for COPD

The following section summarizes current knowledge the effect of theophylline on pulmonary function, exercise capacity, dyspnea, and health status in COPD. While it may be argued that the bronchodilator effect of this medication could explain its effect on exercise, dyspnea, and health status, theophylline, as a systemic drug, clearly has actions that extend beyond the airways. It is quite conceivable that its nonbronchodilator actions, such as its inotropic effect on respiratory muscles, its respiratory stimulant properties, or its effect on the cardiovascular system, may mediate some of these beneficial effects.

A. Pulmonary Function

Theophylline has been a commonly used medication in asthma and COPD for decades. Its effectiveness as maintenance therapy of asthma is firmly established [26], although newer medications, including inhaled corticosteroids, long-acting β-agonists, and antileukotriene drugs, have evolved as more rational agents for this disease. For COPD, randomized, controlled clinical trials have demonstrated that theophylline is a bronchodilator of moderate effectiveness, with FEV_1 increasing by 10–20% over baseline [27–29]. Variations in the degree of bronchodilation probably relate to differences in duration of therapy, patient selection criteria, and the plasma levels of the drug. There is probably a positive dose–response bronchodilator effect [30], although higher plasma levels would be associated with a greater risk of side effects.

While the bronchodilator effect of theophylline is probably not debatable, whether its clinical use is worth its potential side effects is. However, two recent, large, multicenter controlled trials have provided further insight into the role of theophylline in COPD, both as monotherapy and in combination with other bronchodilators. By comparing the effectiveness and side effects of theophylline to those of more commonly used maintenance inhaled bronchodilators, the relative effectiveness of theophylline can be inferred. In the first study, monotherapy with theophylline, monotherapy with the long-acting inhaled β-agonist salmeterol, and the combination of these two drugs were compared in 1185 patients with COPD [31]. Twenty percent in the theophylline group had to withdraw prior to randomization, mostly because of side effects or failure to achieve a target theophylline level. All three treatments resulted in significant increases in FEV_1. However, the theophylline-salmeterol combination had a greater bronchodilator effect than either given as monotherapy, as depicted in Fig. 2. However, another large randomized trial found that the bronchodilator effect of theophylline, although greater than placebo, was less than the long-acting inhaled β-agonist, formoterol [32]. Again, a higher frequency of adverse events was seen with theophylline than with inhaled β-agonists. These studies, therefore, establish the bronchodilator effectiveness of theophylline, place it close to (although probably less than) that of long-acting β-agonists, and suggest that it may be useful added to maintenance inhaled bronchodilators when warranted by an insufficient clinical response to monotherapy. In both of these studies, however, the high frequency of dropouts because of theophylline side effects underscore the difficulties with this drug.

B. Exercise Capacity

Clinical trials evaluating the effectiveness of theophylline on exercise tolerance have shown mixed results [33]. However, several controlled studies have demonstrated a modest beneficial effect of theophylline in this outcome area [30,34–37]. Improvements, which were generally of modest degree, have

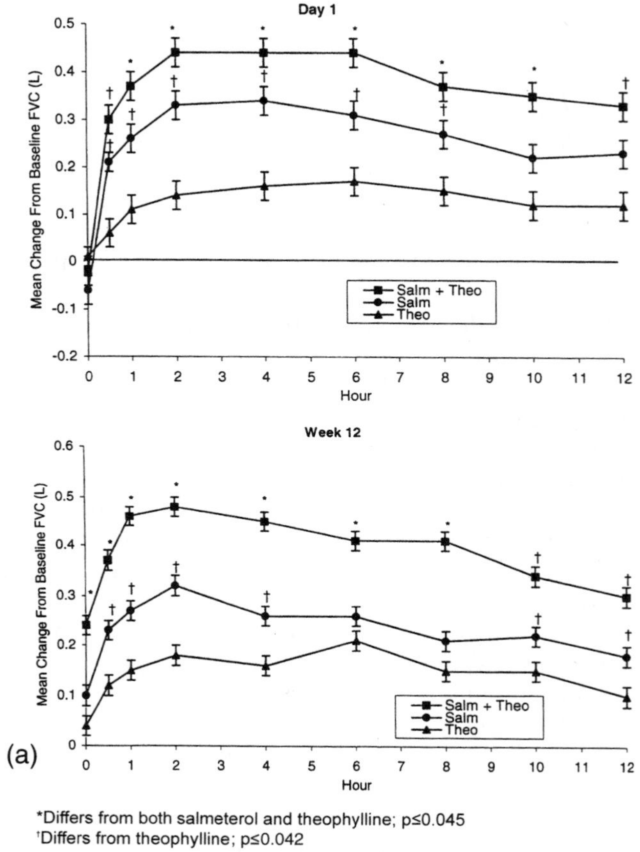

Figure 2 The effect of theophylline, salmeterol, and their combination on serial FEV_1 values and area under the curve for FEV_1 over 12 hr. Twelve-hour serial FEV_1 measurements (a) and area under the curve (b) 12 weeks following randomization to three groups: theophylline titrated to plasma levels between 10 and 20 μg/mL, salmeterol 2 puffs (42 μg) twice daily, or the combination of these bronchodilators. Salmeterol-treated patients had slightly greater FEV_1 values at several time points during serial spirometry than those on theophylline therapy, but the area under the curve representing improvement in this variable for the two groups was similar. The combination of these two bronchodilators was clearly superior in bronchodilator effect than either given as monotherapy. (From Ref. 31, with permission.)

(b)

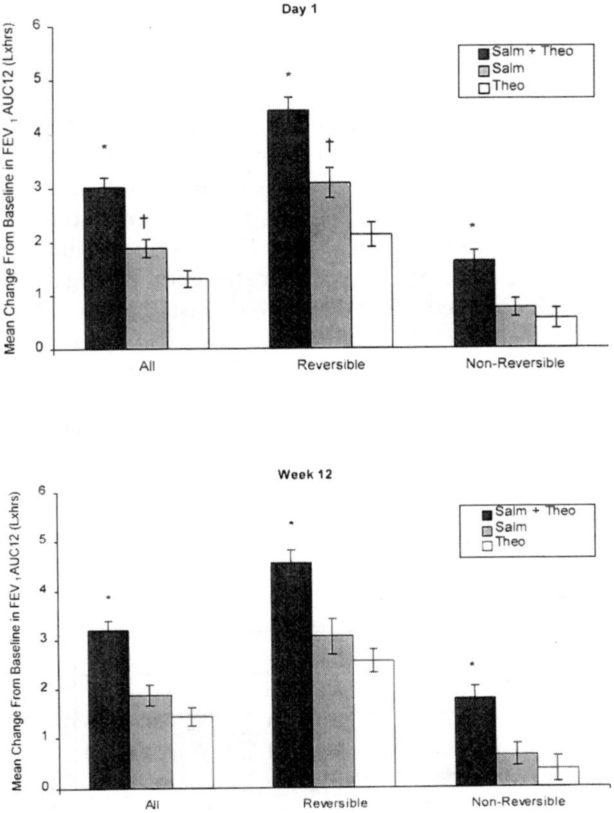

* p≤0.002 S+T vs S and S+T vs T
† p≤0.011 S vs T

Figure 2 Continued.

included statistically significant and clinically meaningful increases in the 6-min walk test, treadmill endurance distance, and maximal work rate on incremental stationary cycle ergometry. Of interest, in some investigations, the improvement in exercise performance was not accompanied by a significant increase in FEV_1 [35,36], leading to speculation that some of theophylline's beneficial effect in this outcome area may be mediated through its effect on lung hyperinflation, respiratory muscles, cardiovascular function, or respiratory drive. Of interest, it appears that aggressive dosing to plasma theophylline levels in the high therapeutic range—with the increased possibility of side effects—are necessary to achieve these results [30,35,37].

C. Dyspnea

Several controlled clinical trials have demonstrated an improvement in dyspnea in COPD patients treated with theophylline. In two early studies, sustained-release theophylline given for 4 weeks [38] and 2 months [28] led to significant improvement in overall dyspnea in COPD patients. In the first study, a reduction in dyspnea was demonstrated by a significant improvement in the Transitional Dyspnea Index and, in the second study, a reduction in visual analog score rated dyspnea from 77 to 58 mm of line length.

In the earlier-described multicenter study comparing the effectiveness of theophylline, the inhaled long-acting β-agonist bronchodilator salmeterol, and their combination [31], theophylline therapy led to a statistically significant improvement in overall dyspnea, as evidenced by a 1.1 unit increase in the Transitional Dyspnea Index focal score (Fig. 3). This positive outcome surpassed the 1.0 unit increase considered clinically meaningful, and was roughly equivalent to that in the salmeterol monotherapy group. Perhaps of more importance and similar to the effect on airways obstruction, the

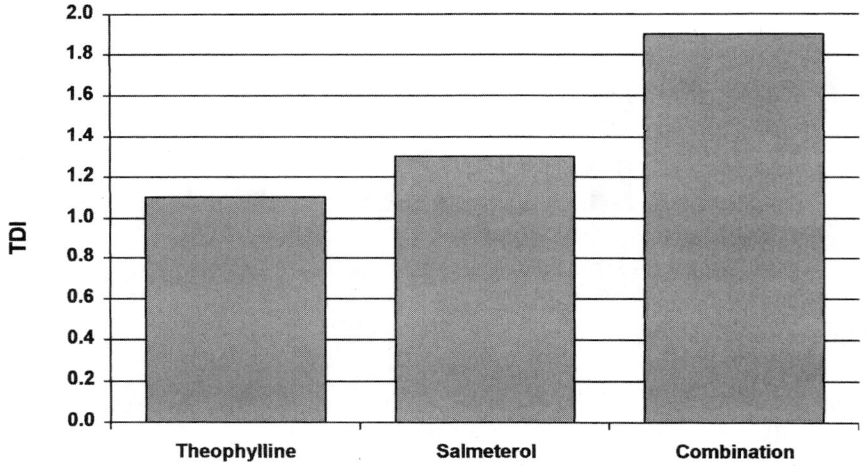

Figure 3 The effect of theophylline, salmeterol, and their combination on dyspnea. This graph depicts the Transitional Dyspnea Index (TDI) focal score at the end of 12 weeks of therapy. A score of zero indicates no change in overall dyspnea; higher scores indicate improvement in dyspnea. A 1-unit change is considered clinically meaningful. Both bronchodilators given as monotherapy and their combination led to statistically significant and clinically meaningful reductions in dyspnea. The TDI score in the group taking the combination of theophylline and salmeterol was significantly higher than in either monotherapy group. (From Ref. 31.)

combined theophylline-salmeterol group had more improvement in dyspnea than either monotherapy group. Thus, combined bronchodilator therapy may offer substantial additive dyspnea relief. It is not clear why theophylline may improve dyspnea, although most likely it is mediated although a reduction in airways obstruction. However, a reduction in static or dynamic hyperinflation or an effect on respiratory muscles may also be important.

D. Health Status

Health status relates to the effect of the disease and its treatment on the patient's sense of well-being. Theophylline, dosed to reach levels of 17 μg/mL, has resulted in clinically meaningful improvement in the dyspnea and fatigue components of the Chronic Respiratory Disease Questionnaire in COPD patients [36]. This effect, which was accompanied by improvement in dyspnea and exercise performance, was not observed when theophylline was dosed to a plasma level of 10 μg/mL. In an unblinded, multicenter study [39], twice-daily theophylline titrated to a level between 10 and 20 mg/L led to significant improvement in all eight components of the SF-36, a generic health status questionnaire. This beneficial effect, however, was significantly less than that of the comparator drug, twice-daily inhaled salmeterol, in the physical functioning, change in health perception, and social functioning components of this questionnaire.

In the earlier-described trial of theophylline, salmeterol, and their combination [31], theophylline therapy resulted in an 8.6-unit increase in the total score of the COPD-specific measure of health status, the Chronic Respiratory Disease Questionnaire at week 12 of treatment. This change was significantly greater than the baseline value and was roughly equivalent to the 7.6-unit increase with salmeterol. Neither monotherapy, however, achieved the 10-unit increase that is considered clinically meaningful with this questionnaire. The combination of these bronchodilators, however, resulted in a 12.7-unit increase in the health status score at 12 weeks, which was significantly better than either bronchodilator taken alone, and did exceed the clinically meaningful threshold. This again attests to the potential importance of combination bronchodilator therapy for COPD.

Theophylline therapy also was proven effective using the respiratory-specific health status instrument, the St. George's Respiratory Questionnaire [32] (Fig. 4). This therapy led to a decrease (i.e., improved health status) in the total score from 47.7 to 41.5 units, which was significantly better than placebo and equivalent to the improvements in the groups given the standard dose or the high dose of the inhaled β-agonist, formoterol. The improvement in health status from all three treatments exceeded the 4-unit threshold considered clinically meaningful for this questionnaire. Of note, the theophylline treat-

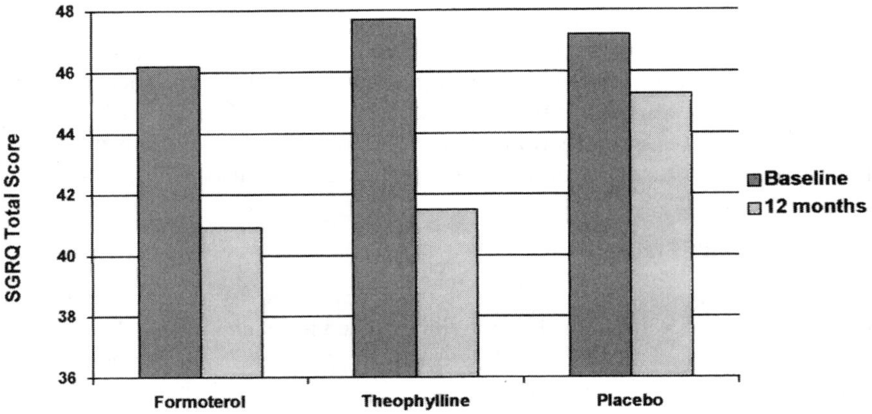

Figure 4 The effect of theophylline on health status. This graph depicts changes in the Saint George's Respiratory Questionnaire (SGRQ) total score from pretreatment to 12 months of therapy. Data from the standard dose (12 μg twice daily) of the inhaled β-agonist, formoterol, theophylline dosed to a target plasma level of 8–20 μg/mL, and placebo are given. A decrease in the SGRQ score indicates improved health status; a 4-unit change is considered clinically meaningful. Both bronchodilators resulted in similar, statistically significant and clinically meaningful improvements in health status compared to placebo. (From Ref. 32.)

ment group was the only one to show significant improvement in the activity component of this questionnaire. This component rates activity limitation from the disease process, and correlates highly with other dyspnea measures.

Thus, chronic dosing of sustained-release theophylline, titrated to therapeutic doses, leads to measurable improvement in health status which is not substantially different from that of the long-acting β-agonist bronchodilators salmeterol and formoterol. This improvement in health status accompanied an improvement in airflow obstruction which, in several studies but not all studies, was somewhat less than regular inhaled bronchodilator therapy. This may reflect beneficial changes from theophylline in areas other than reduced airway resistance.

VIII. Selective Phosphodiesterase Inhibitors in the Treatment of COPD

As previously mentioned, phosphodiesterase is a superfamily of at least 10 genetically distinct isoenzymes. While all inactivate intracellular cyclic AMP and GMP, each has different substrate affinities, tissue distributions, and biological roles. Theophylline, as a relatively nonspecific phosphodiesterase inhibitor, inhibits these isoenzymes with approximately equal potency [40]. However, many of the detrimental actions of this drug may be due to nonselective inhibition of cyclic nucleotide breakdown in nontarget organs [41]. Because of this, the impetus for the development of selective PDE inhibitors for asthma and COPD has been the desirability of a pharmaceutical agent with beneficial anti-inflammatory and/or bronchodilator properties, yet with fewer bothersome side effects resulting from activity in nontarget tissues.

PDE molecules contain three functional domains: a catalytic core, an N-terminus, and a C-terminus, attached to each other by hinge regions [42]. Of these domains, the N-terminus is responsible for much of their heterogeneity of action. PDE isoenzymes also differ in their relative affinities for hydrolyzing cyclic AMP and GMP and in their ability to be regulated by activators or inhibitors [42]. PDE isoenzymes have been isolated in airway smooth muscle, pulmonary arteries, epithelial and endothelial cells, and in several different inflammatory cells found in the airways [40].

While there continues to be intensive research in the development of selective PDE inhibitors for airways disease, none has reached the point of clinical availability. The selective PDE4 inhibitors appear to have the most promise [43]. PDE4 has activity in bronchial smooth muscle and in many cells thought to be involved in inflammation in COPD. It is the predominant isoenzyme expressed in neutrophils, CD8 lymphocytes, and macrophages—cells believed to be particularly responsible for inflammation in COPD. Inhibition of PDE in these target areas might be expected to lead to bronchodilation and downregulation of the inflammatory response in the airways and lung.

Similar to phosphodiesterases in general, side effects (which are in reality extensions of the pharmacology of these drugs) still limit their clinical applicability. This has been especially important in the first-generation PDE4 inhibitors. These side effects include nausea and vomiting, which result from central nervous stimulation, and gastric acid hypersecretion, which results from gastric parietal cell stimulation [44]. Unlike PDE3 inhibitors, the PDE4 inhibitors do not apparently have significant cardiac stimulant properties. Perhaps of considerable importance, recent investigation has identified two distinct conformational states of these isoenzymes, high- and low-affinity binding (HPDE4 and LPDE4, respectively). The central nervous system contains a higher proportion of isoenzyme in the HPDE4 conformation, while inflammatory cells have predominately the LPDE4 conformation.

Selective targeting in newer-generation PDE isoenzyme inhibitors may improve the therapeutic–toxic ratio of this class of drugs [45]. The bronchodilator effects of three oral doses of the second-generation PDE4 inhibitor, cilomilast (Ariflo, SB 207499), were compared to placebo in a large study of COPD patients [46]. Fig. 5 shows sequential changes in prebronchodilator trough FEV_1 (i.e., immediately before the next dose of the study medication) for the four groups. The mean trough FEV_1 in the highest-dose cilomilast group was significantly greater than with placebo, and appeared to be gradually increasing up to the end of the study. At this time, the difference in FEV_1 compared to placebo was 160 mL—a value not much different from long-acting β-agonist trials. Furthermore, the graph shows a gradual increase in FEV_1 over time with the 15-mg dose, which suggests an anti-inflammatory activity of the drug. Quality-of-life scores tended to improve in this group, although the results were not statistically significant. This treatment group, however, had an 11% frequency of nausea, which was described by the investigators as generally mild or moderate and self-limiting. However, 14 of 107 patients assigned to the 15-mg-twice-daily dose group withdrew because of adverse events.

Other trials evaluating PDE4 inhibitors have shown potentially important beneficial effects. Cilomilast led to a 4.1-unit reduction in the St. George's Respiratory Questionnaire, which represented a statistically significant and clinically meaningful improvement in health status. This effect was maintained over 6 months [47]. Use of this drug over a 6-month period was

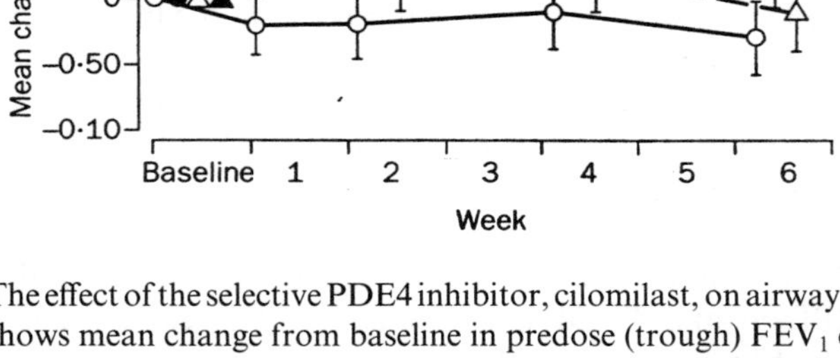

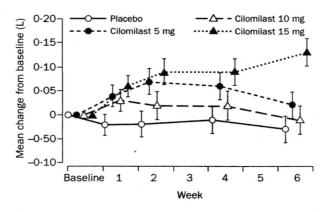

Figure 5 The effect of the selective PDE4 inhibitor, cilomilast, on airway obstruction. This graph shows mean change from baseline in predose (trough) FEV_1 compared to placebo for three doses of cilomilast in patients with COPD. Improvement with the highest dose (15 mg) was significantly greater than with placebo at weeks 1, 2, 4, and 6. The maximum increase in FEV_1 with this dose was 160 mL. The difference between the 15-mg dose and placebo appears to be still increasing by the sixth week. (From Ref. 46, with permission.)

associated with a reduction in health care utilization [48]. Another PDE4 inhibitor, roflumilast, was shown to have a modest bronchodilator effect in a study involving 516 COPD patients [49], with the FEV_1 increasing by 109 mL in its higher dose of 500 μg. Perhaps of considerable importance, the frequency of exacerbation of COPD was reduced by 48% with this dose over the 26 weeks of the study. In preliminary studies, this drug appears to be well tolerated, with a 2% or less incidence of headache, nausea, or diarrhea [50].

Thus, the newer selective PDE4 inhibitors hold promise as potentially useful drugs for COPD. Although their bronchodilator effect appears to be modest, and probably less than that of the inhaled anticholinergic and long-acting β-agonist bronchodilators, they may become valuable as anti-inflammatory drugs for this disease. This latter property is of particular importance because inhaled steroids have been singularly unimpressive as anti-inflammatory agents in COPD.

IX. The Role of Theophylline in the Acute Exacerbation of COPD

The acute exacerbation of COPD is characterized by worsening of dyspnea, an increase in sputum production, and a change in sputum to purulence. Oxygen therapy for hypoxemic patients, noninvasive positive-pressure ventilation, antibiotics, short courses of systemic corticosteroids, and bronchodilator therapy have been proven effective therapy [51]. The use of oral theophylline or intravenous aminophylline as first-line bronchodilator therapy for the exacerbation is not recommended because of limited effectiveness in clinical trials [52] and their potential to produce serious side effects. Furthermore, the addition of a methylxanthine as a second bronchodilator in this setting has proven disappointing [51], and in most cases cannot be recommended.

X. Theophylline and Phosphodiesterase Inhibitor Use in COPD: Where Does It Fit In?

As described above, theophylline has a modest bronchodilator effect in COPD. In addition, the drug may also have other beneficial effects, including a reduction in dyspnea that may be separate from its effect on airway caliber, a downregulation of airway hyperresponsiveness, respiratory stimulation, potentially favorable cardiovascular effects, and protection from diaphragmatic fatigue. The beneficial effect of theophylline and PDE4 inhibitors on indices of airway inflammation is becoming clearer. However, long-term studies testing their usefulness in modifying the course of COPD are lacking at this point. The proven or potential beneficial actions of theophylline and the PDE inhibitors must be weighed against the clear potential for toxicity. A list of arguments for and against the use of theophylline in COPD is given in Table 5. Of practical consideration is the availability of alternate therapy for COPD. This includes the inhaled anticholinergic and long-acting β-agonist bronchodilators, which are at least as effective and probably more effective

Table 5 Pros and Cons of Theophylline as Maintenance Bronchodilator Therapy for COPD

Pro's

1. Theophylline is an inexpensive oral medication that can be taken once or twice daily.
2. Theophylline is a proven bronchodilator for COPD that is roughly equivalent to or somewhat less potent than inhaled anticholinergics or long-acting inhaled β-agonists. It also has other potential useful respiratory effects, including a reduction in static lung volumes and a small improvement in gas exchange.
3. In clinical trials, theophylline has increased exercise capacity, reduced dyspnea, and improved health status.
4. The combination of theophylline with an inhaled bronchodilator such as salmeterol leads to an additive therapeutic effect without substantially increased side effects over monotherapy with theophylline.
5. Theophylline may also have desirable nonrespiratory effects, such as increased respiratory muscle strength and resistance to fatigue, improved mucociliary clearance, enhanced central respiratory drive, a possible anti-inflammatory effect, improved cardiovascular function, and a reduced pulmonary artery pressure.
6. Lower doses of theophylline, with subsequent lower potential for toxicity, may still produce positive effects in some of the above outcome areas.
7. Tachyphylaxis to the bronchodilator effect has not been observed with theophylline use.

Con's

1. The toxic potential of this drug is substantial, and adverse effects can occur even in its so-called therapeutic range.
2. Regular monitoring of theophylline levels is usually necessary, thereby contributing to the inconvenience and cost of this treatment.
3. Theophylline levels are affected by numerous clinical factors and drug interactions. Therefore, the dose of this drug must be adjusted and additional blood levels may be necessary when clinical conditions change or certain other medications are added.
4. Chronological age is the single most important determinant in serious toxicity of this drug, making it less desirable for an elderly COPD population.
5. Alternative therapy with inhaled anticholinergic or long-acting β-agonist bronchodilators is available, and these drugs are probably more effective and have a considerably lower risk of toxicity.

bronchodilators than theophylline, but without the ominous potential for toxicity.

Current practice guidelines for theophylline in COPD [53–57] are fairly consistent in where they place theophylline in the treatment for COPD. Theophylline is clearly not recommended as first-line therapy except in the uncommon setting where the patient cannot or will not use inhaled medications. Instead, theophylline may be considered if the initial response to inhaled anticholinergic or β-agonist therapy is inadequate. Inadequate response is not clearly described in all the guidelines, but refers to persistent, bothersome symptoms or reductions in functional status or health status despite these inhaled medications. In this case, it would be reasonable to consider theophylline as an additional bronchodilator medication to these inhaled drugs. If dyspnea, functional status, or health status improve—with or without concomitant improvement in pulmonary function—the drug should be continued, providing a safe drug level is achieved and bothersome side effects are not present. Selective phosphodiesterase inhibitors, while they hold promise as potential bronchodilator and anti-inflammatory medications, have not been adequately tested and are not available for general clinical use at this time.

References

1. Barnes PJ, Pauwels RA. Theophylline in the management of asthma: time for reappraisal? Eur Respir J 1994; 7:579–591.
2. McFadden ER. Introduction: Methylxanthine therapy and reversible airway obstruction. Am J Med 1985; 79(suppl 6A):1–4.
3. Weinberger M, Hendeles L. Theophylline in asthma. N Engl J Med 1996; 334:1380–1388.
4. Torphy TJ. Phosphodiesterase isozymes: molecular targets for novel antiasthma agents. Am J Respir Crit Care Med 1998; 157:351–370.
5. Barnes PJ. Pharmacology of airway smooth muscle. Am J Respir Crit Care Med 1998; 158:S123–S132.
6. Bukowskyj M, Nakatsu K, Mundt PW. Theophylline reassessed. Ann Intern Med 1984; 101:63–73.
7. Cushley MJ, Tattersfield AE, Holgate ST. Adenosine-induced bronchoconstriction in asthma: antagonism by inhaled theophylline. Am Rev Respir Dis 1984; 129:380–384.
8. Bjork T, Gustafsson LE, Dahlen SE. Isolated bronchi from asthmatics are hyperresponsive to adenosine, which apparently acts intirectly by liberation of leukotrienes and histamine. Am Rev Respir Dis 1992; 145:1087–1091.
9. Ashutosh K, Sedat M, Fragale-Jackson J. Effects of theophylline on respiratory drive in patients with chronic obstructive pulmonary disease. J Clin Pharmacol 1997; 37:1100–1107.

10. Matthay RA. Effects of theophylline on cardiovascular performance in chronic obstructive pulmonary disease. Chest 1985; 88:112S–117S.
11. Decramer M, Janssens S. Theophylline and the respiratory muscles: where are we? Eur Respir J 1989; 2:399–401.
12. Murciano D, Aubier M, Viires N, et al. Effects of theophylline and enprofylline on diaphragmatic contractility. J Appl Physiol 1987; 63:51–57.
13. Murciano D, Aubier M, Lecocguic Y, Pariente R. Effects of theophylline on diaphragmatic strength and fatigue in patients with chronic obstructive lung disease. New Engl J Med 1984; 311:349–353.
14. Aubier M. Effect of theophylline on diaphragmatic muscle function. Chest 1987; 92:27S–31S.
15. Sherman MS, Lang DM, Matityahu A, Campbell D. Theophylline improves measurements of respiratory muscle efficiency. Chest 1996; 110:1437–1442.
16. Snider GL. Theophylline in the ambulatory treatment of chronic obstructive lung disease: resolving a controversy. Cleve Clin J Med 1993; 60:197–201.
17. Vaz CA, Miller MA. Review of the clinical efficacy of theophylline in the treatment of chronic obstructive pulmonary disease. Am Rev Respir Dis 1993; 147:S40–S47.
18. Culpitt SV, de Matos C, Russell RE, Donnelly LE, Rogers DF, Barnes PJ. Effect of theophylline on induced sputum inflammatory indices and neutrophil chemotaxis in chronic obstructive pulmonary disease. Am J Respir Crit Care Med 2002; 165:1371–1376.
19. Roehrs T, Merlotti L, Halpin D, Rosenthal L, Roth T. Effects of thoephylline on nocturnal sleep and daytime sleepiness/alertness. Chest 1995; 108:382–387.
20. Man GCW, Chapman KR, Habib Ali S, Darke AC. Sleep quality and nocturnal respiratory function with once-daily theophylline (Uniphyl) and inhaled salbutamol in patients with COPD. Chest 1996; 110:648–653.
21. Hendeles L, et al. A clinical and pharmacokinetic basis for the selection and use of slow-release theophylline products. Clin Pharmacokinet 1984; 9:95.
22. Richards W, Church JA, Brent DK. Theophylline-associated seizures in children. Ann Allergy 1985; 54:276–279.
23. Zwillich CW, Sutton FD, Neff TA, et al. Theophylline-induced seizures in adults. Correlation with serum concentrations. Ann Intern Med 1975; 82:784–787.
24. Shannon M, Lovejoy FH Jr. The influence of age vs peak serum concentration on life-threatening events after chronic theophylline intoxication. Arch Intern Med 1990; 150:2045–2048.
25. Shannon M. Predictors of major toxicity after theophylline overdose. Ann Intern Med 1993; 119:1161–1167.
26. Weinberger M, Hendeles L. Theophylline in asthma. N Engl J Med 1996:1380–1388.
27. Vaz Fragaso CA, Miller MA. Review of the clinical efficacy of theophylline in the treatment of chronic obstructive pulmonary disease. Am Rev Respir Dis 1993; 147:S40–S47.
28. Murciano D, Auclair MH, Pariente R, Aubier M. A randomized, controlled trial of theophylline in patients with severe chronic obstructive pulmonary disease. N Engl J Med 1989:1521–1525.

29. Nishimura K, Koyama H, Ikeda A, Sugiura N, Kawakatsu K, Izumi T. The additive effect of theophylline on a high-dose combination of inhaled salbutamol and ipratropium bromide in stable COPD. Chest 1995; 107:718–723.
30. Chrystyn H, Mulley BA, Peake MD. Dose response relation to oral theophylline in severe chronic obstructive airways disease. Br Med J 1988; 297:1506–1510.
31. ZuWallack RL, Mahler DA, Reilly D, Church N, Emmett A, Rickard K, Knobil K. Salmeterol plus theophylline combination therapy in the treatment of COPD. Chest 2001; 119:1661–1670.
32. Rossi A, Kristufek P, Levine BE, Thomson MH, Till D, Kottakis J, Della Cioppa G. Comparison of the efficacy, tolerability, and safety of formoterol dry powder and oral, slow-release theophylline in the treatment of COPD. Chest 2002; 121:1058–1069.
33. Liesker JJW, Wijkstra PJ, Ten Hacken NHT, Koeter GH, Postma DS, Kerstjens HAM. A systemic review of the effects of bronchodilators on exercise capacity in patients with COPD. Chest 2002; 121:597–608.
34. Guyatt GH, Townsend M, Pugsley SO, Keller JL, Short HD, Taylor DW, Newhouse MT. Bronchodilators in chronic air-flow obstruction. Am Rev Respir Dis 1987; 135:1069–1074.
35. McKay SE, Howie CA, Thomson AH, Whiting B, Addis GJ. Value of theophylline treatment in patients handicapped by chronic obstructive lung disease. Thorax 1993; 48:227–232.
36. Fink G, Kaye C, Sulkes J, Gabbay U, Spitzer SA. Effect of theophylline on exercise performance in patients with severe chronic obstructive pulmonary disease. Thorax 1994; 49:332–334.
37. Tsukino M, Nishimura K, Ikeda A, Hajiro T, Koyama H, Izumi T. Effects of theophylline and ipratropium bromide on exercise performance in patients with stable chronic obstructive pulmonary disease. Thorax 1998; 53:269–273.
38. Mahler DA, Matthay RA, Snyder PE, et al. Sustained-release theophylline reduces dyspnea in nonreversible obstructive airway disease. Am Rev Respir Dis 1985; 131:22–25.
39. Di Lorenzo G, Morici G, Drago A, Pellitteri ME, Mansueto P, Melluso M, Norrito F, Squassante L, Fasolo A. Efficacy, tolerability, and effects on quality of life of inhaled salmeterol and oral theophylline in patients with mild-to-moderate chronic obstructive pulmonary disease. Clin Ther 1998; 20:1130–1148.
40. Schmidt D, Dent G, Rabe KF. Selective phosphodiesterase inhibitors for the treatment of bronchial asthma and chronic obstructive pulmonary disease. Clin Exp Allergy 1999; 29(suppl 2):99–109.
41. Torphy TJ, Barnette MS, Underwood DC, Griswold DE, Christensen SB, Murdoch RD, Nieman RB, Compton CH. Ariflo (SB 207499), a second generation phosphodiesterase 4 inhibitor for the treatment of asthma and COPD. Pulm Pharmacol 1999; 12:131–135.
42. Torphy TJ. Phosphodiesterase isoenzymes. Molecular targets for novel antiasthma agents. Am J Respir Crit Care Med 1998; 157:351–370.
43. Barnes PJ. Future advances in COPD therapy. Respiration 2001; 68:441–448.
44. Torphy TJ, Barnette MS, Underwood DC, Griswold DE, Christensen SB, Murdoch RD, Nieman RB, Compton CH. Ariflo (SB207499), a second

generation phosphodiesterase 4 inhibitor for the treatment of asthma and COPD: from concept to clinic. Pulm Pharmacol Ther 1999; 12:131–135.
45. Barnette MS. Phosphodiesterase 4 (PDE4) inhibitors in asthma and chronic obstructive pulmonary disease (COPD). Prog Drug Res 1999; 53:193–229.
46. Compton CH, Gubb J, Nieman R, Edelson J, Amit O, Bakst A, Ayres JG, Creemers JPHM, Schulze-Werninghaus G, Brambilla C, Barnes NC. Cilomilast, a selective phosphodiesterase-4 inhibitor for treatment of patients with chronic obstructive pulmonary disease: a randomised, dose-ranging study. Lancet 2001; 358:265–270.
47. Edelson JD, Compton C, Nieman R, Robinson CB, Watt R, Amit O, Bagchi I, Rennard SI, Kelsen S, Strek M. Cilomilast (Airflo) improves health status in patients with COPD: results of a 6-month trial. Am J Respir Crit Care Med 2001;A.
48. Bagchi I, Bakst AW, Edelson JE, Amit O. Cilomilast reduces healthcare resource utilization of chronic obstructive pulmonary disease patients. Am J Respir Crit Care Med 2002;A.
49. Leichtl S, Syed J, Bredenbroker D, Rathgeb F, Wurst W. Efficacy of once-daily roflumilast, a new orally active, selective phosphodiesterase 4 inhibitor, in chronic obstructive pulmonary disease. Am J Respir Crit Care Med 2002;A.
50. Bredenbroker D, Syed J, Leichtl, Rathgeb F, Wurst W. Safety of once-daily roflumilast, a new, orally active, selective phosphodiesterase 4 inhibitor, in patients with COPD. Am J Respir Crit Care Med 2002;A.
51. McCrory DC, Brown C, Gelfand SE, Bach PB. Management of acute exacerbations of COPD. A summary and appraisal of published evidence. Chest 2001; 119:1190–1209.
52. Barr RG, Rowe BH, Camargo CA. Methyl-xanthines for exacerbations of chronic obstructive pulmonary disease. The Cochrane Library. http://www.cochranelibrary.com
53. Anon. Standards for the diagnosis and care of patients with chronic obstructive pulmonary disease. Am J Respir Crit Care Med 1995; 152:S77–S120.
54. Standards of Care Committee for the British Thoracic Society. Standards of care for the treatment of COPD. Thorax 1997; 54(suppl):S1–S22.
55. Siafakas NM, Vermeire P, Pride NB, Paoletti P, Gibson J, Howard P, Yernault JC, Decramer M, Higenbottom T, Postma DS, Rees Jthe Task ForceOptimal assessment and management of chronic obstructive pulmonary disease (COPD). Eur Respir J 1995; 8:1398–1420.
56. Canadian Respiratory Review PanelGuidelines for the treatment of chronic obstructive pulmonary disease (COPD). Toronto: MUMS Guideline Clearinghouse, 1998.
57. National Heart, Lung, and Blood Institute and World Health Organization. Global Strategy for the Diagnosis, Management, and Prevention of Chronic Obstructive Lung Disease: NHLBI/WHO Workshop. Executive summary.
58. Chrystyn H, Mulley BA, Peake MD. Dose response relation to oral theophylline in severe chronic obstructive airways disease. Br Med J 1988; 297:1506–1510.
59. Tedders JG, Thomas AK, Edwards G. A double-blind comparison of a

microcrystalline theophylline tablet and salbutamol in reversible airways obstruction. Br J Clin Pract 1976; 30:212–216.
60. Alexander MR, Dull WL, Kasik JE. Treatment of chronic obstructive pulmonary disease with orally administered theophylline. A double-blind, controlled study. JAMA 1980; 244:2286–2290.
61. Greening AP, Baillie E, Gribbin HR, Pride NB. Sustained release oral aminophylline in patients with airflow obstruction. Thorax 1981; 36:303–307.
62. McKay SE, Howie CA, Thomson AH, Whiting B, Addis GJ. Value of theophylline treatment in patients handicapped by chronic obstructive lung disease. Thorax 1993; 48:227–232.
63. Thomas P, Pugsley JA, Stewart JH. Theophylline and salbutamol improve pulmonary function in patients with irreversible chronic obstructive pulmonary disease. Chest 1992; 101:160–165.
64. Man GC, Champman KR, Ali SH, Darke AC. Sleep quality and nocturnal respiratory function with once-daily theophylline (Uniphyl) and inhaled salbutamol in patients with COPD. Chest 1996; 110:648–653.
65. Fink G, Kaye C, Sulkes J, Gabbay U, Spitzer SA. Effect of theophylline on exercise performance in patients with severe chronic obstructive pulmonary disease. Thorax 1994; 49:332–334.
66. Sherman MS, Lang DM, Matityahu A, Campbell D. Theophylline improves measurements of respiratory muscle efficiency. Chest 1996; 110:1437–1442.
67. Matthys H, Wastag E, Daikeler G, Kohler D. The influence of aminophylline and pindolol on the mucociliary clearance in patients with chronic bronchitis. Br J Clin Pract 1983; 23S:10–15.
68. Ziment I. Theophylline and mucociliary clearance. Chest 1987; 92(suppl 1):38S–43S.
69. Erley CM, Duda SH, Schlepckow S, Koehler J, Huppert PE, Strohmaier WL, et al. Adenosine antagonist theophylline prevents the reduction in glomerular filtration rate after contrast media application. Kidney Int 1994; 45:1425–1431.

15

Corticosteroids in COPD

MARIO CAZZOLA

A. Cardarelli Hospital
Naples, Italy

MARIA GABRIELLA MATERA

Second University of Naples
Naples, Italy

ROMAIN PAUWELS

University Hospital
Ghent, Belgium

I. Introduction

Corticosteroids effectively suppress airway inflammation, but there is considerable debate concerning the utility of these agents in the long-term treatment of patients with chronic obstructive pulmonary disease (COPD) [1,2]. The critiques to their use are: (1) the neutrophilic inflammation, which is characteristic in COPD [3–8], is generally resistant to corticosteroids; (2) corticosteroids prolong the survival of neutrophils by inhibiting apoptosis; and (3) corticosteroid therapy fails to suppress cytokines such as tumor necrosis factor (TNF)-α and interleukin (IL)-8, which are generally considered to be important mediators in neutrophil recruitment and are elevated in patients with COPD [9]. However, the observation that increased numbers of neutrophils are present during acute exacerbations of COPD and acute exacerbations do respond to oral corticosteroids might suggest that neutrophilic inflammation does not per se reflect unresponsiveness to oral or inhaled corticosteroids [10]. Recently, it has been suggested that the lack of efficacy of corticosteroids in attenuating airway inflammation could be due to a reduced corticosteroid sensitivity of macrophages [11]. Macrophages from subjects with COPD are defective in histone deacetylase activity, which is an important

Table 1 Impact of Corticosteroids on Inflammation in COPD

Study	Type of patients enrolled	Treatment, study duration	Outcomes
		Negative studies	
Thompson and co-workers, [15]	Current smokers with chronic bronchitis and at least mild obstruction	Beclomethasone, 1 g/day, 6 weeks	Small increase in FEV_1, small decrease in macroscopic bronchioscopic index of bronchial inflammation, no reduction in the number of neutrophils in BAL
Keatings and co-workers, [16]	Patients with severe COPD (mean FEV_1: 35% of predicted value)	Budesonide, 800 µg twice daily, 2 weeks	No clinical benefit in either lung function or symptom scores, no significant change in the inflammatory indices as measured by total and differential cell counts and concentrations of TNF-α, eosinophil activation markers eosinophilic cationic protein and eosinophil peroxidase, and neutrophil activation markers myeloper-oxidase and human neutrophil lipocalin
		Oral prednisolone, 30 mg daily, 2 weeks	Sputum eosinophil number, eosinophilic cationic protein, and eosinophil peroxidase not modified
Culpitt and co-workers, [17]	Patients with stable COPD	Fluticasone, 500 µg twice daily), 4 weeks	No clinical benefit in terms of lung function or symptom scores, no change in induced sputum inflammatory cells, percentage of neutrophils, IL-8 levels, supernatant elastase activity, matrix metalloproteinase (MMP)-1, MMP-9, and the antiproteases secretory leukoprotease inhibitor and tissue inhibitor of metalloproteinase-1 levels
Loppow and co-workers, [18]	Patients chronic bronchitis (mean FEV_1, 83.4% of predicted value)	Fluticasone 500 µg twice daily, 4 weeks	No improvement in lung function or inflammatory parameters, such as the concentration of exhaled nitric oxide, differential cell counts in induced sputum, and the number of cells positive for inducible nitric oxide synthase, as well as the levels of lactate dehydrogenase, eosinophilic cationic protein, neutrophil elastase and IL-8 in sputum supernatants

		Positive studies	
Llewellyn-Jones and co-workers, [20]	Patients with clinically stable, smoking-related chronic bronchitis and emphysema, mean FEV_1 0.71 L	Fluticasone, 1.5 mg/day, 8 weeks	No effect on peripheral neutrophils or on sputum albumin and myeloperoxidase concentrations, but reduction in the neutrophil chemotactic activity of sputum and beneficial effect on the proteinase/antiproteinase balance
Confalonieri and co-workers, [21]	Patients with stable COPD (mean FEV_1 60.2% of predicted value)	Beclomethasone 500 μg three times daily, 2 months	Reduction in both neutrophils and total cells in induced sputum, no change in spirometry and blood gases
Yildiz and co-workers, [24]	Clinically stable COPD patients	Fluticasone, 1,500 μg/day, 2 months	No significant changes in the number of peripheral blood neutrophils, blood gases and spirometry, but decrease in the total cell number and the number of neutrophils in induced sputum
Balbi and co-workers, [25]	Stable COPD patients with mild disease	Beclomethasone, 1.5 mg/day, 6 weeks	Reductions in the lavage levels of IL-8 and myeloperoxidase, in cell numbers, neutrophil proportion, symptom score, and bronchitis index
Hattotuwa and co-workers, [23]	Patients with mild to severe stable COPD (mean FEV_1 25-80% of predicted value)	Fluticasone, 500 μg twice daily, 3 months	No effect on the major inflammatory cell types in COPD, but reduced epithelial CD8/CD4 ratio and subepithelial mast cell number
Gizycki and co-workers, [26]	Patients with mild to severe COPD (FEV_1 25–80% of predicted value)	Fluticasone, 500 μg twice daily, 3 months	Significant decrease in the numbers of mucosal mast cells, improvement in symptoms

mechanism in switching off proinflammatory genes in cells [12]. Any lack of efficacy of corticosteroids on macrophage activity in COPD could lead to reduced inhibition of neutrophil chemoattractants and increased survival, with perpetuation of pulmonary neutrophilic inflammation [11].

II. Impact of Corticosteroids on Inflammation in COPD

Cigarette smoke, which is the major cause of COPD, reduces histone deacetylase 2 expression, enhances cytokine expression, and inhibits glucocorticoid actions in alveolar macrophages [12]. This mechanism may account for the reduced effectiveness of corticosteroids in COPD [13]. In effect, Cox and co-workers [14] found no benefit of treatment with inhaled beclomethasone dipropionate, 1000 μg/day, on noninvasive measures of airway inflammation in adult smokers with normal spirometry. This finding indicates that cigarette smoke-induced inflammation in its early stages (before a demonstrable airflow obstruction) is not corticosteroid-sensitive. It is not unexpected, therefore, that neither high doses of inhaled nor oral corticosteroid treatment reduce important markers of airway inflammation in induced sputum in patients with COPD.

A volume of evidence, summarized in Table 1, questions the efficacy of inhaled corticosteroids in totally suppressing airway inflammation in COPD. Thompson and co-workers [15] did not find a reduction in the numbers of neutrophils in bronchoalveolar lavage after 6 weeks of treatment with inhaled corticosteroids, although the total cell count was reduced. During two weeks of treatment with inhaled or oral corticosteroids, Keatings and co-workers [16] could not demonstrate any effect on airway inflammation assessed with induced sputum. Even high doses of oral corticosteroids, given in an attempt to reach inflammatory sites, were without any effect. Similarly, Culpitt and co-workers [17] showed that inhaled corticosteroids administered over 4 weeks had no anti-inflammatory effect. Loppow and coworkers [18] documented that a 4-week treatment with inhaled corticosteroids did not improve lung function or inflammatory parameters, such as the concentration of exhaled nitric oxide, differential cell counts and the number of cells positive for inducible nitric oxide synthase (iNOS) in induced sputum, as well as the levels of lactate dehydrogenase (LDH), eosinophilic cationic protein (ECP), neutrophil elastase, and IL-8 in sputum supernatants. More recently, it was observed that dexamethasone did not inhibit basal or stimulated IL-8 release from macrophages obtained from patients with COPD [11].

Nevertheless, the results of several other studies suggest that corticosteroids exert some useful effects on cells and molecular mediators of airway inflammation in COPD. In vitro, for example, they attenuated neutrophil recruitment and activation [19] and reduced neutrophil chemotaxis [20]. In vivo, 12 mg of dexamethasone taken daily by 6 healthy volunteers resulted in a significant reduction in the chemotactic response of neutrophils [19]. Interestingly, the in vivo effect on neutrophil function occurred at a mean serum dexamethasone level that was much lower than that required to exert the same effect in vitro [20]. A 2-month course of treatment with high-dose inhaled corticosteroid reduced significantly sputum neutrophil cell counts and increased the number of sputum macrophages in patients with clinically stable, smoking-related COPD [21]. However, this study was not controlled and there was a high eosinophil count, suggesting that some asthmatic patients may have been included. Llewellyn-Jones and co-workers [22] observed a reduction in the chemotactic activity of sputum after 8 weeks of treatment with 1,500 μg of fluticasone in 17 patients with COPD. Moreover, they found a beneficial effect on the proteinase/antiproteinase balance. Notwithstanding the reduction in neutrophil chemotactic activity, the neutrophils themselves were not likely affected since myeloperoxidase content in sputum was comparable before and after 8 weeks of treatment.

Hattotuwa and co-workers [23] have recently shown that 3 months of treatment with the inhaled corticosteroid fluticasone propionate had no effect on the major inflammatory cell types in COPD, although it reduced the epithelial CD8/CD4 ratio and subepithelial mast cells. Yildiz and co-workers [24] reported that 1,500 μg/day fluticasone for 6 weeks resulted in a small decrease in neutrophil sputum counts, which returned to initial levels after 6 weeks of withdrawal. Inhaled corticosteroids also induced a significant reduction in the lavage levels of IL-8 and myeloperoxidase, in cell numbers, neutrophil proportion, symptom score, and bronchitis index in an open study including a small number of subjects [25]. The documentation that fluticasone propionate given for 3 months to patients with COPD resulted in a significant decrease (on average 65%) in the numbers of mucosal mast cells [26] provides strong support to the opinion that corticosteroids are able to affect the inflammatory cells in the bronchial mucosa of COPD patients. These short-term studies suggest that there is at least some scientific rational for evaluating the clinical role of inhaled corticosteroids in COPD.

III. Clinical Effects of Corticosteroids in COPD

A number of both short-term and long-term controlled trials using oral or inhaled corticosteroids and evaluating clinical and functional parameters have been published. However, these clinical trials on the effects of corticosteroids in COPD had conflicting results.

A. Systemic Corticosteroids in Stable COPD

One systematic review published in 1991 identified 15 randomized, controlled trials of oral corticosteroids in stable COPD [27]. Duration of treatment was generally 2–4 weeks. A meta-analysis from the 10 randomized controlled trials that met all inclusion criteria found that improvement of 20% or more in baseline FEV_1 occurred significantly more often with oral corticosteroids than placebo (weighted mean difference in effect size 10%, 95% confidence interval 2–18%). When the other five randomized, controlled trials were included, the difference in effect size was 11% (4–18%). Oral *corticosteroids* did not change airway hyperresponsiveness [28,29] and bronchodilator response to cumulatively applied doses of a β-agonist or anticholinergic, nor did they alter the protection provided by either drug against histamine [30]. Another retrospective study suggested that systemic oral glucocorticoids administered chronically might be associated with worse survival [31].

Such retrospective analyses are fraught with methodological limitations. For example, it is likely that the most severe patients are those treated with oral glucocorticoids. In effect, some studies of COPD patients taking oral prednisolone suggest that several patients show initial improvement in lung function and a reduction in the subsequent rate of decline [32]. Unfortunately, bronchodilator response is not particularly sensitive in identifying such patients [28]. On the contrary, almost 40% of patients with stable moderate and severe COPD have a bronchodilator response to a 2-week trial of corticosteroids [33]. A response to oral prednisolone occurs as frequently in patients with physiological features of emphysema as in those without such features [34].

Other trials seem to indicate that only those patients with an asthmatic component to their disease appear to benefit most from corticosteroids. Thus, in the study of Chanez and co-workers [35], 12 of 25 unselected patients clinically diagnosed as having COPD responded with an increase in FEV_1 of at least 12% from baseline value and absolute value of 200 ml measured at the end of the treatment to a daily oral dose of 1.5 mg/kg body weight of prednisolone for 15 days. By comparison with nonresponders, responders had a significantly larger number of eosinophils and higher levels of ECP in their bronchoalveolar lavage fluid (BALF); moreover the responders had a thicker reticular basement membrane than the nonresponders. Pizzichini and co-workers [36] reported that an improvement in FEV_1 after a short-term prednisone therapy in smokers with chronic obstructive bronchitis was paralleled by a significant reduction in eosinophilia and eosinophil activation as indicated by sputum ECP levels, but not by changes in neutrophils or neutrophil proteases. Patients without sputum eosinophilia did not show clinical benefit from short-term prednisone therapy. Similar observations were repeated by Fujimoto and co-workers [37], who found that the number of eosinophils at baseline were significantly correlated with the increases in FEV_1 following oral prednisolone treatment for 2 weeks, and the treatment also significantly reduced the eosinophil numbers and ECP level in the sputum. The corticosteroid trial had no effect on the neutrophil numbers or on the sputum neutrophil elastase or IL-8 concentrations.

Only one retrospective long-term study of oral corticosteroids in COPD is available [38]. This study was conducted in 139 patients without any sign of allergy. A favorable effect of prednisolone on FEV_1 over a 14- to 20-year period was documented. At a dose of 10 mg/day or more, FEV_1 remained stable or even increased. A clinically important finding was that a change in the decline of FEV_1 could be observed only after at least 6 to 24 months of therapy. The results of this study seem to support the regular use of oral corticosteroids. However, the retrospective nature of the study, the lack of a true control group and the imprecise definition of COPD are reasons for a cautious interpretation of the data and conclusions.

One randomized trial showed that the addition of a low daily dose (5-mg) of prednisolone to inhaled corticosteroids in patients with relatively mild COPD did not result in additional improvement in pulmonary function, pulmonary symptom scores, or the frequency or duration of COPD exacerbations over a 2-year period [39]. A recent randomized double-blind trial has documented that patients with corticosteroid-dependent COPD who continued oral prednisone daily for 6 months had a similar number of COPD exacerbations as those patients using prednisone on demand [40]. In addition, patients receiving continuous corticosteroids did not have a reduction in dyspnea, improved subjective health ratings, or better spirometric values than patients who gradually stopped taking daily prednisone. Patients who took prednisone only on demand had a significantly lower total exposure to systemic corticosteroids over the 6-month study period. It should be stressed, however, that all the patients received an inhaled corticosteroid.

In any case, Kerstjens [41] has correctly highlighted that even if a relatively short-duration (> 2–4 weeks) use of oral corticosteroids in COPD proved to be useful, this would have to be weighed against its substantial adverse effects and also compare its benefits and harms with those of inhaled corticosteroids.

B. Systemic Corticosteroids in Acute Exacerbation of COPD

Short courses of systemic corticosteroids in acute exacerbations of COPD improve spirometric and clinical outcomes [42].

A recent systematic review of all randomized controlled trials comparing corticosteroids, administered either parenterally or orally, with placebo, in patients with acute exacerbation of COPD documented that subjects who receive corticosteroids compared with control are less likely to fail treatment, but more likely to develop adverse effects. Moreover, it was shown that patients on corticosteroids had a greater increase in FEV_1 within 72 hr (on average 120 mL), but not after, and there was no clear difference in mortality between the two groups [43]. These findings suggest that systemic corticosteroids are beneficial for acute exacerbations of COPD, but at a significantly increased risk of an adverse drug reaction. These recommendations are supported by recent randomized controlled trials. In one study [44], systemic glucocorticoid use significantly reduced the length of initial hospital stay (8.5 versus 9.7 days) and the rate of treatment failure at both 30 days and 90 days. Moreover, it elicited a faster increase in FEV_1, the difference (approximately 100 mL at day 1) having disappeared at day 15. In any case, after the initial 3-day course of intravenous glucocorticoids, a 2-week course of oral glucocorticoids was just as good as an eight-week course, with fewer side effects. Patients with a lower FEV_1 and pre-study use of theophylline had a worse prognosis, whereas those who had already been hospitalized for a COPD exacerbation had a more favorable outcome.

A second study demonstrated that similar benefits can be obtained in patients hospitalized for an acute exacerbation of COPD with a ten day course of 30 mg of prednisolone [45].

A randomized controlled trial studied 27 patients with acute COPD exacerbations not requiring hospitalization [46]. Patients were assigned to receive a 9-day tapering dose of oral prednisone or placebo (in addition to continuing their baseline medications and increasing their β-agonist use). The prednisone group showed a more rapid improvement in PaO_2, FEV_1, and peak expiratory flow (PEF), all of which were statistically significant result. This therapy also resulted in fewer treatment failures (0/13 in the prednisolone group and 8/14 in the placebo group) and a trend toward a more rapid (by day 2) improvement in dyspnea scale scores compared with the placebo group. Unfortunately, the optimal dose and duration of systemic corticosteroids for acute exacerbation of COPD remain unclear, and few data document the efficacy of corticosteroids in outpatient settings.

C. Inhaled Corticosteroids in Stable COPD

Inhaled corticosteroids have a more favorable toxicity profile than oral preparations, making them an attractive alternative. Some data even suggest that replacement of oral by inhaled therapy is possible [47]. However, there remains controversy concerning their use in the chronic management of COPD.

Studies on Airflow Limitation

Most studies of inhaled corticosteroid treatment in patients with COPD have examined its effect on airflow limitation [28,48–56]. Findings have been variable, but several studies have found an increase in FEV_1 after treatment.

Watson and co-workers [54] documented no beneficial effects on the level of lung function in a 9-month single-blind follow-up study with 1200 μg budesonide daily. However, a study by Kerstjens and co-workers [51] showed that a response had already been achieved from 3 months onward. On the contrary, in a self-controlled study in 26 patients with moderate COPD, Dompeling and co-workers [53] observed that the prebronchodilator FEV_1 increased during the first 6 months of the trial with 800 μg beclomethasone, whereas during the next 6 months it decreased again. In both studies, inclusion of COPD patients with some "asthmatic features" such as airway reversibility and allergy might have contributed to this early response. Interestingly, Senderovitz and co-workers [57], who divided their patients into corticosteroid-reversible and corticosteroid-irreversible, using 15% increase over baseline as a dividing point after prednisolone (37.5 mg once daily) for 2 weeks, reported that an initial oral trial was of no value in choosing subsequent long-term inhaled therapy. Another remarkable observation comes from Nishimura and co-workers [58], who found a minority of patients (5 of 30) with significant improvement in FEV_1 receiving 3,000 μg/day of beclomethasone dipropionate after a 4-week treatment period. However, some of these responders had a positive bronchodilator challenge, as well as an elevated serum immunoglobulin (Ig)E level or eosinophil count, suggestive of an asthmatic component to their airflow obstruction.

More recent trials have documented that short-term treatment with inhaled corticosteroids influence lung function. After a 3-month course, fluticasone treatment resulted in a higher prebronchodilator FEV_1 (1.17 L versus 1.07 L) when compared with placebo [59]. In the study of Paggiaro and co-workers [60], the mean baseline FEV_1 changed from 1.52 L to 1.48 L in the placebo group and from 1.60 L to 1.71 L in the fluticasone propionate group, with an adjusted mean change of 0.15 L (9.4%) in favor of fluticasone at the end of six months treatment in patients with moderately severe disease. Forced vital capacity (FVC) improved steadily, with an adjusted mean change of 0.33 L (5.6%) at the end of treatment. An early intervention study with fluticasone propionate 250 μg twice daily in subjects with objective signs of obstructive airway disease, which was a mixture of asthma and COPD patients, documented that during the first 3–6 months, lung function improved, followed by a decline, approximately parallel to that observed in patients receiving [61].

The importance of a regular treatment with inhaled corticosteroids in COPD patients is supported by an interesting trial [62] which documented a deterioration in lung function when patients discontinued their inhaled corticosteroids for 6 weeks.

Therefore, it was not unexpected that a meta-analysis of the original data sets of the randomized controlled trials in patients with clearly defined moderately severe COPD published between 1983 and 1996 showed a beneficial course of FEV_1 during 2 years of treatment with relatively high daily dosages of inhaled corticosteroids [63]. However, the dose to be used, duration of treatment, and the time course of their action remained unresolved. A daily dose of 1,500/1,600 μg of the inhaled corticosteroid was more effective than 800 μg, although it should be noted that only a small number of subjects received the lower dose.

Studies on the Annual Rate of Decline in FEV_1

The same meta-analysis [63] also provided clear evidence that inhaled corticosteroids may modify the rate of decline in FEV_1 in patients with moderately severe COPD. This is a very important effect because, as lung function deteriorates, substantial changes in general health occur [64]. However, Renkema and co-workers [39] who followed for 2 years 58 patients with a $FEV_1 < 80\%$ predicted and treated with 1600 μg daily dose of budesonide, alone or in association with 5 mg oral prednisolone, or placebo, documented that the rate of decline in FEV_1 was not different between the groups, whereas the median FEV_1 slope was more negative in current than in ex-smokers. Moreover, no clear correlation was found between response to oral corticosteroids and FEV_1 slope. Also Weir and co-workers [65] were unable to document a significant difference in the decline in FEV_1 between patients treated with 2,000 μg beclomethasone daily dose or placebo.

In the last few years, several fundamental long-term (3 years or more) controlled clinical trials have been carried out, with a careful selection of patients in order to exclude subjects with an asthmatic component of the disease. The results of the trials are seen in Table 2. These long-term randomized controlled trials [66–69] have been unable to show that chronic use of inhaled corticosteroids reduces the annual rate of decline in FEV_1 when compared with placebo. However, in two of the four studies, the mean FEV_1 remained significantly higher throughout the trial in the corticosteroid therapy group, and all showed an initial improvement in the FEV_1 during the first months of treatment. This was demonstrated in patients with all levels of severity of COPD. van den Boom and co-workers [61] have defined this course of FEV_1 as "inverted hockey-stick."

The European Respiratory Society Study on Chronic Obstructive Pulmonary Disease (EUROSCOP) [66] was a multicenter European study that involved 1227 patients with mild COPD (mean FEV_1 77% of predicted value) who continued to smoke. Active treatment was with 400 μg budesonide twice daily. Although the FEV_1 improved during the first 6 months of active treatment, this increase was not maintained. For the rest of the 3-year study period, FEV_1 declined at a similar rate in both the active and placebo

Table 2 Long-Term Effect of Inhaled Corticosteroids

Study	Number of patients enrolled, study duration	Rate of FEV_1 decline versus placebo	Health Outcomes
EUROSCOP, [66]	1,277 patients with mild COPD (mean FEV_1 77% of predicted value). F/U: 36 months	No change with budesonide, 400 μg twice daily	Not evaluated
Copenhagen City Lung Study, [67]	290 patients with mild-moderate COPD (mean FEV_1 86% of predicted value). F/U: 36 months	No change with budesonide, 800 μg plus 400 μg daily for 6 months followed by 400 μg twice daily for 30 months	No change in exacerbations
ISOLDE, [68]	750 patients, with moderate to severe COPD (mean FEV_1 50% of predicted value). F/U: 36 months	No change with fluticasone, 500 μg twice daily	Decreased exacerbations, reduced rate in decline of the disease-specific St. George's Respiratory Questionnaire
Health Lung Study II, [69]	1,116 patients with mild to moderate COPD (mean FEV_1 64% of predicted value). F/U: 40 months	No change with triamcinolone, 600 μg twice daily	Less airway reactivity; reduced respiratory symptoms; slightly reduced hospitalizations; loss of bone mineral density; increased skin bruising

groups (57 mL/year with inhaled corticosteroids versus 69 mL/year in the placebo group). Budesonide had a more beneficial effect in subjects who had smoked less. Subjects with a history of smoking that was at or below the median of 36 pack-years at enrollment had a decrease in FEV_1 of 190 mL during placebo treatment and of 120 mL during budesonide treatment.The loss of FEV_1 in 3 years among subjects with more than 36 pack-years of smoking was 160 mL during placebo treatment and 150 mL during budesonide treatment. The Copenhagen City Lung study [67] was a 3-year study that involved 290 patients with very mild COPD (mean FEV_1 86% of predicted value), of whom over 70% were smokers. Active treatment was with 800 μg plus 400 μg budesonide daily for 6 months, followed by 400 μg twice daily for 30 months. The study reported no statistically significant difference in the rate of FEV_1 decline between the active and placebo groups. The crude rates of FEV_1 decline were slightly smaller than expected (placebo group 41.8 mL per year; budesonide group 45.1 mL per year). The Inhaled Steroids in Obstructive Lung Disease in Europe (ISOLDE) study [68] was a single-country (UK) study involving 751 patients with moderate to severe COPD (mean FEV_1 50% of predicted value). After a run-in period of 8 weeks, and a 2-week treatment with oral prednisolone, patients were randomized to either 500 μg fluticasone twice daily or placebo for 3 years. Initial treatment with prednisolone elicited an average of about 60-mL improvement in FEV_1 in both groups of patients. However, again, there was no statistically significant difference between the two groups in the annual rate of decline in FEV_1. Patients who did not smoke and those who had initially improved with prednisone did not seem to do any better. The Lung Health Study II [69] was a North American study involving 1,116 patients with mild to moderate COPD (mean FEV_1 64% of predicted value). Active treatment was with triamcinolone 600 μg twice daily for 40 months. There was no statistically significant difference found in the annual rate of decline in FEV_1 between the two groups.

All these studies indicate a lack of effect by inhaled corticosteroids on the decline in FEV_1 in COPD patients. However, Burge [70] has argued that this observed lack of effect might at least in part be a result of the statistical modeling used, which cannot adequately compensate for those with more rapidly progressive disease dropping out earlier.

In any case, notwithstanding this negative finding, evidence is accumulating to support the therapeutic use of these agents, at least in patients with more advanced COPD [71]. In fact, whereas inhaled corticosteroids do not affect the decline in FEV_1, they seem to have a significant effect on other clinical markers depending on severity of the disease, such as symptoms, bronchial hyperresponsiveness, exercise capacity, and acute exacerbations, all influencing the patient's quality of life. Although decline of lung function as measured by FEV_1 is a significant and important determinant of COPD morbidity and even mortality, FEV_1 by itself has relatively weak predictive power for these outcomes [72]. Indeed, clinically relevant changes in health status can occur in the absence of discernible effects on lung function [68]. Unfortunately, the corticosteroid-induced modifications of the first three markers are small, and their value is questionable. On the contrary, the impact of long-term treatment with these agents on acute exacerbations seems to be more important. In fact, symptomatic COPD patients do not complain about their rate of decline of FEV_1 but are worried by disease exacerbations and the impact of COPD on their general well-being [1]. For this reason, many researchers consider it as the true indicator of the efficacy of inhaled corticosteroids in patients suffering from stable COPD, although the beneficial effects have not been entirely consistent between studies.

Impact on Symptoms, Bronchial Hyperresponsiveness, and Exercise Capacity

Several clinical trials have documented a positive effect of inhaled corticosteroids on symptoms, lung function, and exercise capacity. Thompson and co-workers [59] reported that a 3-month treatment with fluticasone resulted in a better exercise-induced dyspnea score (3.70 versus 3.47) when compared with the placebo treatment. Symptom scores for median daily cough and sputum volume were lower with fluticasone propionate than with placebo at the end of a 6-month treatment in patients with moderately severe disease [60]. Moreover, patients receiving fluticasone propionate increased their walking distance significantly more than those receiving placebo. Also Renkema and co-workers [39] observed a small decrease in symptoms score in the corticosteroid-treated groups. However, Dompeling and co-workers [73] demonstrated that when COPD patients were treated with beclomethasone for 2 years, the improvement in symptoms observed during months 7–12 was not confirmed later.

In the Health Lung Study II [69], the incidence of respiratory symptoms over the preceding 12 months did not differ significantly between the treatment groups, with the exception of dyspnea, which was more frequent in the placebo group. However, at 9 and 33 months, the triamcinolone group had less reactivity in response to methacholine than the placebo group. It has been suggested that this happened because airway inflammation decreased. Reduced airway reactivity may have been responsible for the reduced incidence of dyspnea and the lower rate of health care visits for respiratory conditions in this group.

The possibility that long-term therapy with inhaled corticosteroids could modify bronchial hyperresponsiveness is often questioned. Auffarth and co-workers [74] showed that the inhalation of 1,600 μg of budesonide for 2 months did not modify PC_{20} histamine, or the citric acid threshold. Overbeek and co-workers [75] documented that delayed therapy had a lower effect on PC_{20} than immediate therapy with inhaled corticosteroid, and Verhoeven et al [76] observed that, in patients with COPD and bronchial hyperresponsiveness, indices of bronchial hyperresponsiveness were not significantly influenced by six-month treatment with fluticasone.

Impact on Acute Exacerbations

Reducing the number of exacerbations of COPD is an important goal of treatment [77–79]. A recent systematic review of nine randomized trials involving a total of 3,976 patients with COPD demonstrated a beneficial effect of inhaled corticosteroids in reducing rates of COPD exacerbations [80]. The risk ratio was 0.70, with similar benefits in those who were and were not pre-treated with systemic corticosteroids. Reductions in exacerbation severity were seen in the Paggiaro's study [60]. In this study, 37% patients in the placebo group and 32% patients in the fluticasone propionate group had had at least one exacerbation by the end of treatment. Significantly more patients in the placebo group than in the fluticasone propionate group had moderate or severe exacerbations (86% compared with 60%).

The ISOLDE investigators reported a statistically significant reduction of 25% in annual exacerbation rate (an extrapolated variable) with fluticasone [68]. However, the clinical significance of this finding was unclear, as the true number of exacerbations was not reported. A post hoc analysis has recently been carried out to determine whether existing criteria for disease severity identify patients with a different probability of exacerbating and whether the effect of inhaled corticosteroids on acute exacerbations is influenced by disease severity [81]. Patients have been stratified into mild and moderate-to-severe COPD using the American Thoracic Society (ATS) criterion of FEV_1 50% predicted, and the total number of exacerbations and those requiring treatment with oral corticosteroids have been examined. Those with moderate-to-severe disease receiving fluticasone had a median rate of 1.47 exacerbations per year, compared to 1.75 exacerbations per year for those receiving placebo, but not in mild disease (0.67 exacerbations per year for those receiving fluticasone, 0.92 exacerbations per year for those receiving placebo). Fluticasone use was associated with fewer patients with >1 exacerbation per year being treated with oral corticosteroids (mild: fluticasone 8%, placebo 16%; moderate-to-severe: fluticasone 17%, placebo 30%). The authors correctly highlighted that the confined effect to patients with more severe airflow limitation could have represented a genuine difference in efficacy dependent on disease severity. Alternatively, it could have been a reflection of the smaller number of episodes identified in mild disease and hence the risk of a Type 2 statistical error, since the proportional reduction was the same.

Halting treatment with inhaled corticosteroids in patients with COPD is associated with both a higher risk and more rapid onset of exacerbations. Jarad and co-workers [82] studied 272 patients entering the run-in phase of the ISOLDE trial. Inhaled corticosteroids were withdrawn in the first week of the study and during the remaining 7 weeks of the trial 38% of those previously treated with these drugs had an exacerbation, compared to 6% of the chronically untreated group. Patients receiving inhaled corticosteroids reported a longer duration of symptoms, but neither this nor any other recorded variable predicted the risk of exacerbation. van der Valk and co-workers [83] analyzed 244 patients who received 1,000 μg per day of the inhaled corticosteroid fluticasone propionate for 4 months during a run-in phase. They then randomized the patients to continue receiving inhaled corticosteroid treatment or to discontinue treatment and take a placebo for 6 months. In the group that stopped taking inhaled corticosteroid, 57% developed at least one exacerbation compared with 47% of the group that continued taking them. Likewise, 21.5% of patients who discontinued inhaled corticosteroid experienced rapid recurrent exacerbations compared with only 4.9% in the group that continued, indicating a more than a fourfold increased risk in those who discontinued.

The effect of inhaled corticosteroids on the exacerbation frequency in COPD has recently been confirmed in two one-year long studies that compared the effect of regular treatment with a long-acting β_2-agonist, an inhaled corticosteroid or the combination of the two in one inhaler in patients with moderate to severe COPD. Treatment with the inhaled corticosteroid alone had a significant effect on the exacerbation rate [84,85].

Impact on Quality of Life

Health status generally slowly deteriorates in patients with COPD over time. In particular, there is evidence that patient quality of life is related to COPD exacerbation frequency [86]. The impact on quality of life of a regular treatment with inhaled corticosteroids is controversial. Seventy-nine patients with COPD, who did not improve with an initial 2 weeks of treatment with prednisone, were randomized to receive either 1600 μg a day of budesonide or placebo for 6 months. At the end of 6 months, patients who received inhaled corticosteroids did not do any better than those who received placebo in terms of quality of life [87]. Also, the Lung Health Study II showed no benefit in quality-of-life measures [69].

On the contrary, ISOLDE study clearly showed a reduced rate in decline of the disease-specific St George's Respiratory Questionnaire, thought to be partly related to the reduced rate of exacerbations [68]. To determine whether change in health status is detectable over time, Spencer and co-workers [88] analyzed data on 387 patients with COPD participating in the ISOLDE study. Health status was measured using a generic instrument, the SF-36, and a disease-specific instrument, the St George's Respiratory Questionnaire, at baseline and every 6 months for 3 years. Progressive deterioration in all domains of health (symptoms, physical activity, and psychosocial function) was detectable using either instrument. Deterioration was slower in the patients receiving fluticasone (1,000 μg daily) as compared with the patients receiving placebo. FEV_1 was correlated with scores on the respiratory questionnaire at baseline, and the changes in the scores and in FEV_1 over time were correlated. At baseline, smokers had poorer scores on the respiratory questionnaire as compared with the ex-smokers; although this difference was maintained throughout the study, smoking did not influence the rate of decline in health status. The importance of inhaled corticosteroids on health status in COPD patients has been recently confirmed by van der Valk and coworkers [83], who documented that discontinuation of inhaled corticosteroid affects distress due to respiratory symptoms and disturbance of physical activity but does not affect the impact on daily living. These findings suggest that inhaled corticosteroids have greatest influence on deterioration in physical aspects of health rather than psychosocial functions.

Impact on Mortality

Mortality related to COPD has increased worldwide over the last two decades [89]. Some studies [60,66] of inhaled corticosteroids did not show a clear survival advantage with the use of inhaled corticosteroids. However, these studies were conducted mostly in patients with only mild to moderate disease, preventing sufficient accrual of mortality data. Also, in a recent meta-analysis [80], including nine randomized trials which have assessed mortality as an outcome, the authors were not able to demonstrate any significant effect of regular use of inhaled corticosteroids on all-cause mortality. However, a population-based cohort study using administrative databases in Ontario, Canada, which was carried out to determine the association between inhaled corticosteroid therapy and the combined risk of repeat hospitalization and all-cause mortality in elderly patients ($n = 22{,}620$) with COPD [90], showed that patients who were provided inhaled corticosteroid therapy postdischarge (within 90 days) were 29% less likely to experience mortality during 1 year of follow-up after adjustment for various confounding factors. The same investigators [91] later showed that the protective benefit of inhaled corticosteroids in mortality extended to 3 years. Moreover, they have observed that medium- and high-dose therapy were associated with greater reductions in mortality rate than low-dose therapy. Correctly, Vestbo [92] has highlighted that these results are reassuring. In fact, it is well known that as COPD progresses, the risk of an exacerbation resulting in death increases. Since inhaled corticosteroids seem to have an effect on exacerbations, particularly in the more severe stages, this finding can explain the observed reduction in mortality. On the other hand, Bourbeau [93] argues that, based on the available data, we cannot conclude that the use of inhaled corticosteroids reduces mortality in patients with COPD. The completion of prospective trials testing the effect of inhaled corticosteroids on mortality are critically important.

D. Inhaled Corticosteroids in Acute Exacerbation of COPD

Inhaled corticosteroids have not been tested adequately in patients with acute exacerbation of COPD. A preliminary report by Nava and Compagnoni [94] has shown that a very short-term trial of fluticasone propionate in ventilator-dependent patients with COPD may induce a bronchodilator response, mainly related to a reduction in airway resistance, that is not detected by the usual pulmonary function tests. Although the enrolled patients were not suffering from an acute exacerbation, this study seems to indicate the possibility of using inhaled corticosteroids even in extremely compromised patients. In effect, some recent data show that inhaled corticosteroids are as effective as oral corticosteroids in the management of acute exacerbations of COPD. In 199 patients with an acute exacerbation of COPD, Maltais and co-workers [95] completed a double-blind randomized trial of nebulized budesonide (2,000 μg every 6 hr), oral prednisolone (30 mg every 12 hr), and placebo. Compared with placebo, the postbronchodilator FEV_1 was 0.10 L higher with budesonide and 0.16 L higher with prednisolone; the difference between budesonide and prednisolone was not significant. However, more studies are needed to confirm this interesting hypothesis.

IV. Adverse Effects

An analysis of systemic activity and safety of corticosteroids is essential to make appropriate risk–benefit decisions for individual patients with COPD. Adverse effects are thought to be greater with higher doses and duration of therapy. Those attributed to systemic corticosteroid therapy include weight gain, easy bruisability, hypertension, glucose intolerance, epigastric complaints, infections, osteoporosis and fractures, myopathy, adrenal suppression, and cataracts [96]. Corticosteroids have also been shown to have adverse effects on respiratory muscles, which contribute to muscle weakness, decreased functionality, and respiratory failure in patients with advanced COPD [97]. However, the actual incidence of adverse effects has not been studied adequately in patients with COPD, although it has been documented that survival of patients with corticosteroid-induced myopathy was reduced in comparison with control patients with COPD with similar degree of airflow obstruction [98]. In any case, corticosteroid-induced myopathy is a complication of high-dose systemic corticosteroid use. Inhaled corticosteroid therapy is associated with increased rates of oropharyngeal candidiasis, skin bruising, and lower mean cortisol levels [80].

A particular problem that must always be borne in mind is the possibility that corticosteroids could induce osteoporosis. Patients with COPD are at increased risk for osteoporosis. Data from 9,502 people [99] showed the risk of osteoporosis was nearly doubled in people with COPD, and that the risk increased in line with the severity of airflow limitation. Moderate but not mild COPD was also associated with an increased risk of osteoporosis. It is not unexpected, therefore, that some studies have demonstrated lower bone density, primarily in areas with high trabecular bone content such as ribs and vertebrae, in COPD patients who are under chronic corticosteroid use. In a population of older patients taking long-term oral corticosteroids for chronic chest disease, low bone mineral density was a risk factor for fracture, and the magnitude of this relationship was similar to that seen in patients with involutional osteoporosis [100]. The use of oral corticosteroids was associated with a large dose-dependent increase in vertebral fracture rate, which did not appear to be due to a reduction in bone mineral density. When assessing the risk of fracture in such patients, cumulative oral corticosteroid dose is a strong risk factor independent of bone mineral density. McEvoy and co-workers [101] evaluated the prevalence of vertebral fractures among 312 men with smoking-related COPD. At least one radiographic fracture was seen in 49% of patients who had never used corticosteroids, in 57% of inhaled corticosteroid users, and in 63% of systemic corticosteroid users. Thoracic fractures were three times as common as lumbar fractures. An increasing dose and duration of corticosteroid use were associated with a greater number and severity of fractures.

The Lung Health Study II showed a 2% decrease in femoral neck bone density [69]. The EUROSCOP study using lower doses of inhaled corticosteroids showed no changes in bone density [66]. In effect, osteoporosis becomes a concern with daily doses in the range of 1,000 μg/day and higher. In any case, considering that both inhaled corticosteroid therapy and the diagnosis of COPD are risk factors for bone loss, it would be reasonable to screen for osteoporosis in those patients who are receiving long-term, high doses of inhaled corticosteroids. Patients requiring long-term corticosteroids should be treated preventively with calcium and vitamin D supplements, and weight-bearing exercise. Biphosphonates, calcitonin, and hormone replacement therapy are other options for preventing or treating corticosteroid induced osteoporosis and should be considered where appropriate. Efficacy is mainly limited to preventing bone loss at the lumbar spine. They are less efficacious at preventing or treating bone loss at the femoral neck [102].

V. Corticosteroids and Guidelines

Most guidelines for the diagnosis and management of stable COPD, such as those from the European Respiratory Society (ERS) [77], ATS [78], and British Thoracic Society (BTS) [79], emphasize the need to document corticosteroid responsiveness before long-term use. They do not recommend corticosteroids for patients who are not corticosteroid responders, and encourage use of the lowest dose possible in patients who are responders to these compounds and need corticosteroids. The ERS [77] and BTS [79] advocate the use of inhaled corticosteroids to replace or reduce oral corticosteroids in patients who are responders to these agents and require long-term corticosteroids. The ERS [77] also suggests a role for inhaled corticosteroids in patients with mild disease who are "fast decliners" in FEV_1. The ATS [78] does not recommend the use of inhaled corticosteroids until more information is available.

Rudolf [103] examined the use of corticosteroids within and between different European countries and compared it with what is currently recommended in COPD guidelines issued by the ERS [77] and by the BTS [79]. Corticosteroids, which accounted for more than one-fifth of all COPD prescribing in the United Kingdom and one-quarter of all COPD prescriptions in the Netherlands, totaled only one tenth of all prescriptions in Germany and Austria. The author suggested that, despite different national attitudes about the role of inhaled corticosteroids in COPD, this discrepancy could partly be explained by the fact that, at least in the United Kingdom, substantial numbers of COPD patients are misdiagnosed as having asthma, for which the use of inhaled corticosteroids can be regarded as far more appropriate. Interestingly, the use of inhaled corticosteroids in patients with moderate to severe disease by specialist respiratory physicians, who were presumably making informed decisions about the management of correctly diagnosed patients, was larger.

Also, the more recent guidelines for the diagnosis and management of COPD, such as those from the Veterans Health Administration/Department of Veterans Affairs (VHA/DOD) [104] and the Global Obstructive Lung Disease initiative (GOLD) [105], are in general agreement that inhaled corticosteroids should not be used routinely in patients with stable COPD, and that long-term corticosteroid use in still controversial. Both guidelines recommend a short-term trial of corticosteroids to ascertain responsiveness (see Table 3). Response should be measured both clinically and with spirometry. If the patient experiences a definitive improvement, then long-term use may be beneficial for symptoms. A typical trial of oral prednisone is 40–60 mg/day for 10–14 days. The appropriate dose of inhaled corticosteroids has not been determined, but a trial of 14–21 days of the equivalent of 1,500 μg/day beclomethasone or fluticasone 880 μg/day has been suggested [104].

It must be highlighted that VHA/DOD [104] recommends that patients on maximal bronchodilator therapy who have not had a satisfactory response may be considered candidates for a corticosteroid trial. Patients who have a response should be tapered to the lowest possible oral dose. Supplementation or substitution with a high-dose inhaled corticosteroid may allow further reduction or discontinuation of the oral corticosteroid.

GOLD [105] warrants that regular treatment with inhaled corticosteroids is appropriate only for symptomatic COPD patients with a doc-

Table 3 High-Dose Oral Prednisone Trial

Since short-term (2–3 weeks) high-dose steroids do not produce serious toxicities, the ideal use is to administer the glucocorticoids in a short "burst" (up to 40 mg/day for 2–3 weeks).
A positive response includes symptomatic benefit and an increase in FEV1 > 20%.
In nonresponders, discontinue oral steroid.
It should be remembered that it is not known whether a response to short-term, high-dose oral steroid reliably predicts long-term response.
Combination oral and inhaled steroids may be tried as an oral steroid-sparing measure.
Repeatedly evaluate patients to determine if steroid therapy can be discontinued.

umented spirometric response to inhaled corticosteroids or in those with an $FEV_1 < 50\%$ predicted (Stage IIB.; moderate COPD, and Stage III, severe COPD) and repeated exacerbations requiring treatment with antibiotics or oral corticosteroids. Long-term treatment with oral systemic corticosteroids is not recommended for COPD. However, if inhaled corticosteroids have no effect in advanced disease, the use of oral corticosteroids may be considered, but there is no evidence for an effect and a minimal dose must be used [106].

Unfortunately, data that could indicate if these last guidelines have influenced the prescriptive behaviors of physicians are still lacking. Nonetheless, the four fundamental studies that have explored the impact of regular treatment with inhaled corticosteroids on COPD history [66–69] have clearly documented that long-term (3 years) treatment with inhaled corticosteroids is not beneficial in patients with mild or moderate COPD. They have also shown that patients with severe COPD (FEV_1 about 50% of predicted) may feel better with improved quality of life and fewer exacerbations or "flare-ups" if they are treated with a high dose of inhaled corticosteroid, regardless of whether they continue to smoke or not. Anyway, initial improvement with a short course of corticosteroid tablets does not help identify subjects who will benefit from long-term treatment with inhaled corticosteroids.

Both VHA/DOD [104] and GOLD [105] address issues of the use of corticosteroids for the management of acute exacerbations of COPD (Table 4). VHA/DOD [104] suggests utilizing 0.6–0.8 mg/kg prednisone per day to treat outpatient acute exacerbations Once the patient is stabilized, the dose should be tapered carefully, monitoring for relapse of the exacerbation. The goal should be to wean the patient off corticosteroids. This may not be possible in some patients, who should then be treated with the smallest effective dose ideally every other day. GOLD [105] establishes that systemic corticosteroids are beneficial in the management of acute exacerbations of

Table 4 Comparison of Recommendations of VHA/DOD and WHO/NHLBI for the Use of Corticosteroids for the Management of Acute Exacerbation of COPD

VHA/DOD [104]	*Outpatient management*: Certain patients should be considered for systemic corticosteroid treatment. Indications for corticosteroids in COPD exacerbation represent consensus based on expert opinion. Patient groups to consider include the following: On oral corticosteroid or on inhaled corticosteroids Who recently stopped oral corticosteroids Who previously responded to oral corticosteroids With oxygen saturation less than 90% With peak expiratory flow less than 110 L/min Not responding to initial bronchodilator therapy A typical oral dose is 0.6–0.8 mg/kg prednisone per day. Once the patient is stabilized, the dose should be tapered carefully, monitoring for relapse of the exacerbation. The goal should be to wean the patient off corticosteroids. This may not be possible in some patients, who should then be treated with the smallest effective dose, ideally every other day. *Inpatient management*: Corticosteroids should be given early in patients with acute exacerbation of COPD, particularly in patients with severe underlying lung function and those with severe exacerbation. Studies demonstrating the benefits of orticosteroids in acute exacerbation involved a small number of patients and show small improvement in lung function. The recommend dose equivalents of at least 0.5 mg/kg of methylprednisolone every 6 hr for at least 3 days.

Table 4 Continued

GOLD [105]	*Home management*: Systemic corticosteroids are beneficial in the management of acute exacerbations of COPD. They shorten recovery time and help to restore lung function more quickly. They should be considered in addition to bronchodilators if the patient's baseline FEV_1 is less than 50% predicted. A dose of 40 mg of prednisolone per day for 10 days is recommended. *Hospital management*: Oral or intravenous corticosteroids are recommended as an addition to bronchodilator therapy (plus eventually antibiotics and oxygen therapy) in the hospital management of acute exacerbations of COPD. The exact dose that should be given is not known, but high doses are associated with a significant risk of side effects; 30–40 mg of oral prednisolone daily for 10–14 days is a reasonable compromise between efficacy and safety. Prolonged treatment does not result in a greater efficacy and increases the risk of side effects.

COPD. They should be considered in addition to bronchodilators if the symptoms are severe. A dose of 40 mg of prednisolone per day for 10 days is recommended. For the hospital management of acute exacerbation of COPD, VHA/DOD [104] recommends the early administration of corticosteroids in patients, particularly in those with severe underlying lung function and those with severe exacerbation. The suggested dose is equivalent to at least 0.5 mg/kg of methylprednisolone every 6 hr for at least 3 days. Oral or intravenous corticosteroids are recommended by GOLD [105] as an addition to bronchodilator therapy in the hospital management of acute exacerbations of COPD. The exact dose that should be given is not known, but 30–40 mg of oral prednisolone daily tapering over 10–14 days is, a reasonable compromise between efficacy and safety. Prolonged treatment does not result in a greater efficacy and increases the risk of side effects.

VI. Combining an Inhaled Corticosteroid and a Long-Acting β_2-Agonist in COPD

In these last few years, it has become increasingly more evident that the concomitant use of an inhaled corticosteroid and a long-acting β_2-agonist can influence both the airway obstruction and the airway inflammation of COPD patients.

A. Pharmacological Rationale

When a long-acting β_2-agonist is added to an inhaled corticosteroid, it has the potential for countering some of the negative effects of the corticosteroid. For example, several data indicate that long-acting β_2-agonists increase cyclic adenosine 3'5'-monophosphate (cAMP) in neutrophils and therefore inhibit their adhesion, accumulation, and activation, and induce apoptosis [107]. The end result is a possible reduction in the number and activation status of neutrophils in airway tissue and in the airway lumen. They also can cut the number of neutrophils that adhere to the vascular endothelium at sites of inflammation and reduce the amount of plasma leakage [108], but the relevance of these findings to COPD patients is unclear. It is noteworthy to highlight that glucocorticoids have been shown to increase high-affinity β-agonist binding in human neutrophils [109]. The fact that long-acting β_2-agonists increase the peripheral deposition of the inhaled corticosteroid, enhancing the anti-inflammatory activity, constitute another possible mechanism [110]. The apparent benefit in combining agents of these two classes of drugs might be due to a synergistic interaction of the compounds, although the basic molecular mechanism of this interaction is still to be fully identified. Corticosteroids can prevent, at least partially, homologous down-regulation of β_2-adrenoceptor (β_2-AR) number and induce an increase in the rate of receptor synthesis through a process of extended β_2-AR gene transcription [111]. Although airway smooth muscle is among the tissues least susceptible to homologous down-regulation, long-term treatment with a long-acting β_2-agonist may result in tolerance to the bronchodilator effects [112]. Corticosteroids have the potential for enhancing the airway relaxant response to β-adrenergic stimulation. An in-vitro experimental finding suggests that, at least in rabbit, this effect is correlated with increased β-adrenoceptor expression in the tissue [113]. However, the efficiency of coupling between the β_2-AR and G_s (the G protein that mediates stimulation of adenylyl cyclase) has been reported to be modulated by glucocorticoids [114]. As a result, β_2-

AR-stimulated adenylyl cyclase activity and cAMP accumulation increase after glucocorticoid treatment.

An example of interaction between these two classes of drugs that might be useful in COPD is the synergistic inhibition by corticosteroids and long-acting β_2-agonists on TNF-α-induced IL-8 release from cultured human airway smooth-muscle cells [115], and the capacity to counteract the enhancement of long-acting β_2-agonists on TNF-α-induced IL-8 production in cultured human bronchial epithelial cells [116]. IL-8, being a potent chemoattractant and an activator for neutrophils, may result in a persistent inflammatory cycle by establishing a positive feedback loop. Reduction in neutrophil number and function could reduce the severity of disease and degree of airflow obstruction in patients with COPD [115].

Another important finding is the capacity of both inhaled corticosteroids and long-acting β_2-agonists to reduce the total number of bacteria adhering to the respiratory mucosa in a concentration-dependent manner without altering the bacterial tropism for mucosa and to preserve ciliated cells [117]. It is well known that airway colonization and chronic infection contribute to progressive pulmonary damage in COPD patients via the action of proinflammatory substances in what is known as the "vicious circle theory" [118].

B. The Inhaled Combination Therapy in Stable COPD

The addition of an inhaled corticosteroid to a long-acting β_2-agonist was initially studied in a 3-month trial that enrolled 80 COPD patients. The combination therapy progressively improved lung function over the 3-month period compared to the long-acting bronchodilator treatment alone, although the difference between treatments was not statistically significant [119]. However, the combination of salmeterol with fluticasone allowed a significantly greater improvement in lung function after salbutamol than salmeterol alone. This finding is important, because when the airway obstruction becomes more severe, the therapeutic option is to add a fast-acting inhaled β_2-agonist as rescue medication to cause rapid relief of bronchospasm.

The value of regular combination therapy with long-acting β_2-agonists and corticosteroids delivered via a single inhaler to COPD patients has repeatedly been documented. A 24-week treatment with the salmeterol/fluticasone propionate combination explored not only the potential for increasing airflow, but also for reducing symptoms (including dyspnea), and improving health status, compared with the individual components and placebo [120]. The results documented that the salmeterol/fluticasone propionate combination not only improved airflow obstruction, but also provided clinical benefits as manifested by reduced severity of dyspnea, reduced use of rescue salbutamol, and improved health status.

A 52-week multicentre, randomized, double-blind, placebo-controlled trial (Trial of Inhaled Steroids and Long-acting β_2 Agonists, or TRISTAN) compared the safety and efficacy of the salmeterol/fluticasone propionate combination 50/500 μg bid with that of the individual drugs in 1465 patients with COPD (mean FEV_1 45% predicted) [84]. Following 1 year of treatment, the combination of inhaled fluticasone and salmeterol increased FEV_1 and improved health status, as measured by the St. George's Respiratory Questionnaire, to a much greater extent than did placebo or salmeterol alone. Additionally, patients treated with combination therapy had greater reductions in symptom scores compared with all other treatments and greater reductions in activity (limitations) scores compared with placebo and fluticasone. In the total group, salmeterol/fluticasone combination produced a significant reduction in exacerbation rate of 25% compared to placebo. This reduction was 30% in the more severe subgroup ($FEV_1 < 50\%$ predicted), as against a 10% reduction in the less severe subgroup ($FEV_1 \geq 50\%$ predicted).

The combination of budesonide/formoterol has been investigated in a 12-month, randomized, double-blind, placebo-controlled, parallel-group, multicenter study. A total of 812 adults with moderate to severe COPD (mean FEV_1 36% predicted) received two inhalations of either 160/4.5 μg budesonide/formoterol (total dose 320/9 mg), 200 μg budesonide, 4.5 μg formoterol, or placebo bid [85]. Budesonide/formoterol treatment increased FEV_1 by 15% versus placebo, 9% versus budesonide and 1% versus formoterol. These lung function improvements were maintained throughout the 12-month study. Moreover, the combination therapy decreased the mean total symptom score, increased the number of symptom-controlled days and awakening-free nights recorded in the same patients, reduced use of reliever medication, increased reliever-free days when compared to placebo, and improved health-related quality of life. Greater improvements were seen with budesonide/formoterol compared with the other treatments, but these did not achieve statistical significance. Budesonide/formoterol combination also produced statistically and clinically significant reductions in exacerbations in patients with moderate to severe COPD. It reduced the number of severe exacerbations/patient/year by 24% versus placebo, 23% versus formoterol and 11% versus budesonide. Moreover, the combination therapy the number of mild exacerbations compared with placebo (62%), budesonide (35%), and formoterol (15%).

C. Adverse Effects

There is clear evidence that the concentration of inhaled corticosteroids can be reduced when combined with β_2-agonists, thereby minimizing the side effects of the drugs [121]. Nonetheless, there is a real need for establishing whether side effects induced by the combination therapy with long-acting β_2-agonists and corticosteroids are overcome by the clinical advantages.

The combined use of salmeterol and fluticasone propionate in a single formulation provides additive benefit in the treatment of COPD but with comparable safety to the individual components used alone [84,120]. In the TRISTAN study, all treatments were well tolerated [84], although oropharyngeal candidiasis was higher in fluticasone-treated groups (placebo 2%, salmeterol 2%, fluticasone 7%, salmeterol/fluticasone combination 8%). Also, budesonide/formoterol was well tolerated and had a safety profile similar to placebo and the mono-components in patients with moderate to severe COPD during 12 months of treatment [85].

VII. Conclusion

There is a large agreement that very few therapies offer significant benefits to patients with COPD [122]. Since inhaled corticosteroids are potentially beneficial in this disease, their use remains one of the possible therapeutic approaches to the patients with stable COPD [1,70,71]. Because, as the COPE study suggests, close to 40% of patients have no untoward effect from the withdrawal of inhaled corticosteroids [83], there is an urgent need to identify which subgroup of patients with COPD patients responds well to prolonged inhaled glucocorticoid therapy. Therefore, until a test is developed that will distinguish potential corticosteroid responders from nonresponders, it is worthwhile to treat patients with moderate to severe COPD, especially if they manifest repeated exacerbations.

The evidence showing that inhaled corticosteroids are useful agents in the treatment of COPD and the possibility of combining them with long-acting β_2-agonists offer a further therapeutic option that can, in any case, enlarge the number of patients who can be benefited by these agents. The study of Soriano and co-workers [123], which used the UK General Practice Research Database, suggests that the presence of an inhaled corticosteroid in the therapeutic regimen of COPD patients is more effective that the sole bronchodilator in decreasing mortality rate. It can not be forgotten that this study was observational and thus open to all the usual criticisms that can be applied to such studies. However, it seems to indicate that the use of bronchodilators only is the less effective action in the management of COPD patients. This contrasts with the indications of different guidelines [77–79, 104,105], but it is a very important message because, despite recent advances in our understanding for COPD and its treatments, current therapy of COPD is too often based on a nihilistic approach driven by the ineffectiveness of present treatments, other than smoking cessation, to slow the relentlessly progressive loss of lung function that characterizes COPD [122].

References

1. Calverley PM. Inhaled corticosteroids are beneficial in chronic obstructive pulmonary disease. Am J Respir Crit Care Med 2000; 161:341–342.
2. Barnes PJ. Inhaled corticosteroids are not beneficial in chronic obstructive pulmonary disease. Am J Respir Crit Care Med 2000; 161:342–344.
3. Saetta M. Airway inflammation in chronic obstructive pulmonary disease. Am J Respir Crit Care Med 1999; 160:S17–S20.
4. Barnes PJ. Chronic obstructive pulmonary disease. N Engl J Med 2000; 343: 269–280.
5. Saetta M, Turato G, Maestrelli P, et al. Cellular and structural bases of chronic obstructive pulmonary disease. Am J Respir Crit Care Med 2001; 163: 1304–1309.
6. Stanescu D, Sanna A, Veritier C, et al. Airways obstruction, chronic expectoration and rapid decline of FEV_1 in smokers are associated with increased levels of sputum neutrophils. Thorax 1996; 51:267–271.
7. Di Stefano A, Capelli A, Lusuardi M, et al. Severity of airflow limitation is associated with severity of airway inflammation in smokers. Am J Respir Crit Care Med 1998; 158:1277–1285.
8. Jeffery PK. Remodeling in asthma and chronic obstructive lung disease. Am J Respir Crit Care Med 2001; 164:S28–S38.
9. Keatings VM, Collins PD, Scott DM, et al. Differences in interleukin-8 and tumor necrosis factor-á in induced sputum from patients with chronic obstructive pulmonary disease or asthma. Am J Respir Crit Care Med 1996; 153: 530–534.
10. Postma DS, Kerstjens HA. Are inhaled glucocorticosteroids effective in chronic obstructive pulmonary disease? Am J Respir Crit Care Med 1999; 160: S66–S71.
11. Culpitt SV, Rogers DF, Shah P, et al. Impaired inhibition by dexamethasone of cytokine release by alveolar macrophages from patients with chronic obstructive pulmonary disease. Am J Respir Crit Care Med 2003; 167:24–31.
12. Ito K, Lim S, Caramori G, et al. Cigarette smoking reduces histone deacetylase 2 expression, enhances cytokine expression, and inhibits glucocorticoid actions in alveolar macrophages. FASEB J 2001; 15:1110–1112.
13. Ito K, Lim S, Caramori G, et al. A molecular mechanism of action of theophylline: induction of histone deacetylase activity to decrease inflammatory gene expression. Proc Natl Acad Sci USA 2002; 99:8921–8926.
14. Cox G, Whitehead L, Dolovich M, et al. A randomized controlled trial on the effect of inhaled corticosteroids on airways inflammation in adult cigarette smokers. Chest 1999; 115:1271–1277.

15. Thompson AB, Mueller MB, Heires AJ, et al. Aerosolized beclomethasone in chronic bronchitis: improved pulmonary function and diminished airway inflammation. Am Rev Respir Dis 1992; 146:389–395.
16. Keatings VM, Jatakanon A, Worsdell YM, et al. Effects of inhaled and oral glucocorticoids on inflammatory indices in asthma and COPD. Am J Respir Crit Care Med 1997; 155:542–548.
17. Culpitt SV, Maziak W, Loukidis S, et al. Effect of high dose inhaled steroid on cells, cytokines, and proteases in induced sputum in chronic obstructive pulmonary disease. Am J Respir Crit Care Med 1999; 160:1635–1639.
18. Loppow D, Schleiss MB, Kanniess F, et al. In patients with chronic bronchitis a four week trial with inhaled steroids does not attenuate airway inflammation. Respir Med 2001; 95:115–121.
19. Lomas DA, Ip M, Chamba A, Stockley RA. The effect of in vitro and in vivo dexamethasone on human neutrophil function. Agents Actions 1991; 33:279–285.
20. Llewellyn-Jones CG, Hill SL, Stockley RA. Effect of fluticasone propionate on neutrophil chemotaxis, superoxide generation, and extracellular proteolytic activity in vitro. Thorax 1994; 49:207–212.
21. Confalonieri M, Mainardi E, Della Porta R, et al. Inhaled corticosteroids reduce neutrophilic bronchial inflammation in patients with chronic obstructive pulmonary disease. Thorax 1998; 53:583–585.
22. Llewellyn-Jones CG, Harris TA, Stockley RA. Effect of fluticasone propionate on sputum of patients with chronic bronchitis and emphysema. Am J Respir Crit Care Med 1996; 153:616–621.
23. Hattotuwa KL, Gizycki MJ, Ansari TW, et al. The effects of inhaled fluticasone on airway inflammation in chronic obstructive pulmonary disease: a double-blind, placebo-controlled biopsy study. Am J Respir Crit Care Med 2002; 165:1592–1596.
24. Yildiz F, Kaur AC, Ilgazli A, et al. Inhaled corticosteroids may reduce neutrophilic inflammation in patients with stable chronic obstructive pulmonary disease. Respiration 2000; 67:71–76.
25. Balbi B, Majori M, Bertacco S, et al. Inhaled corticosteroids in stable COPD patients: do they have effects on cells and molecular mediators of airway inflammation? Chest 2000; 117:1633–1637.
26. Gizycki MJ, Hattotuwa KL, Barnes N, et al. Effects of fluticasone propionate on inflammatory cells in COPD: an ultrastructural examination of endobronchial biopsy tissue. Thorax 2002; 57:799–803.
27. Callahan CM, Dittus RS, Katz BP. Oral corticosteroid therapy for patients with stable chronic obstructive pulmonary disease: a meta-analysis. Ann Intern Med 1991; 114:216–223.
28. Weir DC, Burge PS. Effects of high dose inhaled beclomethasone dipropionate, 750 μg and 1500 μg twice daily and 40 mg per day oral prednisolone on lung function, symptoms and brochial hyper-reactivity in patients with non-asthmatic chronic airflow obstruction. Thorax 1993; 48:309–316.
29. Wempe JB, Postma DS, Breederveld N, et al. Separate and combined effects of

corticosteroids and bronchodilators on airflow obstruction and airway hyperresponsiveness in asthma. J Allergy Clin Immunol 1992; 89:679–687.
30. Wempe JB, Postma DS, Breederveld N, et al. Effects of corticosteroids on bronchodilator action in chronic obstructive lung disease. Thorax 1992; 47: 616–621.
31. Schols AM, Wesseling G, Kester AD, et al. Dose dependent increased mortality risk in COPD patients treated with oral glucocorticoids. Eur Respir J 2001; 17:337–342.
32. Davies L, Nisar M, Pearson MG, et al. Oral corticosteroid trials in the management of stable chronic obstructive pulmonary disease. QJM 1999; 92: 395–400.
33. Nisar M, Walshaw MJ, Earis JE, et al. Assessment of airway reversibility of airway obstruction in patients with chronic obstructive airways disease. Thorax 1990; 45:190–194.
34. Weir DC, Gove RI, Robertson AS, et al. Response to corticosteroids in chronic airflow obstruction: relationship to emphysema and airway collapse. Eur Respir J 1991; 4:1185–1190.
35. Chanez P, Vignola AM, O'Shaugnessy T, et al. Corticosteroid reversibility in COPD is related to features of asthma. Am J Respir Crit Care Med 1997; 155:1529–1534.
36. Pizzichini E, Pizzichini MM, Gibson P, et al. Sputum eosinophilia predicts benefit from prednisone in smokers with chronic obstructive bronchitis. Am J Respir Crit Care Med 1998; 158:1511–1517.
37. Fujimoto K, Kubo K, Yamamoto H, et al. Eosinophilic inflammation in the airway is related to glucocorticoid reversibility in patients with pulmonary emphysema. Chest 1999; 115:697–702.
38. Postma DS, Peters I, Steenhuis EJ, et al. Moderately severe chronic airflow obstruction: can corticosteroids slow down obstruction? Eur Respir J 1988; 1: 22–26.
39. Renkema TEJ, Schouten JP, Koeter GH, Postma DS. Effects of long-term treatment with corticosteroids in COPD. Chest 1996; 109:1156–1162.
40. Rice KL, Rubins JB, Lebahn F, et al. Withdrawal of chronic systemic corticosteroids in patients with COPD: a randomized trial. Am J Respir Crit Care Med 2000; 162:174–178.
41. Kerstjens HA. Stable chronic obstructive pulmonary disease. Br Med J 1999; 319:495–500.
42. Bach PB, Brown C, Gelfand SE, et al. Management of acute exacerbations of chronic obstructive pulmonary disease: a summary and appraisal of published evidence. Ann Intern Med 2001; 134:600–620.
43. Wood-Baker R, Walters EH, Gibson P. Oral corticosteroids for acute exacerbations of chronic obstructive pulmonary disease. Cochrane Database Syst Rev 2001; 2:CD001288.
44. Niewoehner DE, Erbland ML, Deupree RH, et al. Effect of systemic glucocorticoids on exacerbations of chronic obstructive pulmonary disease. Department of Veterans Affairs Cooperative Study Group. N Engl J Med 1999; 340, 1941–1947.

45. Davies L, Angus R, Calverley PM. Oral corticosteroids in patients admitted to hospital with exacerbations of chronic obstructive pulmonary disease: a prospective randomized controlled trial. Lancet 1999; 354:456–460.
46. Thompson WH, Nielson CP, Carvalho P, et al. Controlled trial of oral prednisone in outpatients with acute COPD exacerbation. Am J Respir Crit Care Med 1996; 154:407–412.
47. Shim CS, Williams MHAerosol beclomethasone in patients with steroid-responsive chronic obstructive pulmonary disease. Am J Med 1985; 78:655–658.
48. Engel T, Heinig JM, Madsen O, et al. A trial of inhaled budesonide on airway responsiveness in smokers with chronic bronchitis. Eur Respir J 1989; 2:935–939.
49. Bergstrand H, Bjornson A, Blaschke E, et al. Effects of an inhaled corticosteroid, budesonide, on alveolar macrophage function in smokers. Thorax 1990; 45:362–368.
50. Auffarth B, Postma DS, de Monchy JG, et al. Effects of inhaled budesonide on spirometric values, reversibility, airway responsiveness, and cough threshold in smokers with chronic obstructive lung disease. Thorax 1991; 46:372–377.
51. Kerstjens HAM, Brand PLP, Hughes MD, et al. A comparison of bronchodilator therapy with or without inhaled corticosteroid therapy for obstructive airways disease. N Engl J Med 1992; 327:1413–1419.
52. Thompson AB, Mueller MB, Heires AJ, et al. Aerosolized beclomethasone in chronic bronchitis: improved pulmonary function and diminished airway inflammation. Am Rev Respir Dis 1992; 146:389–395.
53. Dompeling E, van Schayck CP, Molema J, et al. Inhaled beclomethasone improves the course of asthma and COPD. Eur Respir J 1992; 5:945–952.
54. Watson A, Lim TK, Joyce H, et al. Failure of inhaled corticosteroids to modify bronchoconstrictor or bronchodilator responsiveness in middle-aged smokers with mild airflow obstruction. Chest 1992; 101:350–355.
55. Weiner P, Weiner M, Azgad Y, et al. Inhaled budesonide therapy for patients with stable COPD. Chest 1995; 108:1568–1571.
56. Wilcke JT, Dirksen A. The effect of inhaled glucocorticosteroids in emphysema due to alpha1-antitrypsin deficiency. Respir Med 1997; 91:275–279.
57. Senderovitz T, Vestbo J, Frandsen J, et al. Steroid reversibility test followed by inhaled budesonide or placebo in outpatients with stable chronic obstructive pulmonary disease. Danish Society of Respiratory Medicine. Respir Med 1999; 93:715–718.
58. Nishimura K, Koyama H, Ikeda A, et al. The effect of high-dose inhaled beclomethasone dipropionate in patients with stable COPD. Chest 1999; 115: 31–37.
59. Thompson WH, Carvalho P, Souza JP, et al. Controlled trial of inhaled fluticasone propionate in moderate to severe COPD. Lung 2002; 180:191–201.
60. Paggiaro PL, Dahle R, Bakran I, et al. Multicentre randomised placebo-controlled trial of inhaled fluticasone propionate in patients with chronic obstructive pulmonary disease. Lancet 1998; 351:773–780.
61. van den Boom G, Rutten-van Molken MPMH, Molema J, et al. The cost ef-

fectiveness of early treatment with fluticasone propionate 250 μg twice a day in subjects with obstructive airway disease. Results of the DIMCA program. Am J Respir Crit Care Med 2001; 164:2057–2066.
62. O'Brien A, Russo-Magno P, Karki A, et al. Effects of withdrawal of inhaled steroids in men with severe irreversible airflow obstruction. Am J Respir Crit Care Med 2001; 164:365–371.
63. van Grunsven PM, van Schayck CP, Derenne JP, et al. Long term effects of inhaled corticosteroids in chronic obstructive pulmonary disease: a meta-analysis. Thorax 1999; 54:7–14.
64. Jones PW, Quirk FH, Baveystock CM. The St George's respiratory questionnaire. Respir Med 1991; 85(suppl B):25–31.
65. Weir DC, Bale GA, Bright P, et al. A double-blind placebo-controlled study of the effect of inhaled beclomethasone dipropionate for 2 years in patients with nonasthmatic chronic obstructive pulmonary disease. Clin Exp Allergy 1999; 29(Suppl 2):125–128.
66. Pauwels RA, Löfdahl CG, Laitinen LA, et al. Long-term treatment with inhaled budesonide in persons with mild chronic obstructive pulmonary disease who continue smoking: European Respiratory Society Study on Chronic Obstructive Pulmonary Disease. N Engl J Med 1999; 340:1948–1953.
67. Vestbo J, Sorensen T, Lange P, et al. Long-term effect of inhaled budesonide in mild and moderate chronic obstructive pulmonary disease: a randomized controlled trial. Lancet 1999; 353:1819–1823.
68. Burge PS, Calverley PMA, Jones PW, et al. Randomized, double blind, placebo controlled study of fluticasone propionate in patients with moderate to severe chronic obstructive pulmonary disease. The ISOLDE trial. Br Med J 2000; 320:1297–1303.
69. The Lung Health Study Research GroupEffect of inhaled triamcinolone on the decline in pulmonary function in chronic obstructive pulmonary disease. N Engl J Med 2000; 343:1902–1909.
70. Burge S. Should inhaled corticosteroids be used in the long term treatment of chronic obstructive pulmonary disease? Drugs 2001; 61:1535–1544.
71. Pauwels R. Inhaled glucocorticosteroids and chronic obstructive pulmonary disease: how full is the glass? Am J Respir Crit Care Med 2002; 165:1579–1580.
72. Anthonisen NR, Wright EC, Hodgkin JE. Prognosis in chronic obstructive pulmonary disease. Am Rev Respir Dis 1986; 133:14–20.
73. Dompeling E, van Schayck CP, van Grunsven PM, et al. Slowing the deterioration of asthma and chronic obstructive pulmonary disease observed during bronchodilator therapy by adding inhaled corticosteroids. A 4-year prospective study. Ann Intern Med 1993; 118:770–778.
74. Auffarth B, Postma DS, de Monchy JG, et al. Effects of inhaled budesonide on spirometric values, reversibility, airway responsiveness, and cough threshold in smokers with chronic obstructive lung disease. Thorax 1991; 46:372–377.
75. Overbeek SE, Kerstjens HA, Bogaard JM, et al. Is delayed introduction of inhaled corticosteroids harmful in patients with obstructive airways disease

(asthma and COPD)? The Dutch CNSLD Study Group. The Dutch Chronic Nonspecific Lung Disease Study Groups. Chest 1996; 110:35–41.
76. Verhoeven GT, Hegmans JPJJ, Mulder PGH, et al. Effects of fluticasone propionate in COPD patients with bronchial hyperresponsiveness. Thorax 2002; 57:694–700.
77. Siafakas NM, Vermeire P, Pride NB, et al. Optimal assessment and management of chronic obstructive pulmonary disease (COPD). The European Respiratory Society Task Force. Eur Respir J 1995; 8:1398–1420.
78. American Thoracic Society. Standards for the diagnosis and care of patients with chronic obstructive pulmonary disease. Am J Respir Crit Care Med 1995; 152:S77–S121.
79. British Thoracic SocietyGuidelines for the management of chronic obstructive pulmonary disease. Thorax 1997; 52(suppl 5):1–28.
80. Alsaeedi A, Sin DD, McAlister FA. The effects of inhaled corticosteroids in chronic obstructive pulmonary disease: a systematic review of randomized placebo-controlled trials. Am J Med 2002; 113:59–65.
81. Jones PW, Willits LR, Burge PS, et al. Disease severity and the effect of fluticasone propionate on chronic obstructive pulmonary disease exacerbations. Eur Respir J 2003; 21:68–73.
82. Jarad NA, Wedzicha JA, Burge PS, et al. An observational study of inhaled corticosteroid withdrawal in stable chronic obstructive pulmonary disease. ISOLDE Study Group. Respir Med 1999; 93:161–166.
83. van der Valk P, Monninkhof E, van der Palen J, et al. Effect of discontinuation of inhaled corticosteroids in patients with chronic obstructive pulmonary disease: The COPE Study. Am J Respir Crit Care Med 2002; 166: 1358–1363.
84. Calverley P, Pauwels R, Vestbo J, et al. Combined salmeterol and fluticasone in the treatment of chronic obstructive pulmonary disease: a randomised controlled trial. Lancet 2003; 361:449–456.
85. Szafranski W, Cukier A, Ramirez A, et al. Efficacy and safety of budesonide/formoterol in the management of chronic obstructive pulmonary disease. Eur Respir J 2003; 21:74–81.
86. Seemungal TA, Donaldson GC, Paul EA, et al. Effect of exacerbation on quality of life in patients with chronic obstructive pulmonary disease. Am J Respir Crit Care Med 1998; 157:1418–1422.
87. Bourbeau J, Rouleau MY, Boucher S. Randomised controlled trial of inhaled corticosteroids in patients with chronic obstructive pulmonary disease. Thorax 1998; 53:477–482.
88. Spencer S, Calverley PM, Burge SP, et al. Health status deterioration in patients with chronic obstructive pulmonary disease. Am J Respir Crit Care Med 2001; 163:122–128.
89. Murray CJ, Lopez AD. Alternative projections of mortality and disability by cause 1990–2020: Global Burden of Disease Study. Lancet 1997; 349:1498–1504.
90. Sin DD, Tu JV. Inhaled corticosteroids and the risk of mortality and readmission in elderly patients with chronic obstructive pulmonary disease. Am J Respir Crit Care Med 2001; 164:580–584.

91. Sin DD, Man SF. Inhaled corticosteroids and survival in chronic obstructive pulmonary disease: does the dose matter? Eur Respir J 2003; 21:260–266.
92. Vestbo J. Another piece of the inhaled corticosteroids-in-COPD puzzle. Am J Respir Crit Care Med 2001; 164:514–515.
93. Bourbeau J. Inhaled corticosteroids and survival in chronic obstructive pulmonary disease. Eur Respir J 2003; 21:202–203.
94. Nava S, Compagnoni ML. Controlled short-term trial of fluticasone propionate in ventilator-dependent patients with COPD. Chest 2000; 118:990–999.
95. Maltais F, Ostinelli J, Bourbeau J, et al. Comparison of nebulized budesonide and oral prednisolone with placebo in the treatment of acute exacerbations of chronic obstructive pulmonary disease: a randomized controlled trial. Am J Respir Crit Care Med 2002; 165:698–703.
96. Lipworth BJ. Systemic adverse effects of inhaled corticosteroid therapy: a systematic review and meta-analysis. Arch Intern Med 1999; 159:941–955.
97. Gallagher CG. Respiratory steroid myopathy. Am J Respir Crit Care Med 1994; 150:4–6.
98. Decramer M, de Bock V, Dom R. Functional and histologic picture of steroid-induced myopathy in chronic obstructive pulmonary disease. Am J Respir Crit Care Med 1996; 153:1958–1964.
99. Sin DD, Man JP, Man SF. The risk of osteoporosis in Caucasian men and women with obstructive airways disease. Am J Med 2003; 114:10–14.
100. Walsh LJ, Lewis SA, Wong CA, et al. The impact of oral corticosteroid use on bone mineral density and vertebral fracture. Am J Respir Crit Care Med 2002; 166:691–695.
101. McEvoy CE, Ensrud KE, Bender E, et al. Association between corticosteroid use and vertebral fractures in older men with chronic obstructive pulmonary disease. Am J Respir Crit Care Med 1998; 157:704–709.
102. Homik JE, Cranney A, Shea B, et al. A meta-analysis on the use of biphosphonates in corticosteroid induced osteoporosis. J Rheumatol 1999; 26:1148–1157.
103. Rudolf M. The reality of drug use in COPD: the European perspective. Chest 2000; 117(suppl 2):29S–32S.
104. Veterans Health Administration (VHA). Clinical practice guideline for the management of chronic obstructive pulmonary disease. Version 1.1a. Washington (DC): Department of Veterans Affairs (US), Veterans Health Administration, 1999.
105. Global Initiative for Chronic Obstructive Lung Disease (GOLD), World Health Organization (WHO), National Heart, Lung and Blood Institute (NHLBI) Global strategy for the diagnosis, management, and prevention of chronic obstructive pulmonary disease. Bethesda (MD): Global Initiative for Chronic Obstructive Lung Disease, World Health Organization, National Heart, Lung and Blood Institute, 2001.
106. Pauwels RA. National and international guidelines for COPD: the need for evidence. Chest 2000; 117(suppl 2):20S–22S.
107. Johnson M, Rennard S. Alternative mechanisms for long-acting β_2-adrenergic agonists in COPD. Chest 2001; 120:258–270.

108. Bowden JJ, Sulakvelidze I, McDonald DM. Inhibition of neutrophil and eosinophil adhesion to venules of rat trachea by β_2-adrenergic agonist formoterol. J Appl Physiol 1994; 77:397–405.
109. Davies A, Lefkowitz R. Agonist-promoted high affinity state of β-adrenergic receptor in human neutrophils: modulation by corticosteroids. J Clin Endocrinol Metab 1981; 53:703–708.
110. Saari SM, Vidgren MT, Herrala J, et al. Possibilities of formoterol to enhance the peripheral lung deposition of the inhaled liposome corticosteroids. Respir Med 2002; 96:999–1005.
111. Barnes PJ. Efficacy of inhaled corticosteroids in asthma. J Allergy Clin Immunol 1998; 102:531–538.
112. Lipworth BJ. Airway subsensitivity with long-acting β_2-agonists. Is there cause for concern? Drug Saf 1997; 16:295–308.
113. Schramm CM. β-Adrenergic relaxation of rabbit tracheal smooth muscle: a receptor deficit that improves with corticosteroid administration. J Pharmacol Exp Ther 2000; 292:280–287.
114. Mak JCW, Nishikawa M, Shirasaki H, et al. Protective effects of a glucocorticoid on downregulation of pulmonary β_2-adrenergic receptors in vivo. J Clin Invest 1995; 96:99–106.
115. Pang L, Knox AJ. Synergistic inhibition by β_2-agonists and corticosteroids on tumour necrosis factor α induced interleukin-8 release from cultured human airway smooth muscle cells. Am J Respir Cell Mol Biol 2000; 23:79–85.
116. Korn SH, Jerre A, Brattsand R. Effects of formoterol and budesonide on GM-CSF and IL-8 secretion by triggered human bronchial epithelial cells. Eur Resp J 2001; 17:1070–1077.
117. Dowling RB, Johnson M, Cole PJ, et al. Effect of fluticasone propionate and salmeterol on Pseudomonas aeruginosa infection of the respiratory mucosa in vitro. Eur Respir J 1999; 14:363–369.
118. Wilson R. Infections of the airways. Curr Opin Infect Dis 1991; 4:166–177.
119. Cazzola M, Di Lorenzo G, Di Perna F, et al. Additive effects of salmeterol and fluticasone or theophylline in COPD. Chest 2000; 118:1576–1581.
120. Mahler DA, Wire P, Horstman D, et al. Effectiveness of fluticasone propionate and salmeterol combination delivered via the Diskus device in the treatment of chronic obstructive pulmonary disease. Am J Respir Crit Care Med 2002; 166:1084–1091.
121. Roth M, Johnson PR, Rudiger JJ, et al. Interaction between glucocorticoids and β_2 agonists on bronchial airway smooth muscle cells through synchronised cellular signalling. Lancet 2002; 360:1293–1299.
122. Rennard SI. COPD: treatments benefit patients. Lancet 2003; 361:444–445.
123. Soriano JB, Vestbo J, Pride NB, et al. Survival in COPD patients after regular use of fluticasone propionate and salmeterol in general practice. Eur Respir J 2002; 20:819–825.

16

Antioxidants and Protease Inhibitors

MARIO CAZZOLA

A. Cardarelli Hospital
Naples, Italy

MARIA GABRIELLA MATERA

Second University of Naples
Naples, Italy

I. Introduction

The recent Global Initiative for Chronic Obstructive Lung Disease (GOLD) guidelines [1] have highlighted that, in addition to inflammation, two other processes may be important in the pathogenesis of chronic obstructive pulmonary disease (COPD). They are oxidative stress (OS), and an imbalance between proteases and endogenous antiproteases in the lung (Fig. 1). These processes may themselves be consequences of inflammation, or they may result from environmental (e.g., oxidant compounds in cigarette smoke) or genetic (e.g., α_1-antitrypsin (α_1-AT) deficiency) factors.

II. Oxidative Stress and COPD

Oxidative stress, widely recognized as a central feature of many diseases, may result from an increased exposure to oxidants and/or decreased antioxidant capacity [2]. Table 1 summarizes the most important reactive oxygen species capable of inducing OS.

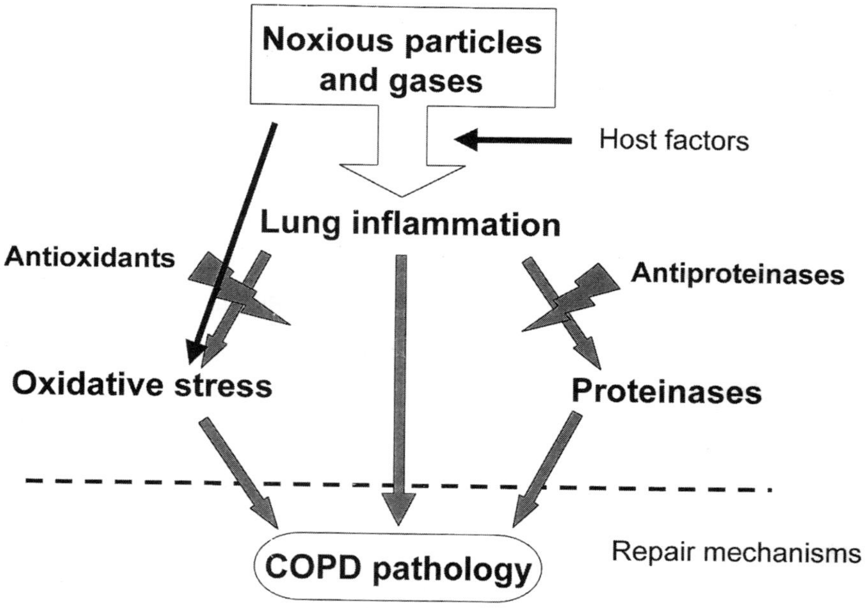

Figure 1 Pathogenesis of COPD.

Table 1 Major Reactive Oxygen Species of Oxidative Stress

Free radicals[a]	
Hydroxyl radical	$HO\cdot$
Superoxide radical	$O_2^{\cdot -}$
Peroxyl[b]	$ROO\cdot$
Alkoxyl[b]	$RO\cdot$
Nonradical oxygen species	
Hydrogen peroxide	H_2O_2
Singlet oxygen	$^1O_2$

[a] Free radicals contain an unpaired electron.
[b] Peroxyl and alkoxyl radicals result from lipid peroxidation of polyunsaturated fatty acids (ROOH).

Activated phagocytic cells (neutrophils, eosinophils, monocytes, and macrophages) produce large amounts of reactive oxygen species (ROS) that may degrade many biological molecules, resulting in damages to cell membrane and structural proteins, inactivation of enzymes, and altered cellular metabolism [3]. In particular, it has been demonstrated that $O_2^{\cdot -}$ has some proinflammatory properties, such as recruitment of neutrophils at sites of inflammation, formation of chemotactic factors [3], DNA damage, depolymerization of hyaluronic acid and collagen [3], lipid peroxidation, and formation of peroxinitrite ($ONOO^-$), another highly reactive oxidant produced by the combination of $O_2^{\cdot -}$ and NO. There is evidence that oxidants can also operate as signaling molecules [4]. In fact, OS increases nuclear factor (NF)-κB and activator protein-1 (AP-1) activity in many different cells, including inflammatory and epithelial cells [4]. NF-κB and AP-1 are critical transcription factors for maximal expression of many cytokines, including interleukin (IL)-8, a potent chemotactic factor and activator for neutrophils and tumour necrosis factor (TNF)-α, enzymes (e.g., iNOS, cyclo-oxygenase-2 and γ-glutamylcysteine synthetase), and adhesion molecules involved in inflammatory responses (e.g., intercellular adhesion molecule-1, E-selectin, and vascular cell adhesion molecule-1) [5,6].

The inhalation of exogenous compounds like ozone, cigarette smoke, and other chemicals and dust, can also lead to the formation of ROS in the lungs [6]. All biochemical and cellular changes caused by ROS increase permeability of alveolar-capillary membrane, alter pulmonary vascular reactivity, and decrease surface activity of pulmonary surfactant, all of which can ultimately alter airway function (Table 2).

Oxidative stress is a feature of both asthma and COPD, but is thought to be more prominent in COPD, where it results in inactivation of antiproteases, airspace epithelial injury, mucus hypersecretion, increased neutrophils in the pulmonary microvasculature, transcription factor activation, gene expression of pro-inflammatory mediators, and reversible airway narrowing [7] (Fig. 2).

In patients with COPD the increased OS results from the increased burden of oxidants present in cigarette smoke or from the increased amounts of ROS released from leukocytes in the airspace and in the blood [8]. It has been demonstrated that cigarette smoke initiates a superoxide-dependent mechanism that, through activating NF-κB and increasing IL-8 mRNA expression, produces infiltration of neutrophils into the airways in vivo [9]. Therefore, inflammation itself induces OS in the lungs.

Whether inhaled in the form of cigarette smoke or released from activated neutrophils, oxidants inactivate α_1-AT by oxidating the methionine residue at its active site, producing a functional deficiency of α_1-AT in the airspaces, an event that is considered critical in the pathogenesis of emphysema [10].

Table 2 Effects of Reactive Oxygen Species on Airway Cells and Tissues

Direct contraction
Increased contractile response to
Acetylcholine or methacholine
Histamine
5-Hydroxytryptamine
Bradykinin
Substance P
Decreased numbers and function of β-adrenergic receptors
Proliferation of myocytes
Increased permeability
Increased mucus production
Decreased numbers and function of epithelial cilia
Damaged epithelial cells
Altered expression of adhesion molecules
Influx of inflammatory cells
Altered release of inflammatory mediators

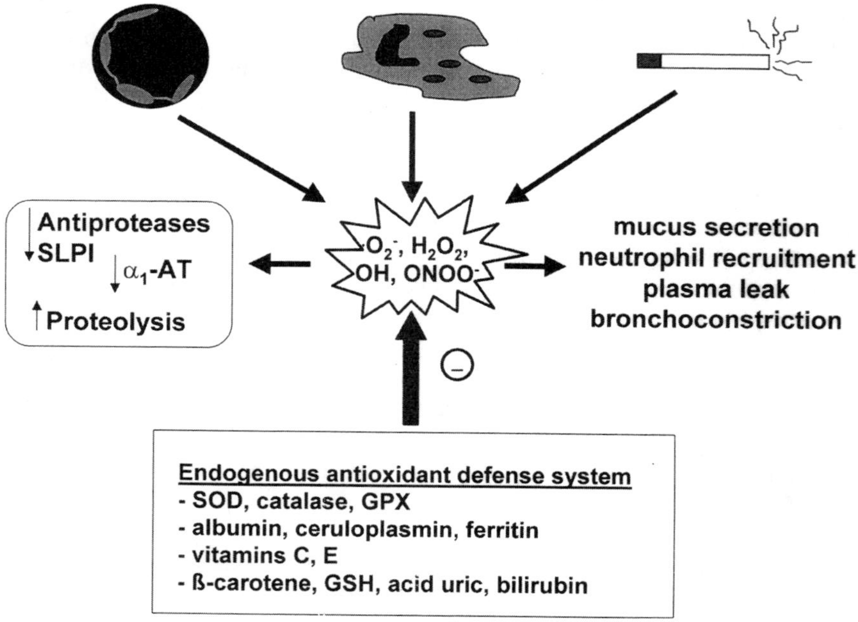

Figure 2 Increased oxidative stress in COPD.

The toxicity of oxidants is normally balanced by the protective activity of an array of endogenous antioxidant defence systems that include enzymes such as superoxide dismutase (SOD), catalase, and glutathione peroxidase (GPX); macromolecules such as albumin, ceruloplasmin, and ferritin; and a variety of low molecular weight antioxidants, including ascorbic acid (vitamin C), α-tocopherol (vitamin E), β-carotene, reduced glutathione (GSH), uric acid, and bilirubin [11] (Fig. 2). These antioxidants act at the molecular and cellular level by modulating gene expression and regulating apoptosis and signal transduction [12].

Free radicals are generated as a part of normal cellular activity, and thus the intracellular enzymatic antioxidant defences are paramount to the protection of organ function (Fig. 3). Under normal circumstances, formation of $O_2^{\cdot -}$ is kept under tight control by SOD enzymes. Three forms of SOD may be important: Mn SOD, which is located in the mitochondria; Cu-Zn SOD, which resides in the cytoplasm; and extracellular (EC) SOD, which is localized predominantly in the extracellular matrix of tissues as well as in extracellular fluids [2]. EC-SOD is the only known extracellular

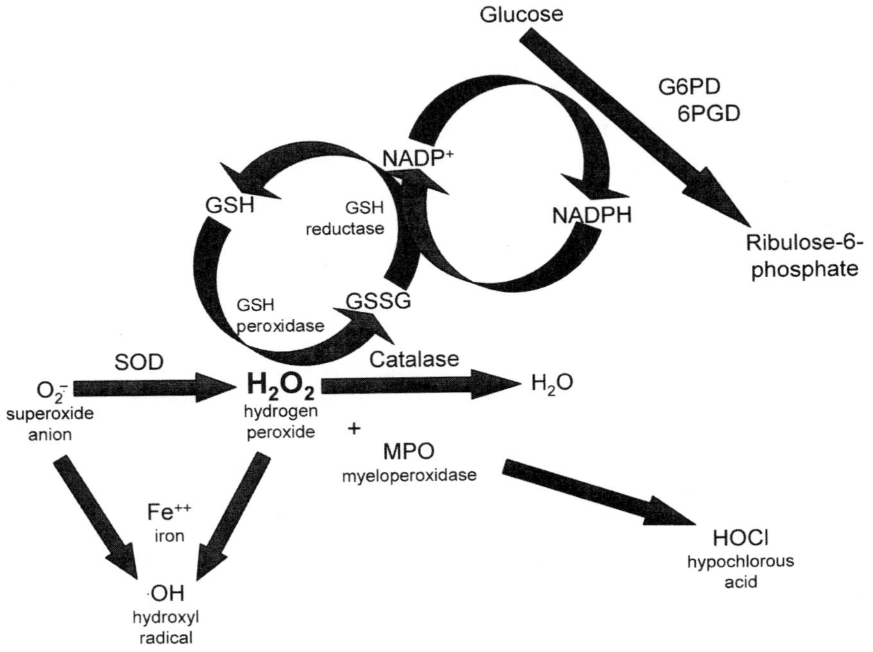

Figure 3 Basic oxygen radical and antioxidant chemistry.

antioxidant enzyme that scavenges superoxide in the lungs and therefore may be a critical component in both the responses to increased OS and preservation of NO-dependent processes. In acute and chronic inflammation, the production of $O_2^{\cdot -}$ is increased at a rate that overwhelms the capacity of the endogenous SOD enzyme defence system to remove them.

Reduced glutathione (L-glutamyl-L-cysteinyl-glycine [GSH]), a ubiquitous sulphydryl-containing tripeptide that is found in very high concentrations in normal respiratory epithelial lining fluid [13], is another important component of the lung antioxidant defences. The GSH system efficiently scavenges oxidants, thereby protecting cells and tissues from damage by oxidants released by inflammatory cells or delivered from other exogenous sources [14]. GSH serves as an antioxidant by reacting directly with free radicals and by providing substrate for GPX. Both direct and enzymatic oxidation of GSH results in the formation of oxidised glutathione (GSSG), which is reconverted to GSH by glutathione reductase (GR) [15].

In addition to its direct antioxidant role, GSH may act to preserve antiprotease activity in theses conditions. It inhibits myeloperoxidase-mediated inactivation of α_1-AT [16] and in combination with GSH peroxidase inhibits loss of lipid peroxidation-induced α_1-AT activity [17]. Additionally, catalase-suppressible inhibition of α_1-AT by gas-phase cigarette smoke is reduced by GSH [18]. GSH may also help maintain α_1-AT activity by allowing reduction of the inactivated mixed-disulphide form of this molecule [19].

There is increasing evidence for an oxidant/antioxidant imbalance in COPD [2]. A recent study documented decreased antioxidant capacity in smokers and patients with COPD, although no relationship was found between plasma antioxidant capacity and measurements of airflow limitation in either smokers or in patients with COPD [20]. Knowledge of the mechanisms of the effects of OS should in the future allow the development of potent antioxidant therapies.

A. Therapeutic Options to Improve the Oxidant/Antioxidant Imbalance in COPD

The putative use of antioxidants as preventive agents for the development of COPD has been promulgated based on the proposed relationships among oxidants, tissue injury, and disease [21].

Currently, there is no effective antioxidant therapy that has both good bioavailability and potency [20]. Nevertheless, various approaches have been proposed (Table 3). MacNee [22] has suggested targeting the inflammatory response by reducing the sequestration or migration of leukocytes from the pulmonary circulation into the airspaces. Alternatively, he has proposed the

Table 3 Therapeutic Options for Redressing the Oxidant/Antioxidant Imbalance in COPD

Dietary supplementation
Antioxidant nutrients (blueberries, spinach, fruits)
Vitamin C, vitamin E, β-carotene, catechins
Glutathione
Glutathione precursors
N-acetylcysteine
N-acystelyn
HMS90
Carbocysteine lysine salt monohydrate
Ambroxol
Apocynin
Superoxide dismutase mimetics
Anti-inflammatory agents
Corticosteroids
Phosphodiesterase inhibitors
Long-acting β_2-agonists
Spin-trap antioxidants
α-phenyl-*N*-*tert*-butyl nitrone (PBN)
Sodium 2-sulfophenyl-N-tert-butyl nitrone (S-PBN)
Disodium 2,4-disulfophenyl-N-tert-butyl nitrone (NXY-059)

molecular manipulation of antioxidant genes, such as GPX or genes involved in the synthesis of glutathione, such as γ-glutamylcysteine synthetase or the development of molecules with activity similar to those of antioxidant enzymes such as catalase and SOD.

Another approach would simply be to administer antioxidant therapy or to develop molecules with activity similar to those of antioxidant enzymes, such as catalase and SOD. Most of the suggested approaches though are theoretical and have never been tested in humans. Consequently, an effective antioxidant therapy for COPD patients is still lacking.

Dietary Supplementation

There has been considerable interest in the association between dietary intake of antioxidants and measurements of systemic OS and lung function/symptoms in the general population and in smokers. A possible protective effect against the development of respiratory symptoms or a decline in pulmonary function has been observed for dietary antioxidants [23] and/or fruit, [24] and for N-3 fatty acids and/or fish intake [25]. Antioxidants and foods rich in antioxidants are thought to protect the airways against oxidant mediated damage [26], while the N-3 fatty acids mainly present in fish are thought to have anti-inflammatory effects through their influence on the metabolism of arachidonic acid [27]. It has been found that blueberries and spinach had high antioxidant capacities [28], which were 20–50 times higher that those of some other fruits and vegetables.

Epidemiological evidence indicates that low intake of antioxidant nutrients such as vitamins C, E, and A may be associated with reduced lung function [29,30] and chronic respiratory symptoms [31]. Vitamin C, a versatile water-soluble antioxidant, protects against lipid peroxidation by scavenging ROS in the aqueous phase before they can initiate lipid peroxidation. Vitamin E resides in the lipid domain of biological membranes and plasma lipoprotein, where it prevents lipid peroxidation of polyunsaturated fatty acids.

Smokers have a higher requirement for vitamin C than do nonsmokers [32]. In fact, vitamin C concentrations are lower in smokers than in nonsmokers and are inversely related to cigarette consumption [33]. The lower vitamin C status of smokers is most likely due to increased turnover of the vitamin as a result of increased OS [34]. In one study, vitamin C supplementation (2,000 mg/day for 5 days) significantly reduced the amount of urinary F_2-isoprostanes, an indicator of OS that is elevated in smokers, whereas vitamin E had no effect [35]. It has been proposed that smokers require a $\geq$2–3 fold the current recommended dietary allowance of 60 mg/day to maintain plasma vitamin C concentrations comparable with those in nonsmokers [36].

It has been suggested that dietary vitamin C and β-carotene, but not vitamin E, elicit a protective effect on lung function but not on respiratory symptoms [23]. A recent population based study of 3,714 males and 4,256 females supports a protective role for vitamin C against the risk of obstructive airways disease [37]. However, a more recent study has demonstrated that vitamin E and β-cryptoxanthin, a carotenoid, appear to be stronger correlates of lung function than vitamin C [38]. Another study attempted to measure the differences in diet between subjects with a defined smoking history who have developed COPD and subjects with the same exposure to cigarette smoke who have not developed the disease. The findings in this study indicate that it is more likely to be the combined effect of various fruits and vegetables that protects against lung obstruction than high levels of vitamin C, as previously suggested [39].

Recently, it has been suggested that a high intake of catechins, which are polyphenolic compounds from green tea and solid fruits, protects against the development of COPD [40].

Using data from the Third National Health and Nutrition Examination Survey comprising a sample representative of the United States population in 1988–1994, Hu and Cassano [41] found that serum selenium had a more positive association with FEV_1 in smokers. Although data in COPD patients are not available, this finding might have implications for further research, because selenium supplementation to the diet of asthmatic patients has been found to enhance the activity of the selenium-dependent enzyme glutathione peroxidase and to improve clinical symptoms in these patients [42].

Ebselen [2-phenyl-1,2-benz-isoselenazol-3(2*H*)-one], a seleno-organic compound that has both antioxidant and anti-inflammatory properties and also possesses thiol peroxidase activity, is another compound that might be of interest for the treatment of inflammatory reactions in airways. It exhibits its anti-oxidant activity mainly as a GPX mimic, but has also been shown to act as a scavenger of peroxynitrite [43].

A GPX mimic, BXT-51072 (2,3-dihydro-4,4-dimethyl-benzisoselenazine), is able to protect endothelial cells from OS, to reduce cytokine-induced up-regulation of adhesion molecules and to diminish neutrophil adhesion to these endothelial cells [44].

Glutathione

Many reports support that depletion of endogenous GSH enhances the cytotoxic effects of ROS [3]. Consequently, attempts to supplement lung GSH have been tried using GSH or its precursors [45]. Unfortunately, cells cannot take up extracellular GSH [45]. In effect, it must first be hydrolyzed to glutamic acid, cysteine, and glycine, which are subsequently transported into the cell and serve as substrates for GSH synthesis. GSH is synthesized in the cell in two steps. The first step, the synthesis of γ-glutamylcysteine, is limited by the availability of intracellular cysteine [45]. The γ-glutamylcysteine, as a γ-glutamyl amino acid, can easily be transported into the cell where it combines with glycine in the second step of GSH synthesis [45]. There are, however, doubts that the normal intracellular concentration of GSH could be affected by the administration of exogenous GSH or amino acids and the peptide precursors for GSH because of feedback inhibition of γ-glutamylcysteine synthetase by GSH [46]. The administration of GSH monoethyl ester that has been used to increase intracellular reduced GSH in vitro and has been shown in some studies to be more effective than GSH itself [45], may allow augmentation of intracellular GSH, but this may be toxic to cells at higher doses. Although many patients have been treated with GSH safely, no clinical trials have been conducted with the cell membrane-permeable derivative GSH esters [46]. The dose necessary to maintain elevated lung GSH levels in inflammatory lung diseases is also unknown [46]. Nevertheless, there are reports that exogenous GSH does increase intracellular GSH in vitro [47]. In any case, the absorption of oral GSH remains controversial, with animal studies suggesting significant absorption and some human studies showing little to none [48, 49]. Based on these findings, it appears that inhalation might be the preferred route of administration for respiratory and perhaps systemic effect.

Some clinical trials of nebulized reduced GSH have demonstrated the bioavailability and safety of up to 600 mg twice daily [50,51]. In patients with idiopathic pulmonary fibrosis, exogenous nebulized GSH provoked an increase in total ELF GSH and oxidized GSH, with a decrease in spontaneous superoxide anion release by alveolar macrophages [50]. However, in asthmatic patients, nebulized GSH has been shown to induce bronchial hyperreactivity [52]. Inhalation of sulphites that come from GSH solution could be involved in these effects. Nevertheless, in a small group of patients suffering from emphysema, 120 mg inhaled GSH twice daily improved breathing [53].

Glutathione Precursors

At present, GSH precursor amino acids are the best means of manipulating GSH biosynthesis intracellularly. Cysteine is a thiol that is the rate limiting amino acid in GSH synthesis. Cysteine administration is not possible since it is oxidized to cystine (the oxidized form of cysteine), which is neurotoxic, but in the form of glutamylcystine moieties more readily enters into cells. There are many other GSH precursors, notably *n*-acetylcysteine (NAC), which is currently used to enhance GSH levels in the lung.

N-Acetylcysteine (NAC)

NAC is a thiol-containing compound that is used to reduce viscosity and elasticity of mucus. Moreover, it is able to scavenge H_2O_2, $HO^{\cdot}$, and HOCl [54]. Pretreatment of human alveolar and bronchial epithelial cells with NAC protects both cell types against injurious effects of H_2O_2 [55]. Also, it has been shown that NAC protects against HOCl-induced contraction of guinea-pig tracheal smooth muscles [56] and inhibits lipopolysaccharide-induced leukocyte accumulation in rat lung [57]. Although NAC is a free radical scavenger, its more important antioxidant role is providing an intracellular source of cysteine. In fact, it can easily be deacetylated to cysteine, an important precursor of cellular glutathione synthesis, and thus stimulate the cellular glutathione system.

Bridgeman et al. [58] showed that after five days of a daily dose up to 1,800 mg, there was a significant increase in plasma levels of GSH. However, there was no associated rise in the levels of GSH in the BALF or ELF nor was there a significant increase in lung tissue cysteine or GSH [58]. This suggests that it may be difficult to produce a large enough change in GSH with NAC to increase the antioxidant capacity of the lungs in subjects who are not already depleted in GSH [46]. In spite of this, some studies have shown that NAC reduces the number of exacerbation days in patients with COPD [59,60]. Eklund et al. [61], who investigated the effect of NAC in healthy smokers after an eight week period of 200 mg three times daily, observed a reduction in the BALF of eosinophilic cationic protein, lactoferrin, antichymotrypsin, and chemotactic activity for neutrophils. In vitro experiments have shown that thiol compounds block the release of inflammatory mediators from epithelial cells and macrophages by a mechanism involving increasing intracellular GSH and decreasing NF-κB activation [62,63]. Several other findings support the view that NAC attenuates the degree of inflammation and lung injury [64]. It exerts its effect both as a source of sulphydryl groups (repletion of intracellular GSH) and through a direct reaction with hydroxyl radical [65]. In addition, NAC may reduce oxyradical-related oxidant processes by directly interfering with the oxidants, up-regulating antioxidant systems such as SOD [66] or enhancing the catalytic activity of glutathione peroxidase [67]. Kasielski and Novak [68] demonstrated that long-term oral administration of NAC attenuates H_2O_2 formation in the airways of COPD subjects. However, this treatment had no influence on concentrations of exhaled and circulatory end products of lipid peroxidation. It is likely that administration of NAC may not sufficiently increase the serum and/or extracellular fluid anti-oxidant capacity to prevent lipid peroxidation [68]. On the other hand, NAC and cysteine hardly penetrate into the hydrophobic microenvironment of lipids and therefore are not able to protect them from peroxidative damage.

It must be stressed that animal studies have suggested that NAC produces deleterious effects on the lung epithelium in response to hyperoxia exposure [69]. Moreover, NAC is associated with a number of adverse effects that detract from its utility as antioxidant agent. These include blurred vision, dysphoria, and gastrointestinal discomfort [70].

N-Acystelyn (NAL)

NAL is a mucolytic and antioxidant thiol compound consisting of an equimolar mixture of L-lysine and NAC and possesses a free thiol group. The advantage of NAL over NAC is that it has a neutral pH, whereas NAC is acidic. NAL can be aerosolized into the lung without causing increased airway responsiveness [71]. It may represent an interesting alternative approach to augmenting the antioxidant screen in the lungs. In fact, NAL, at concentrations obtainable in vivo by inhalation, impairs the chemiluminescence response of human neutrophils related to highly cytotoxic hydroxyl and hypohalite radicals' production [71]. Gillissen et al. [72] compared the effect of NAL and NAC and found that both drugs enhanced intracellular

GSH in alveolar epithelial cells and inhibited H_2O_2 and $O_2^{\cdot -}$ released from human blood-derived neutrophils from smokers with COPD. NAL also inhibited ROS generation by human neutrophils induced by serum-opsonized zymosan. This inhibitory response was comparable to the effects of NAC [71]. Moreover, NAL inhibited oxidant-mediated IL-8 expression and NF-κB nuclear binding in human alveolar epithelial cells [73].

Other Cysteine Donors

HMS90 (Immunocal) is a bovine whey protein consisting of several compounds, including albumin, lactoferrin, and α-lactalbumin that are rich in cystine residues. Albumin and lactoferrin are also rich in γ-glutamylcystine, which is easily transported into cells, making it a more readily available substrate for GSH biosynthesis [74]. It has been documented that one month of supplementation with HMS90 is able to induce a significant and dramatic increase in whole blood GSH levels and pulmonary function [75].

Certain other thiol-releasing agents such as GSH ethyl ester and l-thiozolidine-4-carboxylate are potentially useful compounds for cysteine/GSH delivery. However, studies are needed to validate the bioavailability of these compounds in lung inflammation [45].

Carbocysteine Lysine Salt Monohydrate (CLS), Ambroxol, Apocynin, and Superoxide Desmutase Mimetics

CLS is a mucoactive drug. In vitro, in BALF from patients affected by COPD, CLS was more effective as scavenger in comparison to GSH and NAC [76]. It has been suggested that CLS could act by interfering with the conversion of xanthine dehydrogenase into $O_2^{\cdot -}$-producing xanthine oxidase [76].

Ambroxol is another mucoactive drug. Ambroxol, unlike NAC and GSH, reduces $O_2^{\cdot -}$. In contrast, GSH and NAC scavenge H_2O_2, while ambroxol has no anti-H_2O_2 effect [77]. An antioxidative effect of ambroxol may also be associated with the reduction of pro-oxidative metabolism in inflammatory cells [78]. Moreover, it can inhibit migration and activation of leukocytes [79]. The application of ambroxol into culture media containing BALF cells inhibited spontaneous and stimulated generation of ROS by BALF cells harvested from COPD patients and control subjects in an ambroxol concentration–dependent manner [80].

Apocynin, a nontoxic compound isolated from the medicinal plant *Picrorhiza kurroa*, is a NADPH-oxidase inhibitor that completely prevents production of ROS by granulocytes and macrophages [81] and inhibits both $O_2^{\cdot -}$ and $ONOO^-$ formation by macrophages [82]. It also increases GSH synthesis through activation of AP-1 in human type II alveolar epithelial cells [83].

Overexpressing Mn SOD protects lung epithelial cells from oxidant injury in vitro [3]. In particular, inhalation of SOD reduces cigarette smoke-induced neutrophil infiltration and airway hyperresponsiveness in guinea pigs in vivo [3]. Unfortunately, there are drawbacks and issues associated with the use of the native enzymes as therapeutic agents [3]. To overcome the limitations associated with native enzyme therapy, a series of SOD mimetics (SODm) that catalytically remove $O_2^{\cdot-}$ has been developed. Recently, a low-molecular weight, synthetic Mn SODm, M40403, has been shown to be active in rat models of inflammation in vivo where $O_2^{\cdot-}$ has been postulated to play a role [84]. It is not known yet if such mimetics may also have beneficial effects in COPD.

Anti-Inflammatory Agents: Corticosteroids, Leukotriene B_4 (LTB_4) Antagonists, Phosphodiesterase (PDE) Inhibitors, Long-Acting β_2-Agonists, and Spin-Trap Antioxidants

MacNee [85] proposed to target the inflammatory response by reducing the sequestration or migration of leukocytes from the pulmonary circulation into the airspaces. Alternatively, it should also be possible to use anti-inflammatory agents to prevent the release of ROS from activated leukocytes or to quench those oxidants once they are formed, by enhancing the antioxidant screen in the lungs.

Corticosteroids inhibit the action of transcription factors such as AP-1 and NF-κB leading to decreased levels of pro-inflammatory cytokines and mediators, chemokines, inflammatory enzymes, and adhesion molecules [86], and, subsequently, to a reduced influx of leukocytes from the blood into the airways and to less activation of inflammatory cells present in the airways. Both blood into processes will reduce the amount of ROS generated by these kinds of cells. However, high amounts of ROS can reduce the effectiveness of steroids to suppress the release of cytokines by macrophages [87] by the suppression of the functional activity of the glucocorticoid receptor under oxidative condition [88]. These findings may explain the failure of glucocorticoids to function effectively in COPD where a high OS is present.

The capacity for LTB_4, to amplify neutrophil activity has supported the drive to develop compounds with an anti-inflammatory activity that is mediated through the inhibition of LTB_4 and thereby undermines neutrophil activity in inflammatory conditions [89]. Currently, there are long-acting and potent LTB_4 receptor antagonists, such as BIIL 284 that have shown efficacy against inflammation and neutrophilia in primates. ZK158252 and ZK183838 are two other new LTB_4 receptor antagonists.

Inhibitors of PDE isoenzymes have been shown to attenuate human neutrophil functions including $O_2^{\cdot-}$ production [90]. This action is selective for those pro-inflammatory stimuli that elevate cAMP resulting in enhanced activity of protein kinase A and inhibition of the production of potentially harmful reactive oxidants by these cells [91].

The long-acting β_2-agonist salmeterol inhibits the respiratory burst of human neutrophils in a dose-dependent manner. The inhibitory activity of salmeterol is not reversed in the presence of the β-blocker propranolol, and does not correlate with its ability of increasing cAMP levels. Albuterol is without response [92]. Oxidant production by FMLP- and calcium ionophore (A23187)-activated neutrophils is particularly sensitive to inhibition by low concentrations (0.3–3 μM) of salmeterol [93].

Spin-trap antioxidants, such as α-phenyl-*N-tert*-butyl nitrone (PBN), sodium 2-sulfophenyl-N-tert-butyl nitrone (S-PBN) and disodium 2,4-disulfophenyl-N-tert-butyl nitrone (NXY-059), are potent and inhibit intracellular reactive oxygen species formation by forming stable compounds [94]. Interestingly, PBN inhibits formation of H_2O_2 at the level of complex I in mitochondrial preparations, which suggests a direct interaction with mitochondria in vivo [95].

B. Possible Limitation to Antioxidant Therapy in COPD

A large body of evidence suggests that OS contributes in the pathogenesis of COPD. Unfortunately, a documentation of the real impact of antioxidant therapy in modifying the natural history of COPD is still lacking. Recent studies have indicated that genetic polymorphisms of antioxidant genes are associated more commonly with the presence of COPD than predicted from the control population. [96]. It must be highlighted that van Schayck et al. [97] suggested that anti-oxidant treatment might be relatively more effective among those COPD patients who do not respond as well to inhaled steroids (low reversibility and heavy smoking).

III. Proteases and COPD

Neutrophils migrate into the lungs by chemotaxis in response to an inflammatory stimulus. They then degranulate and release destructive proteolytic enzymes, such as neutrophil elastase (NE). However, for NE to have these effects, it has to overcome the anti-elastases that protect the tissues [98]. In healthy individuals, the most important proteinase inhibitors are members of the serpin superfamily typified by α_1-AT and α_1-antichymotrypsin [99] (Fig. 4). Secretory leukoprotease inhibitor (SLPI), a 12-kD serpin that appears to be a major inhibitor of elastase activity in the airways, and tissues inhibitors of metalloproteinases (TIMPs) are other endogenous antiproteases. Other serpins, such as elafin, may be important in counteracting protease activity in the lung [100]. Elafin, an elastase-specific inhibitor, is found in bronchoalveolar lavage and is synthesized by epithelial cells in response to inflammatory stimuli [101].

Several proteases, such as NE, proteinase-3, cathepsin B and G, could directly produce many of the features of smoking-related COPD. Although NE is likely to be the major mechanism mediating elastolysis in patients with α_1-AT deficiency, it may not be the major elastolytic enzyme in smoking-related COPD, and it is important to consider other enzymes as targets for inhibition [102]. In effect, the idea that the neutrophil is the effector cell of the crucial protease NE, and that cigarette smoke also inactivates α_1-AT, the major antiproteolytic substance in the lung parenchyma, has become controversial. In fact, the numbers of neutrophils present in human tissue do not correlate with the degree of lung destruction, whereas correlations are

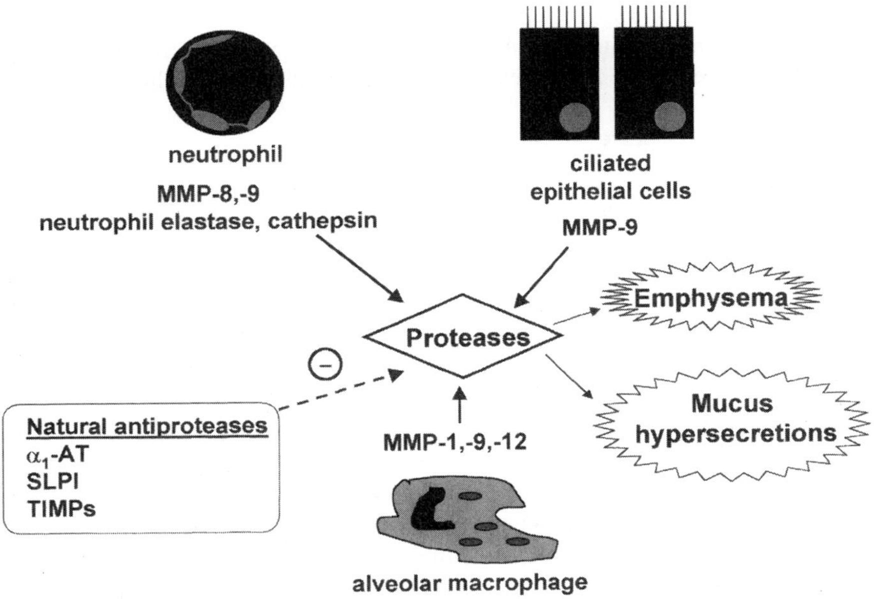

Figure 4 Inflammatory mechanisms in COPD. Cigarette smoke (and other irritants) activate macrophages and neutrophils. These cells then release proteases, such as neutrophil elastase, metalloproteinases (MMPs), and cathepsin, that break down connective tissue in the lung parenchyma, resulting in emphysema, and also stimulate mucus hypersecretion. These enzymes are normally counteracted by protease inhibitors, including α_1-antitrypsin (α_1-AT), secretory leukoprotease inhibitor (SLPI), and tissue inhibitor of MMPs (TIMPs).

obtained with numbers of macrophages [103]. A variety of macrophage-derived matrix metalloproteinases (MMPs), or matrixins, act on extracellular matrix [104]. Neutrophils, eosinophils, and airway epithelial cells also produce these endopeptidases. Interestingly, increased levels of various metalloproteinases, including MMP-1 (collagenase), MMP-2, MMP-8, and MMP-9 (gelatinase B) have been found in human lungs with emphysema compared with lungs without emphyoema [105].

Several lines of evidence suggest that in COPD there is excessive activity of proteases, and an imbalance between proteases and endogenous antiproteases [99]. This condition results in excess proteolytic activity and damage to the lung parenchyma.

A. Therapeutic Options for Creating Balance Between Proteases and Protease Inhibitors Imbalance in COPD

One approach to intervention in lung-destruction process in COPD is to supply inhibitors to suppress protease activity (Table 4). Another approach could be to supply a natural inhibitor of proteases in sufficient quantity to create a balance between extracellular proteases and protease inhibitors [106].

Neutrophil Elastase Inhibitors

Peptide NE inhibitors, such as ICI 200355 and nonpeptide inhibitors, such as ONO-5046 (sivelistat) inhibit NE-induced lung injury in experimental animals [107,108], and inhibit NE-induced secretion of mucus in vitro. FR901277 is another NE inhibitor that inhibits the elastase activity potently both in vitro and in vivo [108]. The cephalosporin-based compound L-658,758 inhibits elastinolysis by NE and proteiase-3 in sputum samples from adult cystic fibrosis patients [110].

There are few clinical studies of NE inhibitors in COPD. A clinical study of oral MR889 (midesteine) administered for four weeks in patients with COPD showed reduced urinary desmosine levels in a subset of patients [111]. ZD-0892 is in phase I clinical trials for COPD [112].

NE inhibitors could also be administered as an aerosol into the airway. This requires considerably less inhibitor than systemic administration, allows a more efficient delivery of active inhibitor, and is easier to administer to patients [113]. GR243214 is a prototype inhibitor that could be administered by aerosol [114]. Other agents, such as FR901277, MDL 201,404YA (alternatively, CE-1037), ICI 200 880, ICI 200 880, and TEI-8362, seem to act when administered directly into the airways, but this has been observed only in the experimental setting. EPI-HNE-4, engineered from the Kunitz domain, is another new, rapidly acting, potent, and specific human NE inhibitor that, when directly administered into trachea of rats induces effective,

Table 4 Therapeutic Options for Creating Balance Between Proteases and Protease Inhibitors Imbalance in COPD

Neutrophil elastase inhibitors	
	ICI 200355
	Sivelistat
	FR901277
	L-658,758
	Midesteine
	ZD-0892
	GR243214
	MDL 201,404YA
	ICI 200 880
	TEI-8362
	EPI-HNE-4
	Recombinant monocyte/neutrophil elastase inhibitor
	GW311616A
	DMP 777
Matrix metalloproteinase inhibitors	
	Batimastat
	Marimastat
	RS-113456
	RS-132908
Retinoic acid	
Serpins	
	Lex032
	SQN-5
	Pre-elafin
Cathepsin inhibitors	
	Suramin
α_1-Antitrypsin	
Recombinant human secretory leukoprotease inhibitor	

dose-dependent protection of the lungs [116]. Recombinant monocyte/NE inhibitor has the ability to inhibit NE in inflammatory pulmonary exudates [117]. The local use of recombinant monocyte/NE applied directly to the airway as an aerosol offers promise for preventing or reducing at least the lung injury component of cystic fibrosis.

All these inhibitors act extracellularly and may not inhibit the enzyme at the site of release when neutrophils adhere to connective tissue. Intracellular NE inhibitors, such as GW311616A and DMP 777, might therefore be more effective in preventing lung destruction [114]. They penetrate neutrophils and inactivate NE within the azurophil granule. This limits the area of damage produced during cell migration and degranulation.

Serpins

LEX032 is a recombinant serpin in which the properties of two very similarly structured protease inhibitors, α_1-AT and α_1-antichymotrypsin, were combined by replacing six equivalent amino acids of α_1-antichymotrypsin with the critical amino acids, which gives α_1-AT its human NE-inhibiting property. It retains enzyme inhibition and secondary anti-inflammatory actions of α_1-antichymotrypsin and gains the ability to inhibit NE [117].

SQN-5, a mouse serpin that is highly similar to the human serpins SCCA1 and SCCA2, inhibits cathepsins K, L, S, and V but not cathepsin B or H, like SCCA1. Moreover, like SCCA2, it inhibits the chymotrypsin-like enzymes, mast cell chymase and cathepsin G [118].

Pre-elafin, also known as trappin-2, is a 117-amino acid (including a 22-amino acid signal peptide) elastase-specific inhibitor. Recombinant human pre-elafin exerts a significant protective effect against NE-induced acute lung injury in hamsters [119]. Also recombinant human proteinase inhibitor 9 (PI9), an intracellular 42-kDa member of the ovalbumin family of serpins, is a potent inhibitor of human NE in vitro [120].

Cathepsin Inhibitors

Suramin, a hexasulfonated naphthylurea that has been used as an antitumor drug, is a potent inhibitor of cathepsin G, proteinase 3, and NE [121], but there have been no reported clinical trial with this drug. Novel and more specific cathepsin inhibitors are now in development [106].

Matrix Metalloproteinase Inhibitors

It may be possible to inhibit the induction of MMPs in COPD with specific transcription inhibitors [122]. Another approach to inhibiting MMPs is to develop specific enzyme inhibitors, but it is still not clear whether there is one predominant MMP in COPD or whether a broad-spectrum inhibitor will be necessary [122]. Tetracyclines and hydroxamates, such as batimastat (BB-94) that can inhibit the in vivo increase in MMP induced by lipopolysaccharide and, consequently, modulate airway remodelling [123], and the orally active marimastat (BB-2516), are nonselective MMP inhibitors [122]. RS-113456 and RS-132908 are two orally bioavailable synthetic hydroxamate-based MMP inhibitors. Both markedly inhibited the smoke-induced airspace enlargement in mice, and reduced macrophage accumulation within the lung tissue [124]. More selective inhibitors of individual MMPs, such as MMP-9 and MMP-12, are now in development and are likely to be better tolerated in chronic therapy.

Retinoic Acid

Retinoic acid attenuates the induction and activation of MMP-1 and MMP-3 [125]. All-*trans*-retinoic acid selectively down-regulates MMP-9 and up-regulates TIMP-1 in human bronchoalveolar lavage cells [126]. This effect of retinoic acid is due to transcriptional regulation. Dramatic results have been obtained when retinoic acid has been administered daily to young adult rats 25 days after they have been instilled in the lungs with elastase. Twelve days after treatment with all-*trans*-retinoic acid, evidence of lung damage and symptoms of experimental emphysema have been reversed [127].

α_1-Antitrypsin

Danazol [128] and tamoxifen [129] can increase the concentrations of α_1-AT in subjects with normal α_1-AT because the secretory process is not impaired in these patients [99]. In a different way, patients with a α_1-AT deficiency can be supplemented with α_1-AT extracted from human plasma that must be given intravenously but has a half-life of only five days [122]. However, since only 2% of intravenously infused drug reaches the lung, direct delivery by inhalation is an attractive alternative [130]. In effect, human α_1-AT can be aerosolized to a respirable size while preserving biochemical function and augmenting the epithelial lining fluid above protective levels without ill effects [131]. Recombinant α_1-AT with amino acid substitutions to increase stability may result in a more stable product. Replacement of the active site methionine by valine results in an elastase inhibitor that cannot be inactivated by oxidants [132]. Gene therapy is another possibility, using an adenovirus vector or liposomes, but there have been major problems in developing efficient delivery systems [106].

Secretory Leukoprotease Inhibitor

Recombinant human SLPI (rSLPI) given by aerosolization increases anti-NE activity in epithelial lining fluid for more than 12 hours, indicating potential therapeutic use for this agent [133]. It is likely that aerosol therapy with rSLPI will be most beneficial for well-ventilated lung tissue that needs protection against NE [134]. It has been suggested that inhaled rSLPI could prove beneficial in partnership with α_1-AT [135] or apocynin [136] in the treatment of COPD.

B. Limitations to Antiprotease Therapy

Both macrophages and neutrophils, which are increased in the smoker's lung, are now clearly implicated in the development of emphysema. These cells express distinct proteases, implying more than one enzyme system is clinically relevant to the injury incurred in COPD. Distinguishing features of patients with COPD may reveal subsets of individuals in whom one or another protease system is dominant. This could prove to be the basis for targeted drug therapy to prevent progression to end-stage lung disease, especially for individuals who quit smoking at later stages of emphysematous damage. Unfortunately, MMPs degrade α_1-AT, and NE degrades TIMPs. These enzymes, by neutralizing each other's natural inhibitors, can not only amplify overall proteolytic activity, but also deactivate supplied natural inhibitors of proteases.

IV. Conclusions

A large body of evidence indicates that in patients with COPD, oxidants and proteases complement each other in their potential to destroy lung parenchyma. It is therefore appealing to combine therapeutic strategies aimed at augmenting or complementing the antioxidant and antiproteolytic activities. Unfortunately, this type of therapeutic approach is still in its infancy. None of the drugs that clinicians have at their disposal are really effective. On the other hand, almost all agents that are in development are in very early phases of pharmacological analysis and it is likely that only few of them, or none, will enter clinical practice. It is clear that there is a need for a real commitment from researchers and drug companies to further explore the field in the future. The need is evident considering that in the last 30 years the treatment of the COPD has been based primarily on bronchodilators and secondarily on corticosteroids. This approach has been unable to modify the course of the disease.

References

1. NHLBI/WHO Global strategy for the diagnosis, management and prevention of chronic obstructive pulmonary disease. Global Initiative for Chronic Obstructive Lung Disease (GOLD). NHLBI/WHO workshop report. Bethesda: National Heart, Lung and Blood Institute, April 2001. *http://www.goldcopd.com.*
2. Repine JE, Bast A, Lankhorst I and The Oxidative Stress Study Group. Oxidative stress in chronic obstructive pulmonary disease. Am J Respir Crit Care Med 1997; 156:341–357.

3. Cuzzocrea S, Riley DP, Caputi AP, et al. Antioxidant therapy: a new pharmacological approach in shock, inflammation, and ischemia/reperfusion injury. Pharmacol Rev 2001; 53:135–159.
4. Rahman I, MacNee W. Role of transcription factors in inflammatory lung diseases. Thorax 1998; 53:601–612.
5. Gius D, Botero A, Shah S, et al. Intracellular oxidation/reduction status in the regulation of transcription factors NF-κB and AP-1. Toxicol Lett 1999; 106:93–106.
6. Henricks PAJ, Nijkamp FP. Reactive oxygen species as mediators in asthma. Pulm Pharmacol Ther 2001; 14:409–421.
7. MacNee W. Oxidants/antioxidants and chronic obstructive pulmonary disease: pathogenesis to therapy. Novartis Found Symp 2001; 234:169–185.
8. Rahman I, MacNee W. Role of oxidants/antioxidants in smoking-induced airways diseases. Free Radic Biol Med 1996; 21:669–681.
9. Nishikawa M, Kakemizu N, Ito T, et al. Superoxide mediates cigarette smoke-induced infiltration of neutrophils into the airways through nuclear factor-κB activation and IL-8 mRNA expression in guinea pigs in vivo. Am J Respir Cell Mol Biol 2000; 20:189–198.
10. Kramps JA, Rudolphus A, Stolk J, et al. Role of antileukoprotease in the lung. Ann NY Acad Sci USA 1991; 624:97–108.
11. Jamieson D. Oxygen toxicity and reactive oxygen metabolites in mammals. Free Radic Bio Med 1989; 7:87–108.
12. Frei B. Molecular and biological mechanisms of antioxidant action. FASEB J 1999; 13:963–964.
13. Cantin AM, North SL, Hubbard RC, et al. Normal alveolar epithelial lining fluid contains high levels of glutathione. J Appl Physiol 1987; 63:152–157.
14. Davis WB, Pacht ER. Extracellular antioxidant defenses. In: Crystal RG, West JB, Weibel ER, Barnes PJ, eds. The Lung: Scientific Foundations. 2d ed. Philadelphia: Lippincott-Raven, 1997:2271–2278.
15. Meister A. Glutathione metabolism. Methods Enzymol 1995; 251:3–7.
16. Borregaard N, Jensen HS, Bjerrum OW. Prevention of tissue damage: inhibition of myeloperoxidase-mediated inactivation of α_1-proteinase inhibitor by *N*-acetyl cysteine, glutathione, and methionine. Agents Actions 1987; 22:255–260.
17. Mohsenin V, Gee JL. Oxidation of α_1-protease inhibitor: role of lipid peroxidation products. J Appl Physiol 1989; 66:2211–2215.
18. Pryor WA, Dooley MM, Church DF. The inactivation of α_1-proteinase inhibitor by gas-phase cigarette smoke: protection by antioxidants and reducing species. Chem Biol Interact 1986; 57:271–283.
19. Tyagi SC. Reversible inhibition of neutrophil elastase by thiol-modified α_1-protease inhibitor. J Biol. Chem. 1991; 266:5279–5285.
20. Rahman I, Swarska E, Henry M, et al. Is there any relationship between plasma antioxidant capacity and lung function in smokers and in patients with chronic obstructive pulmonary disease? Thorax 2000; 55:189–193.
21. MacNee W, Rahman I. Oxidants and antioxidants as therapeutic targets in

chronic obstructive pulmonary disease. Am J Respir Crit Care Med 1999; 160: 8S–65S.
22. MacNee W. Oxidative stress and lung inflammation in airways disease. Eur J Pharmacol 2001; 429:195–207.
23. Grievink L, Smit HA, Ocké MC, et al. Dietary intake of antioxidant (pro)-vitamins, respiratory symptoms and pulmonary function: the MORGEN study. Thorax 1998; 78:166–171.
24. Carey IM, Strachan DP, Cook DG. Effect of changes in fresh fruit consumption on ventilatory function in healthy British adults. Am J Respir Crit Care Med 1998; 158:728–733.
25. Sharp DS, Rodriquez BL, Shahar E, et al. Fish consumption may limit the damage of smoking on the lung. Am J Respir Crit Care Med 1994; 150:983–987.
26. Sridhar MK. Nutrition and lung health: should people at risk of chronic obstructive lung disease eat more fruit and vegetables? BMJ 1995; 310:75–76.
27. Simopoulos AP. Omega-3 fatty acids in health and disease and in growth and development. Am J Clin Nutr 1991; 54:438–463.
28. Cao G, Sofic E, Prior RL. Antioxidant capacity of tea and common vegetables. J Agric Food Chem 1996; 44:3426–3431.
29. Strachan DP, Cox BD, Erzinclioglu SW, et al. Ventilatory function and winter fresh fruit consumption in a random sample of British adults. Thorax 1991; 46:624–629.
30. Schwartz J, Weiss ST. Relationship between dietary vitamin C intake and pulmonary function in the first national health and nutrition examination survey (NHANES 1). Am J Clin Nutr 1994; 59:110–114.
31. Miedema I, Feskens EJM, Heederik D, et al. Dietary determinants of long-term incidence of chronic nonspecific lung diseases: the Zutphen study. Am J Epidemiol 1993; 138:37–45.
32. Weber P, Bendich A, Schalch W. Vitamin C and human health—a review of recent data relevant to human requirements. Int J Vitam Nutr Res 1996; 66: 19–30.
33. Lykkesfeldt J, Prieme H, Loft S, Poulsen HE. Effect of smoking cessation on plasma ascorbic acid concentration. BMJ 1996; 313:91.
34. Lykkesfeldt J, Loft S, Nielsen JB, et al. Ascorbic acid and dehydroascorbic acid as biomarkers of oxidative stress caused by smoking. Am J Clin Nutr 1997; 65:959–963.
35. Reilly M, Delanty N, Lawson JA, et al. Modulation of oxidant stress in vivo in chronic cigarette smokers. Circulation 1996; 94:19–25.
36. Smith JL, Hodges RE. Serum levels of vitamin C in relation to dietary and supplemental intake of vitamin C in smokers and nonsmokers. Ann NY Acad Sci 1987; 498:144–152.
37. Sargeant LA, Jaeckel A, Wareham NJ. Interaction of vitamin C with the relation between smoking and obstructive airways disease in EPIC Norfolk. European Prospective Investigation into Cancer and Nutrition. Eur Respir J 2000; 16:397–403.
38. Schunemann HJ, Grant BJ, Freudenheim JL, et al. The relation of serum levels of antioxidant vitamins C E and, retinol and carotenoids with pulmonary func-

tion in the general population. Am J Respir Crit Care Med 2001; 163:1246–1255.
39. Watson L, Margetts B, Howarth P, et al. The association between diet and chronic obstructive pulmonary disease in subjects selected from general practice. Eur Respir J 2002; 20:313–318.
40. Tabak C, Arts ICW, Smit HA, et al. Chronic obstructive pulmonary disease and intake of catechins, flavonols, and flavones. The MORGEN Study. Am J Respir Crit Care Med 2001; 164:61–64.
41. Hu G, Cassano PA. Antioxidant nutrients and pulmonary function: the Third National Health and Nutrition Examination Survey (NHANES III). Am J Epidemiol 2000; 151:975–981.
42. Hasselmark L, Malmgren R, Zetterström O, et al. Selenium supplementation in intrinsic asthma. Allergy 1993; 48:30–36.
43. Sies H, Masumoto H. Ebselen as a glutathione peroxidase mimic and as a scavenger of peroxynitrite. Adv Pharmacol 1997; 38:229–246.
44. Moutet M, D'Alessio P, Malette P, et al. Glutathione peroxidase mimics prevent TNF-α- and neutrophil-induced endothelial alterations. Free Radic Biol Med 1998; 25:270–281.
45. Rahman I, MacNee W. Oxidative stress and regulation of glutathione in lung inflammation. Eur Respir J 2000; 16:534–554.
46. Rahman I, MacNee W. Lung glutathione and oxidative stress: implications in cigarette smoke-induced airway disease. Am J Physiol 1999; 277:L1067–L1088.
47. Deneke SM, Susanto I, Vogel KA, et al. Mechanisms of use of extracellular glutathione by lung epithelial cells and pulmonary artery endothelial cells. Am J Respir Cell Mol Biol 1995; 12:662–668.
48. Hagen TM, Wierzbicka GT, Sillau AH, et al. Bioavailability of dietary glutathione: effect on plasma concentration. Am J Physiol 1990; 259:G524–G529.
49. Witschi A, Reddy S, Stofer B, et al. The systemic availability of oral glutathione. Eur J Clin Pharmacol 1992; 43:667–669.
50. Borok Z, Buhl R, Grimes GJ, et al. Effect of glutathione aerosol on oxidant-antioxidant imbalance in idiopathic pulmonary fibrosis. Lancet 1991; 338:215–216.
51. Holroyd KJ, Buhl R, Borok Z, et al. Correction of glutathione deficiency in the lower respiratory tract of HIV seropositive individuals by glutathione aerosol treatment. Thorax 1993; 48:985–989.
52. Marrades RM, Roca J, Barbera A, et al. Nebulized glutathione induces bronchoconstriction in patients with mild asthma. Am J Respir Crit Care Med 1997; 156:425–430.
53. Lamson DW, Brignall MS. The use of nebulized glutathione in the treatment of emphysema: a case report. Altern Med Rev 2000; 5:429–431.
54. Aruoma OI, Halliwell B, Hoey BM, et al. The antioxidant action of N-acetylcysteine: its reaction with hydrogen peroxide, hydroxyl radical, superoxide, and hypochlorous acid. Free Radic Biol Med 1989; 6:593–597.
55. Mulier B, Rahman I, Watchorn T, et al. Hydrogen peroxide-induced epithelial

injury: the protective role of intracellular nonprotein thiols NPSH. Eur Respir J 1998; 11:384–391.
56. Bast A, Haenen G, Doelman CJA. Oxidants and antioxidants: state of the art. Am J Med 1991; 91(suppl 3C):2S–13S.
57. Moldéus P, Cotgreave IA. *N*-acetylcysteine. Meth Enzymol 1994; 234:482–492.
58. Bridgeman MME, Marsden M, Selby C, et al. Effect of N-acetyl cysteine on the concentrations of thiols in plasma, bronchoalveolar lavage fluid and lining tissue. Thorax 1994; 49:670–675.
59. Bowman G, Backer U, Larsson S, et al. Oral acetylcysteine reduces exacerbation rate in chronic bronchitis. Eur J Respir Dis 1983; 64:405–415.
60. Rasmusse JB, Glennow C. Reduction in days of illness after long-term treatment with N-acetylcysteine controlled-release tablets in patients with chronic bronchitis. Eur J Respir Dis 1988; 1:351–355.
61. Eklund A, Eriksson O, Hakansson L, et al. Oral N-acetylcysteine reduces selected humoral markers of inflammatory cell activity in BAL fluid from healthy smokers: correlation to effects on cellular variables. Eur Respir J 1988; 1:832–838.
62. Rahman I, Mulier B, Gilmour PS, et al. Oxidant-mediated lung epithelial cell tolerance: the role of intracellular glutathione and nuclear factor-κB. Biochem Pharmacol 2001; 62:787–794.
63. Parmentier M, Hirani N, Rahman I, et al. Regulation of lipopolysaccharide-mediated interleukin-1β release by N-acetylcysteine in THP-1 cells. Eur Respir J 2000; 16:933–939.
64. Cuzzocrea S, Mazzon E, Dugo L, et al. Protective effects of *n*-acetylcysteine on lung injury and red blood cell modification induced by carrageenan in the rat. FASEB J 2001; 15:1187–1200.
65. Schillier HJ, Reilly PM, Bulkley GB. Tissue perfusion in critical illnesses. Antioxidant therapy. Crit Care Med 1993; 21:92–102.
66. Pouwell RJ, Machiedo GW, Rush BJ, et al. Effect of oxygen-free radical scavengers on survival in sepsis. Am Surg 1991; 57:86–88.
67. Aruoma OI, Halliwell B, Hoey BM, et al. The antioxidant action of n-acetylcysteine: its reaction with hydrogen peroxide, hydroxyl radical, superoxide, and hypochlorous acid. J Free Radic Biol Med 1989; 6:593–597.
68. Kasielski M, Nowak D. Long-term administration of N-acetylcysteine decreases hydrogen peroxide exhalation in subjects with chronic obstructive pulmonary disease. Respir Med 2001; 95:448–456.
69. van Klaveren RJ, Dinsdale D, Pype JL, et al. *N*-acetylcysteine does not protect against type II cell injury after prolonged exposure to hyperoxia in rats. Am J Physiol 1997; 273:L548–L555.
70. Traveline JM, Sudarshan S, Roy BG, et al. Effect of *N*-acetylcysteine on human diaphragm strength and fatigability. Am J Respir Crit Care Med 1997; 156: 1567–1571.
71. AM, Vanderbist F, Parij N, et al. Effect of the mucoactive drug nacystelyn on the respiratory burst of human blood polymorphonuclear neutrophils. Pulm Pharmacol Ther 1997; 10:287–292.

72. Gillissen A, Jaworska M, Orth M, et al. Nacystelyn, a novel lysine salt of *N*-acetylcysteine, to augment cellular antioxidant defence in vitro. Respir Med 1997; 91:159–168.
73. Antonicelli F, Parmentier M, Drost EM, et al. Nacystelyn inhibits oxidant-mediated interleukin-8 expression and NF-kappaB nuclear binding in alveolar epithelial cells. Free Radic Biol Med 2002; 32:492–502.
74. Lands LC, Grey VL, Smountas AA. Effect of supplementation with a cysteine donor on muscular performance. J Appl Physiol 1999; 87:1381–1385.
75. Lothian B, Grey V, Kimoff RJ, et al. Treatment of obstructive airway disease with a cysteine donor protein supplement: a case report. Chest 2000; 117:914–916.
76. Pinamonti S, Venturoli L, Leis M, et al. Antioxidant activity of carbocysteine lysine salt monohydrate. Panminerva Med 2001; 43:215–220.
77. Gillissen A, Scharling B, Jaworska M, et al. Oxidant scavenger function of ambroxol in vitro: a comparison with *N*-acetylcysteine. Res Exp Med (Berl) 1997; 196:389–398.
78. Gillissen A, Nowak D. Characterisation of N-acetylcysteine and ambroxol in anti-oxidant therapy. Respir Med 1998; 92:609–623.
79. Suzuki M, Teramoto S, Matsuse T, et al. Inhibitory effect of ambroxol on superoxide anion production and generation by murine lung alveolar macrophages. J Asthma 1998; 35:267–272.
80. Teramoto S, Suzuki M, Ohga E, et al. Effects of ambroxol on spontaneous or stimulated generation of reactive oxygen species by bronchoalveolar lavage cells harvested from patients with or without chronic obstructive pulmonary disease. Pharmacology 1999; 59:135–141.
81. van den Worm E, Beukelman CJ, Van den Berg AJ, et al. Effects of methoxylation of apocynin and analogs on the inhibition of reactive oxygen species production by stimulated human neutrophils. Eur J Pharmacol 2001; 433:225–230.
82. Muijsers RB, van Den Worm E, Folkerts G, et al. Apocynin inhibits peroxynitrite formation by murine macrophages. Br J Pharmacol 2000; 130:932–993.
83. Laperre TS, Jimenez LA, Antonicelli F, et al. Apocynin increases glutathione synthesis and activates AP-1 in alveolar epithelial cells. FEBS Lett 1999; 443: 235–239.
84. Salvemini D, Mazzon E, Dugo L, et al. Pharmacological manipulation of the inflammatory cascade by the superoxide dismutase mimetic. M40403. Brit J Pharmacol 2001; 132:815–827.
85. MacNee W. Antioxidants. In: Hansel TT, Barnes PJ, eds. New Drugs for Asthma, Allergy and COPD. Karger: Prog Respir Res. Basel, 2001(31):151–155.
86. Barnes PJ. Molecular mechanisms of corticosteroids in allergic diseases. Allergy 2001; 56:928–936.
87. Ito K, Lim S, Caramori G, et al. Cigarette smoke reduces histone deacetylase 2 expression, enhances cytokine expression, and inhibits glucocorticoid actions in alveolar macrophages. FASEB J 2001; 15:1110–1112.

88. Wang HC, Zentner MD, Deng HT, et al. Oxidative stress disrupts glucocorticoid hormone-dependent transcription of the amiloride-sensitive epithelial sodium channel α-subunit in lung epithelial cells through ERK-dependent and thioredoxin-sensitive pathways. J Biol Chem 2000; 275:8600–860.
89. Kilfeather S. 5-Lipoxygenase inhibitors for the treatment of COPD. Chest 2002; 121:197S–200S.
90. Nielson CP, Vestal RE, Sturm RJ, et al. Effects of selective phosphodiesterase inhibitors on the polymorphonuclear leukocyte respiratory burst. J Allergy Clin Immunol 1990; 86:801–808.
91. Mahomed AG, Theron AJ, Anderson R, et al. Anti-oxidative effects of theophylline on human neutrophils involve cyclic nucleotides and protein kinase A. Inflammation 1998; 22:545–55.
92. Ottonello L, Morone P, Dapino P, et al. Inhibitory effect of salmeterol on the respiratory burst of adherent human neutrophils. Clin Exp Immunol 1996; 106: 97–102.
93. Anderson R, Feldman C, Theron AJ, et al. Anti-inflammatory, membrane-stabilizing interactions of salmeterol with human neutrophils in vitro. Brit J Pharmacol 1996; 117:1387–1394.
94. Thomas CE, Ohlweiler DF, Carr AA, et al. Characterization of the radical trapping activity of a novel series of cyclic nitrone spin traps. J Biol Chem 1996; 271:3097–310.
95. Hensley K, Pye QN, Maidt ML, et al. Interaction of □-phenyl-N-tert-butyl nitrone and alternative electron acceptors with complex I indicates a substrate reduction site upstream from the rotenone binding site. J Neurochem 1998; 71:2549–2557.
96. Smith CAD, Harrison DJ. Association between polymorphism in gene or microsomal epoxide hydralase and susceptibility to emphysema. Lancet 1997; 350:630–633.
97. van Schayck CP, Dekhuijzen PNR, Gorgels WJ, et al. Are anti-oxidant and anti-inflammatory treatments effective in different subgrops of COPD? A hypothesis. Respir Med 1998; 92:1259–1264.
98. Stockley RA. Biochemical and cellular mechanisms. In: Calverley P, Pride N, eds. Chronic Obstructive Pulmonary Disease. London: Chapman & Hall, 1995:93–133.
99. Stockley RA. Proteases and antiproteases. Novartis Found Symp 2001; 234: 189–199.
100. Reid PT, Marsden ME, Cunningham GA, et al. Human neutrophil elastase regulates the expression and secretion of elafin (elastase-specific inhibitor) in Type II alveolar epithelial cells. FEBS Letts 1999; 457:33–37.
101. Sallenave JM, Shulmann J, Crossley J, et al. Regulation of secretory leukocyte proteinase inhibitor (SLPI) and elastase-specific inhibitor (ESI/elafin) in human airway epithelial cells by cytokines and neutrophilic enzymes. Am J Respir Cell Mol Biol 1994; 11:733–741.
102. Barnes PJ. Mechanisms in COPD: differences from asthma. Chest 2000; 117: 10S–14S.

103. Finkelstein R, Fraser R, Ghezzo H, et al. Alveolar inflammation and its relation to emphysema in smokers. Am J Respir Crit Care Med 1995; 152:1666–1672.
104. Senior R, Connolly N, Cury J, et al. Elastin degradation by human alveolar macrophages. Am Rev Respir Dis 1989; 139:1251–1256.
105. Ohnishi K, Takagi M, Kurokawa Y, et al. Matrix metalloproteinase-mediated extracellular matrix protein degradation in human pulmonary emphysema. Lab Invest 1998; 78:1077–1080.
106. Leckie MJ, Bryan SA, Hansel TT, et al. Novel therapy for COPD. Exp Opin Invest Drugs 2000; 9:3–23.
107. Williams JC, Falcone RC, Knee C, et al. Biologic characterization of ICI 200,880 and ICI 200,355, novel inhibitors of human neutrophil elastase. Am Rev Respir Dis 1991; 144:875–883.
108. Kawabata K, Suzuki M, Sugitani M, et al. ONO-5046, a novel inhibitor of human neutrophil elastase. Biochem Biophys Res Commun 1991; 177:814–820.
109. Fujie K, Shinguh Y, Yamazaki A, et al. Inhibition of elastase-induced acute inflammation and pulmonary emphysema in hamsters by a novel neutrophil elastase inhibitor FR901277. Inflamm Res 1999; 48:160–167.
110. Rees DD, Brain JD, Wohl ME, et al. Inhibition of neutrophil elastase in CF sputum by L-658,758. J Pharmacol Exp Ther 1997; 283:1201–1206.
111. Luisetti M, Sturani C, Sella D, et al. MR889, a neutrophil elastase inhibitor, in patients with chronic obstructive pulmonary disease: a double-blind, randomized, placebo-controlled clinical trial. Eur Respir J 1996; 9:1482–1486.
112. Ohbayashi H. ZD-0892 AstraZeneca. Curr Opin Investig Drugs 2000; 1:227–229.
113. Burdon JGW, Knight KR, Brenton S, et al. Antiproteinase deficiency, emphysema and replacement therapy. Aust N Z J Med 1996; 26:769–771.
114. Smith RA, Stockley RA, Hodgson ST. Neutrophil elastase inhibitors. In: Hansel TT, Barnes PJ, eds. New Drugs for Asthma, Allergy and COPD. Vol. 31. Prog Respir Res Basel, Karger, 2001:173–176.
115. Delacourt C, Herigault S, Delclaux C, et al. Protection against acute lung injury by Intravenous or intratracheal pretreatment with EPI-HNE-4, a new potent neutrophil elastase inhibitor. Am J Respir Cell Mol Biol 2002; 26:290–297.
116. Rees DD, Rogers RA, Cooley J, et al. Recombinant human monocyte/neutrophil elastase inhibitor protects rat lungs against injury from cystic fibrosis airway secretions. Am J Respir Cell Mol Biol 1999; 20:69–78.
117. Sands H, Hook JB. Pharmacology and pharmacokinetics of LEX 032, a bioengineered serpin: the first of a potential new class of drugs. Drug Metab Rev 1997; 29:309–328.
118. Al-Khunaizi M, Luke CJ, Askew YS, et al. The serpin SQN-5 is a dual mechanistic-class inhibitor of serine and cysteine proteinases. Biochemistry 2002; 41:3189–3199.
119. Tremblay GM, Vachon E, Larouche C, et al. Inhibition of human neutrophil elastase-induced acute lung injury in hamsters by recombinant human pre-elafin (Trappin-2). Chest 2002; 121:582–588.

120. Dahlen JR, Foster DC, Kisiel W. Inhibition of neutrophil elastase by recombinant human proteinase inhibitor 9. Biochim Biophys Acta 1999; 1451: 233–241.
121. Cadene M, Duranton J, North A, et al. Inhibition of neutrophil serine proteinases by suramin. J Biol Chem 1997; 272:9950–9955.
122. Barnes PJ. Novel approaches and targets for treatment of chronic obstructive pulmonary disease. Am J Respir Crit Care Med 1999; 160:S72–S79.
123. Corbel M, Lanchou J, Germain N, et al. Modulation of airway remodeling-associated mediators by the antifibrotic compound, pirfenidone, and the matrix metalloproteinase inhibitor, batimastat, during acute lung injury in mice. Eur J Pharmacol 2001; 426:113–121.
124. Martin RL, Shapiro SD, Tong SE, et al. Macrophage metalloelastase inhibitors. In: Hansel TT, Barnes PJ, eds. New Drugs for Asthma, Allergy and COPD. Vol. 31. Prog Respir Res Basel, Karger, 2001:177–180.
125. Zhu YK, Liu X, Ertl RF, et al. Retinoic acid attenuates cytokine-driven fibroblast degradation of extracellular matrix in three-dimensional culture. Am J Respir Cell Mol Biol 2001; 25:620–627.
126. Frankenberger M, Hauck RW, Frankenberger B, et al. All trans-retinoic acid selectively down-regulates matrix metalloproteinase-9 (MMP-9) and up-regulates tissue inhibitor of metalloproteinase-1 (TIMP-1) in human bronchoalveolar lavage cells. Mol Med 2001; 7:263–270.
127. Massaro GD, Massaro D. Retinoic acid treatment abrogates elastase-induced pulmonary emphysema in rats. Nat Med 1997; 3:675–677.
128. Gadek JE, Fulmer JD, Gelfand JA, et al. Danazol-induced augmentation of serum α_1-antitrypsin levels in individuals with marked deficiency of this antiprotease. J Clin Invest 1980; 66:82–87.
129. Wewers MD, Brantly ML, Casolaro MA, et al. Evaluation of tamoxifen as a therapy to augment α_1-antitrypsin concentrations in Z homozygous α_1-antitrypsin-deficient subjects. Am Rev Respir Dis 1987; 135:401–402.
130. Crystal RG. α_1-Antitrypsin deficiency: pathogenesis and treatment. Hosp Pract 1991; 2:81–94.
131. Hubbard RC, Crystal RG. Strategies for aerosol therapy of α_1-antitrypsin deficiency by the aerosol route. Lung 1990; 168(suppl):565–578.
132. Rosenberg S, Barr PJ, Najarian RC, et al. Synthesis in yeast of a functional oxidation-resistant mutant of human α_1-antitrypsin. Nature 1984; 312:77–80.
133. McElvaney NG, Doujaiji B, Moan MJ, et al. Pharmacokinetics of recombinant secretory leukoprotease inhibitor aerosolized to normals and individuals with cystic fibrosis. Am Rev Respir Dis 1993; 148:1056–1060.
134. Stolk J, Camps J, Feitsma HI, et al. Pulmonary deposition and disappearance of aerosolised secretory leucocyte protease inhibitor. Thorax 1995; 50:645–650.
135. Bingle L, Tetley TD. Secretory leukoprotease inhibitor: partnering α_1-proteinase inhibitor to combat pulmonary inflammation. Thorax 1996; 51:1273–1274.
136. Stolk J, Rossie W, Dijkman JH. Apocynin improves the efficacy of secretory leukocyte protease inhibitor in experimental emphysema. Am J Respir Crit Care Med 1994; 150:1628–1631.

17

An Integrated Approach to the Pharmacological Therapy of COPD

BARTOLOME R. CELLI

St. Elizabeth's Medical Center and Tufts University
Boston, Massachusetts, U.S.A.

I. Introduction

All of the major scientific respiratory societies have defined chronic obstructive pulmonary disease (COPD) as a disease state characterized by airflow limitation that is not fully reversible [1–3]. The Global Initiative for Lung Disease (GOLD) has expanded the concept to include that airflow limitation is usually progressive and associated with an abnormal inflammatory response to inhaled particles or gases [1].

Although precise, all of the definitions are full of negative connotations to those less familiar with the great advances that have been made in the treatment of COPD. This "negative" approach to the characterization of the disease, coupled with the fact that COPD is the fastest-rising major cause of death in the United States and will be the third most frequent cause of death in the world by the year 2020 [4], provide a negative picture that promotes a fatalistic attitude toward the disease and its therapy. Even more important is the fact that this concept and such an attitude are far from being real. In this chapter, I hope to convince the reader that we have effective therapy and COPD is not only preventable but also treatable and that pharmacotherapy is a highly effective component of the overall treat-

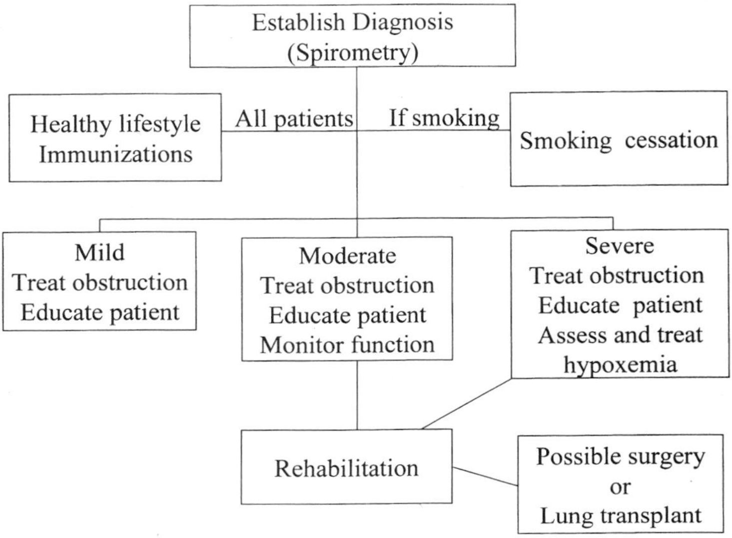

Figure 1 Algorithm summarizing the general approach to the patient with possible chronic obstructive pulmonary disease.

ment plan in that disease. An overall algorithm describing the general treatment of patients with COPD is shown in Fig. 1.

II. Change in Paradigm: A Constructive Analogy with Systemic Hypertension

In this work, we review why we must change this attitude and promote the concept that COPD is a preventable and treatable disease, one for which more research and the application of currently available and rational treatment can not only prolong the life of the patients afflicted with the disease but also improve the quality of their life.

Let us start with the definition of COPD per se and examine how we have come to use the defining physiology as the outcome to evaluate the effectiveness of interventions. COPD is defined spirometrically as airflow limitation that is "not" fully reversible. The limitation to airflow is documented with the use of the forced expiratory volume in 1 sec (FEV_1), which fails to improve with bronchodilator. In a contradictory way, we have then planned many studies attempting to reverse what we have defined as being "not" fully reversible. It is no surprise that the lack of large response in

FEV_1 to many different therapeutic agents [5–15] has resulted in a nihilism that is not deserved. The same data can be viewed entirely different if we interpret the facts using a new paradigm. For this, let us make an analogy with the diagnosis and treatment of hypertension, an area with great and significant progress over the last decades.

Where would the treatment of hypertension be if hypertension had been defined as high blood pressure that did not respond to antihypertensives? The analogy can be expanded with a careful analysis of how cardiologists and nephrologists have addressed the problem of systemic hypertension. Although the primary aim of the studies evaluating therapeutic response to antihypertensives is to reduce the blood pressure in hypertensive patients, the actual magnitude of the achieved decrease is rather modest. A review of several trials of medications for high blood pressure showed that the mean drop in systolic blood pressure with treatment was 12–14 mmHg (9–10%), and it was 5 mmHg or 5% for the diastolic pressure [16]. The change in those and other more recent trials [17] are very modest and not different from the magnitude of change in FEV_1 reported in many bronchodilator trials in patients with COPD [5–10]. If we were to try to convince the medical community at large and the patients themselves that changes of blood pressure of that magnitude are important and significant, very few persons would accept the long-term treatment for hypertension. It is because the outcomes that really matter, such as incidence of death from coronary heart disease, cerebrovascular accidents, and vascular death decreased 34%, 19%, and 23%, respectively, in patients receiving treatment compared with controls, that the medical world has adopted a positive attitude to the treatment of hypertension. Currently, the field of COPD is where the field of hypertension was not too long ago, a field requiring a change in the way we think about it so that we can move forward with optimism and confidence.

It is time to change the way in which we think about COPD. It is time for a new paradigm. The disease can be defined with and easy tool, the FEV_1/FVC ratio, very similar to the definition of hypertension with the sphigmomanometer. Just like hypertension, we need to examine the effect of therapy not only on the degree of airflow limitation, but in outcomes that resemble those affected by hypertension. In the analogy developed here, dyspnea with exercise would be the equivalent to angina, exacerbation with that of unstable angina, respiratory insufficiency with that of heart failure or pulmonary edema, and the need for mechanical ventilation with that of a myocardial infarction with cardiogenic shock. In this new paradigm, mortality would also be an outcome to evaluate. Indeed, recent evidence suggests that the survival of patients with COPD has improved over the last two decades [18]. In this book we have given outcomes different from the FEV_1, the same if not more importance than lung function itself.

III. Proof of Concept

As discussed in this book, there have been several trials of different bronchodilators and glucocorticosteroids [5–10,13–15] that have shown a large and significant decrease in functional and exercise dyspnea in patients receiving treatment compared with placebo, with improvement in FEV_1 that is similar in magnitude to the changes frequently reported as positive by trials of antihypertensive therapy in systemic hypertension. Furthermore, several of those trials have documented a decrease in the number of exacerbations and a prolongation in the time to hospitalization due to exacerbation [6,7,9–13]. COPD is the one respiratory disease in which multiple randomized trials have resulted in strong evidence of improvement in other outcomes. The administration of oxygen prolongs the survival of patients with hypoxemia [19,20], and supplemental oxygen to patients with less degree of hypoxemia not only improves exercise endurance but also improves dyspnea [21] and respiratory breathing pattern [22]. Pulmonary rehabilitation with exercise training has resulted not only in improvement in dyspnea, but also in quality of life and utilization of health care resources [23,24]. The evidence sup-

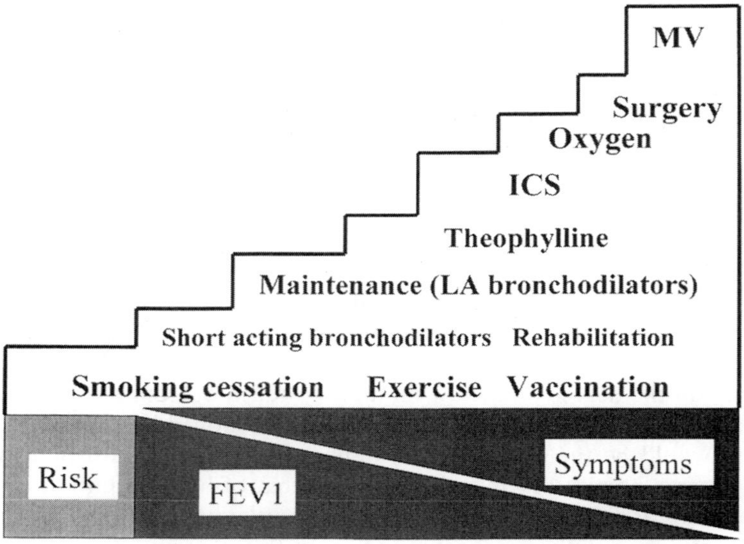

Figure 2 For patients at risk and already diagnosed with COPD, there is a large number of therapeutic options, including effective pharmacotherapy. As the disease progresses (more airflow limitation and more symptoms), therapy becomes more complex and the use of multiple modalities become the rule.

porting pulmonary rehabilitation is so overwhelming that it has become the gold standard against which new therapies such as lung pneumoplasty are being compared. The popularization of noninvasive mechanical ventilation as a first-line therapy for patients with exacerbation of COPD presenting with incipient respiratory failure is backed by several well-conducted randomized trials that documented improvement not only in the rate of intubations but also in length of hospital stay and, more important, in mortality [25–27]. For patients with special lung pathological phenotype such as inhomogenous emphysema and hyperinflation, the possibility of temporary benefit with lung-volume reduction surgery is a reality [28]. Finally, the progress obtained in lung transplant has allowed many patients previously condemned to a miserable death at a relatively young age to achieve fully active lifestyle.

The large range of therapies available to patients with COPD is summarized in Fig. 2. The advent of new pharmacological therapies will expand the horizon even more. It is exciting to realize how much we can do for our patients, and a nihilistic attitude is not justified.

IV. COPD: A Pulmonary Disease with Systemic Consequences

Currently, the disease severity is graded using a single objective physiological measure of lung function, the FEV_1 [1–3]. However, COPD is associated with a range of other local and systemic clinical manifestations, which are not closely related to the severity of airflow limitation, such as a worsening dyspnea [1–3], reduction in exercise capacity [29], pulmonary hypertension [30], peripheral muscle weakness [29], and malnutrition [31]. Furthermore, several large studies have shown that the FEV_1 is not the only determinant of mortality in this population [32–34] and a number of other risk factors have now been identified. These include the presence in clinically stable patients of persistent hypoxemia or hypercapnia [19,20], the timed walk distance after completing pulmonary rehabilitation [35], and a low body mass index [31,36].

Therefore, grading COPD solely on the FEV_1 limits our capacity to express fully the degree of severity and does not reflect the clinical manifestations of the disease and its ultimate prognosis. Indeed, in its latest statement on COPD, the American Thoracic Society (ATS) expressed the need for a multicomponent staging system that, in addition to the degree of impairment, incorporates the perceptive and the systemic consequences of COPD. It was felt that such a grading system could help categorize and grade the heterogeneous manifestations of patients with this common disorder [3].

COPD can be described as affecting at least three domains, the respiratory, the perceptive and the systemic domain, as summarized in Fig. 3. Each of these domains has validated expressions that can be measured. Among others, the variables shown in Fig. 1 have been validated over time. The first domain, that of impairment, is adequately described by the degree of airflow limitation. In this regard, the stages proposed by the ATS have proven useful in separating groups with various degrees of impairment in health status [37], incidence of exacerbations [38], pharmacoeconomic costs [14], and mortality [32,33]. The second domain, that of perception, is described by dyspnea [39,40]. Dyspnea is an independent predictor of survival in patients after pulmonary rehabilitation [41], and dyspnea correlates well with health status scores [42]. The third domain, that due to the systemic consequences of COPD, can be evaluated with simple exercise tests such as the 6-min walk test (6MWD). This simple test has been shown to be the best predictor of mortality in patients with COPD after pulmonary rehabilitation [35] and after lung-volume reduction surgery [43], and also in patients with cardiomyopathy [44] and in patients with primary pulmonary hypertension [45]. In COPD, 6MWD is a better predictor of survival than the FEV_1 and, for each 100-m difference, mortality increases proportionally [46]. The 6MWD is an excellent predictor of health-care resources utilization [47]. Another expression of systemic involvement is the body mass index (BMI).

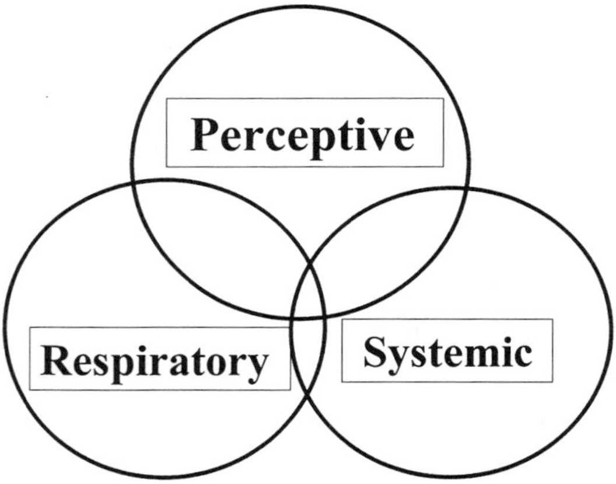

Figure 3 Chronic obstructive pulmonary disease may be represented as involving at least three domains, a perceptive domain (best expressed by dyspnea), a respiratory domain (usually expressed by the lung function), and a systemic domain (as expressed by the body mass index or exercise capacity). Pharmacological therapy has been shown to improve all three domains.

Several studies have documented an inverse relationship between body mass index (weight/height^2) and survival in COPD [31,36].

This sum of the pulmonary and nonpulmonary compromise characteristic of patients with COPD profoundly affects the functional and perceptive domains of patients with the disease, and those changes result in alterations in the overall health status of the patient. The development and validation of disease-specific questionnaires [48] that adequately reflect the impact of disease on health status has provided even more insight as to the true effect of our therapeutic armamentarium. Indeed, using these tools, we have come to realize the positive impact of pharmacotherapeutic agents on patients with COPD.

V. General Principles of Pharmacological Therapy in COPD

The evidence provided by this book indicates that effective medications for COPD are available and that all patients who are symptomatic merit a trial of drug treatment. Therapy with currently available medications can reduce or abolish symptoms, increase exercise capacity, reduce the number and severity of exacerbations, and improve health status.

The inhaled route is preferred when both inhaled and oral formulations are available. Smaller doses of active treatment can be delivered directly, with equal or greater efficacy and with fewer side effects, when administered by inhalation. However, clinical experience also shows that patients must be educated in the correct use of whatever inhalation device is employed. Significant numbers of patients cannot effectively coordinate their inspiratory maneuver with a metered-dose inhaler but can use a breath-activated inhaler, a dry-powder device, or a spacer chamber. The latter may be especially useful when inhaled corticosteroids are administered, as it reduces the oropharyngeal deposition and subsequent local side effects associated with these drugs.

Compliance with treatment is variable, but when assessed in large clinical trials, at least 85% of patients take 70% of the prescribed doses [11]. This probably reflects the fact that most patients with COPD suffer from persistent symptoms. Adherence to treatment is helped by a clear explanation of the purposes and likely outcome of therapy, together with reinforcement and review of both of these aspects of management.

Although spirometry is needed to make an accurate diagnosis, the change in lung function occurring after a brief treatment with any drug is not helpful in predicting other clinically related outcomes. Describing patients as treatment "responders" or "nonresponders" by whether the patient is "reversible" or "irreversible" using spirometric criteria alone is not useful. As has been described in the previous chapters, significant responses can occur in outcomes different from the FEV_1, and those may be more clinically relevant to patients than the mere change in lung function.

VI. Initiation of Drug Therapy

As shown in Fig. 1, the numbers of therapeutic tools available to treat patients with COPD are many. The clinician should always keep in mind that the overall goals of treatment are to prevent further deterioration in lung function, to alleviate symptoms, and to treat complications as they arise. Therefore, once the diagnosis of COPD is confirmed, the patient should be encouraged to participate actively in disease management. This concept of *collaborative management* may improve self-reliance and esteem. All patients should be encouraged to lead a healthful lifestyle and to exercise regularly. Preventive care is extremely important at this time, and all patients should receive immunizations including pneumococcal vaccine [49,50] and yearly influenza vaccines [1–3].

The most important principle governing the initiation of pharmacological therapy is the development of symptoms, namely dyspnea, cough, and/or phlegm. The symptoms may initially be intermittent but then become more persistent and progressive. Trials aimed at patients with asymptomatic milder forms of COPD need to be conducted before we can conclusively recommend therapy at earlier stages of the disease (GOLD stage 0 or patients at risk). Results from the Lung Health Trial I, comparing regular use of ipratropium with placebo, failed to show a difference in rate of FEV_1 decline between active and control groups [5]. This has been interpreted as a negative study, but unfortunately, no outcomes different from the FEV_1 were evaluated and the question remains whether the inclusion of other outcomes would have modified our conclusion.

All of the COPD guidelines [1–3] agree that as soon as patients begin to complain of intermittent symptoms, the administration of bronchodilators is indicated. Despite substantial differences in their site of action within the cell and some evidence for nonbronchodilator activity with some classes of drug, the most important consequence of bronchodilator therapy appears to be airway smooth muscle relaxation and improved lung emptying during tidal breathing. The resultant increase in FEV_1 may be small. However, as reviewed by Ferguson and O'Donnell in the appropriate chapters, these changes are often accompanied by larger changes in lung volumes with a reduction in residual volume and/or a delaying of the onset of dynamic hyperinflation during exercise. Both of these changes contribute to a reduction in perceived breathlessness. In general, the more advanced the COPD, the more important the changes in lung volume become relative to those in FEV_1.

The most accepted therapeutic regimes include the administration of short-acting selective β-agonists because they provide fast relief, are economical, and have proven relatively safe over the years. The administration of short-acting anticholinergics is an appropriate alternative. Once symptoms become more frequent and limiting, such as increasing dyspnea or night awakening, the administration of a combination of a short-acting β-agonist such as albuterol or ipratroprium bromide has proven useful and cost-effective [51,52]. One possible algorithm describing the progressive use of pharmacological therapy is shown in Fig. 4.

The advent of long-acting bronchodilators has beneficially influenced the way in which we can treat our patients, and once the patient has persistent symptoms, the regular use of long-acting bronchodilators is justified [1]. Long-acting inhaled β-agonists improve health status, possibly to a greater degree than using regular short-acting bronchodilators [53]. Additionally, these drugs reduce symptoms, rescue medication use, and increase the time between exacerbations compared with placebo [7,53]. Combining short-acting agents such as ipratropium with a longer-acting β-agonist produces a greater change in spirometry over 3 months than either agent alone [54]. Combining long-acting inhaled β-agonists and ipratropium leads to fewer

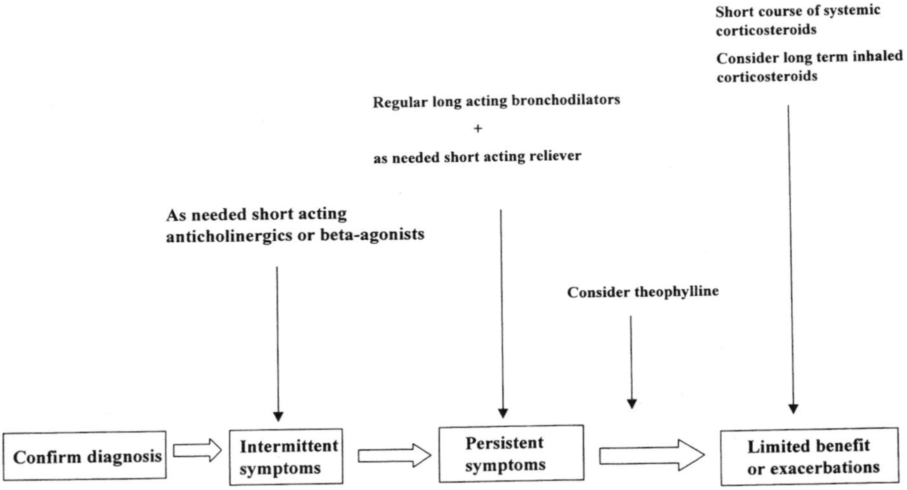

Figure 4 Pharmacological treatment of patients with COPD.

exacerbations than either drug alone. No good comparative data between different long-acting inhaled β-agonists is presently available, although it is likely that their effects will be similar.

The recent addition of tiotropium to the pharmacological armamentarium available for the treatment of patients with COPD provides clinicians with the first once-a-day bronchodilator. Indeed, the published trials indicate significant effects not only on FEV_1 [6] but also on important outcomes such as dyspnea and health status [9]. The large effects on the degree of airflow limitation that have been reported with this agent are matched by even larger changes in resting lung volumes [55] and exercise-induced dynamic hyperinflation. Figure 5 shows the changes on all lung function after 6 weeks of tiotropium compared with placebo. The remarkable decrease in functional residual capacity is similar in magnitude to that reported for lung-volume reduction surgery [56]. Indeed, this effect has been termed pharmacological pneumectomy, which may be more important than the improvement in airflow limitation as an explanation for the improvement in functional dyspnea and health status reported in the larger randomized trials of tiotropium [6,9].

Once the treatment with inhaled bronchodilators is optimized, a possible alternative addition may be the administration of theophylline. This medication has the advantage of being available in oral forms and therefore easy to administer. Although theophylline is a weak bronchodilator, other actions have been proposed. How important they are clinically remains to be established. The narrow therapeutic margin and complex pharmacokinetics

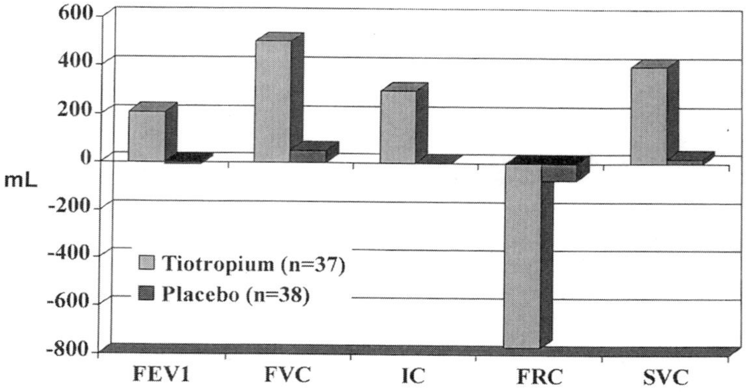

Figure 5 The long-acting anticholinergic tiotropium improves airflow limitation (FEV_1). In addition, it also improves resting lung volume such as the functional residual capacity (FRC), inspiratory capacity (IC), and the forced (FVC) and slow (SVC) vital capacity.

make their use difficult, but modern slow-release preparations have greatly improved this problem and lead to a stable plasma level throughout the day. Generally, therapeutic levels should be measured and patients should be kept on the lowest effective dose. Recommended serum are level between 8 and 14 μg/dL. Theophylline is commonly taken in the morning and the evening, but 24-hr formulations are available. The slow onset of action makes these agents suitable for maintenance but not rescue therapy. There is some evidence of a dose–response effect, which is limited by toxicity [57]. Combining long-acting β-agonists and theophylline appears to produce a greater spirometric change than either drug alone [10]. Plasma levels of theophylline are decreased by cigarette smoking, anticonvulsant drugs, and rifampicin and increased by respiratory acidosis, congestive cardiac failure, liver cirrhosis, and other therapies such as erythromycin and ciprofloxacin.

VII. Use of Corticosteroids

Glucocorticosteroids are usually considered in individual patients who fail to improve on adequate bronchodilator therapy [58,59]. Glucocorticoids act at multiple points within the inflammatory cascade, although their effects in COPD are more modest compared with bronchial asthma. Data from large patient studies suggest that inhaled corticosteroids can produce a small increase in postbronchodilator FEV_1 and a small reduction in bronchial reactivity in stable COPD [11,12,60,61]. In outpatients, exacerbations necessitate a course of oral steroids [62], but it is important to wean patients quickly since the older COPD population is susceptible to complications such as skin damage, cataracts, diabetes, osteoporosis, and secondary infection. These risks do not accompany standard doses of inhaled corticosteroid aerosols, which may cause thrush but pose a negligible risk for causing pulmonary infection. Most studies suggest that only 10–30% of patients with COPD improve if given chronic oral steroid therapy [58]. The dangers of steroids require that careful documentation of the effectiveness of such therapy before a patient is placed on prolonged daily or alternate-day dosing. The latter regimen may be safer, but its effectiveness has not been adequately evaluated in COPD. Several recently reported large multicenter trials evaluated the role of inhaled corticosteroids in preventing or slowing the progressive course of symptomatic COPD [11,12,60,61]. The results showed minimal if any benefits in the rate of decline of lung function. On the other hand, in the one study in which it was evaluated, inhaled fluticasone decreased the rate of loss of health-related quality of life that is characteristic of patients with severe COPD [11]. In addition, its regular use was also associated with a decrease in the rate of exacerbations. Finally, recent retrospective analyses of large databases suggest a possible effect of inhaled corticosteroids on increased mortality [63,64]. This has prompted the initiation of a large prospective trial to explore the effect of inhaled corticosteroids on mortality. Results of this trial could influence how and when to use corticosteroids. The concurrent use of inhaled steroids with albuterol and ipratropium has to be evaluated on an individual basis. Patients with moderate to severe COPD who have had repeated episodes of acute exacerbation may be the best candidates for this form of therapy. The onset of action is slow and there is little data to support a dose–response relationship. Most studies have been performed using relatively high doses as "proof of principle" rather than to define the effective dose of treatment. High-dose inhaled glucocorticoids can be systemically available due to absorption from the pulmonary circulation, but the effect is also less than that of oral corticosteroids (prednisolone).

VIII. Other Medications

Mucokinetics are a loosely defined group of drugs that aim to decrease sputum viscosity and adhesiveness in order to facilitate expectoration. The only controlled study in the United States suggesting a value for these drugs in the chronic management of bronchitis was a multicenter evaluation of organic iodide [65]. This study demonstrated symptomatic benefits. The values of other agents, including water, have not been clearly demonstrated. Some agents (such as oral acetylcysteine) are favored in Europe for their antioxidant effects in addition to their mucokinetic properties. Several small controlled trials have shown some effect of these agents on FEV_1 and in recurrence of acute exacerbations of the disease [66,67]. A large trial now underway may help define the possible role of these agents. Genetically engineered ribonuclease seems to be useful in cystic fibrosis, but is of no value in COPD.

Although supplemental weekly or monthly administration of alpha 1-antitrypsin may be indicated in nonsmoking, younger patients with genetically determined emphysema, in practice such therapy is difficult to initiate. There is evidence that the administration of alpha-1 antitrypsin is relatively safe, but the appropriate selection of the candidate for such therapy is not clear [68]. Patients with very severe and crippling COPD, or those with good lung function, are not good candidates for therapy. Likewise, deficient nonsmoking patients are at low risk to develop airflow obstruction. Therefore, the most likely candidates for replacement therapy would be smoking patients with mild to moderate COPD. The cost of therapy is prohibitive, especially considering that the safety of this enzyme and its long-term effects remain unknown.

IX. Management of Acute Exacerbations

An exacerbation of COPD is an event in the natural course of the disease characterized by a change in the patient's baseline dyspnea, cough, and/or sputum beyond day-to-day variability and sufficient to warrant a change in management. In the case of an acute exacerbation the pharmacological therapy is initiated with the same therapeutic agents available for its chronic management [1–3]. Care must be taken to rule out heart failure, myocardial infarction, arrhythmias and pulmonary embolism, all of which may present with clinical signs and symptoms similar to exacerbation of COPD.

The most important agents for acute exacerbation of COPD are anticholinergic and β-agonist aerosols. Ipratropium may be administered via a metered-dose inhaler (MDI), sometimes with a spacer if the administration is erratic, or as an inhalant solution by nebulization. Although the upper limit of dosage has not been established, the drug is safe, and higher dosages can be given to a poorly responsive patient. However, the prolonged half-life means that repeat doses should not be given more often than every 4–8 hr. The β_2-agonists should also be administered using the same techniques. These drugs have a reduced functional half-life in exacerbations of COPD, and thus may be given every 30–60 min if tolerated. The safety and value of continuous nebulization have not been established, but in selected cases this may be worth a trial. Subcutaneous or intramuscular dosing is recommended only if aerosol use is not feasible; intravenous administration is not an acceptable practice.

Combination therapy is often needed, and systemic corticosteroids should be added to the regimen. Several randomized trial [69–71] proved the usefulness of corticosteroids. It is important to avoid prolonged (over 2 weeks) or high-dose therapy, since older patients are susceptible to severe complications such as psychosis, fluid retention, and a vascular necrosis of bones. In addition, data from the large randomized trial in which 2 versus 8 weeks of steroids were compared showed no benefits from the longer administration of the medication [70]. Weaning must be accomplished as soon as possible.

If the sputum is purulent and/or increased in volume, bacterial infection must be treated. The major bacteria to be considered are *Streptococcus pneumoniae*, *Hemophilus influenzae*, and *Moraxella catarrhalis*. The antibiotic choice will depend on local experience, supported by sputum culture and sensitivities if the patient is moderately ill or needs to be admitted to hospital. The recent introduction of oral fluoroquinolones and macrolides has increased our capacity to treat patients with acute respiratory tract infections effectively. Quinolones may be favored in the more severe patients, for whom Gram-negative bacteria with resistance to many antibiotics seem to be a growing problem [72–75]. Mucokinetic agents, such as iodides, given systemically have not been shown to be effective in exacerbations of COPD, although some patients report subjective improvement when given these agents.

In those cases in which the exacerbation leads to the development of ventilatory failure, characterized by hypercapnia and moderate acidosis (serum pH 7.25–7.35), treatment with noninvasive positive-pressure ventilation (NIPPV) as a first-line therapy is supported by several well-conducted randomized trials that documented improvement notonly in the rate of intubations but also in length of hospital stay and, more important, in mortality [25,27]. Although a full review of NIPPV in acute on chronic respiratory failure is beyond the scope of this book, NIPPV is a great new adjunct to pharmacological therapy of exacerbation. The integration of all of these modalities in the management of exacerbation is shown in Fig. 6.

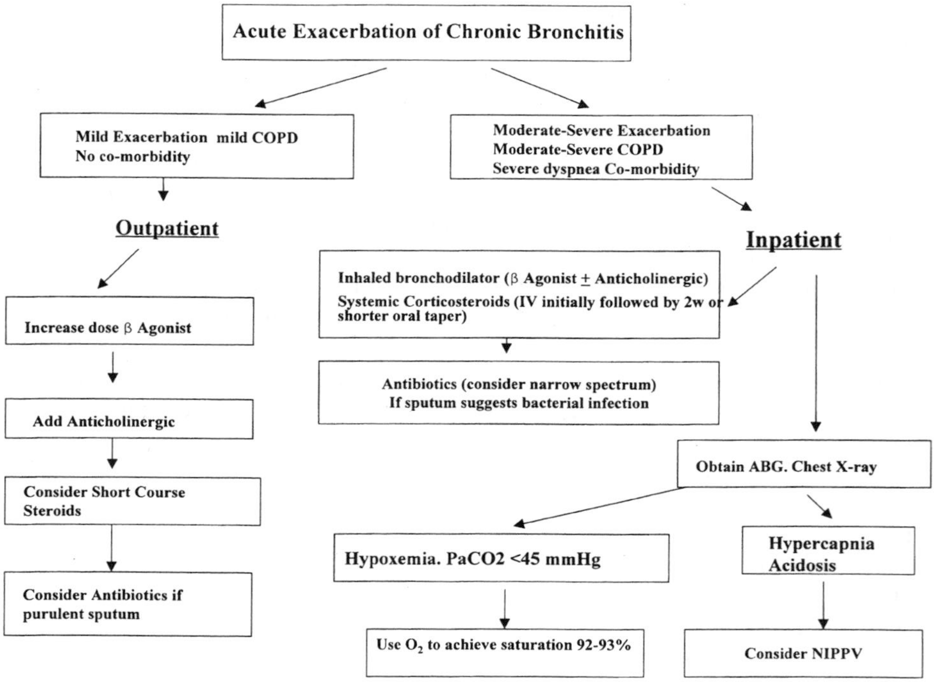

Figure 6 Algorithm describing the comprehensive approach to the treatment of patients with COPD exacerbation.

X. Summary and Conclusion

In summary, in this work we describe why COPD has been associated with a nihilistic attitude. Based on current evidence, this nihilistic attitude is totally unjustified. The disease has to be viewed under a new paradigm, one that accepts COPD is not only as a pulmonary disease, but also as one with important measurable systemic consequences. COPD is not only preventable but also treatable. Caregivers should familiarize themselves with the multiple complementary forms of treatment and individualize the therapy to each patient's particular situation. The future for patients with this disease is bright as its pathogenesis, clinical, and phenotypic manifestations are unraveled. The evidence accumulated over the recent past indicate that evaluation of outcomes different from pure airflow limitation provides firm evidence about the beneficial effect of drugs on those outcomes. The advent of newer and even more effective therapies, including novel drug groups, will lead to a decline in the contribution of this disease to poor world health.

References

1. Pawels R, Sonia Buist A, Calverley P, Jenkins C, Hurd S. Global strategy for the diagnosis, management and prevention of chronic obstrtuctive pulmonary disease. NHLBI/WHO Global Initiative for Chronic Obstructive Lung Disease (GOLD). Workshop summay. Am J Respir Crit Care Med 2001; 163:1256–1276.
2. Siafakas NM, Vermeire P, Pride NB, Paoletti P, Gibson J, Howard P, Yernault JC, Decramer M, Higenbottam T, Postma DS, Rees Jon behalf of the Task ForceOptimal assessment and management of chronic obstructive pulmonary disease (COPD). Eur Respir J 1995; 8:1398–1420.
3. American Thoracic Society. Definitions, epidemiology, pathophysiology, diagnosis and staging. Am J Respir Crit Care Med 1995; 152:S78–S83.
4. Murray CJL, Lopez AD. Mortality by cause for eight regions of the world: Global Burden of Disease Study. Lancet 1997; 349:1269–1276.
5. Anthonisen NR, Connett JE, Kiley JP, Altose M, Bailey W, Sonia Buist A, Conway W, Enright P, Kanner R, O'Hara P, Owens G, Scanlon P, Tashkin D, Wise R. Effect of smoking intervention and the use of an inhaled anticholinergic bronchodilator on the rate of decline of FEV1: the Lung Health Study. JAMA 1994; 272:1497–1505.
6. Casaburi R, Mahler D, Jones P, Wanner A, SanPedro G, ZuWallack R, Menjoge S, Serby C, Witek T. A long term evaluation of once-daily inhaled tiotropium in chronic obstructive pulmonary disease. Eur Respir J 2002; 19:217–224.
7. Mahler D, Donohue J, Barbee R, Goldman M, Gross N, Wisnewiski M, Yancey S, Zakes B, Rickard K, Anderson W. Efficacy of salmeterol xinoafate in the treatment of COPD. Chest 1999; 115:957–965.

8. Jones P, Bosh T. Quality of life changes in COPD patients treated with salmeterol. Am J Respir Crit Care Med 1997; 155:1283–1289.
9. Vincken W, van Noord J, Greefhorst A, Bantje Th, Kesten S, Korducki L, Cornelissen Pon behalf of the Dutch/Belgian tiotropium study groupImproved health outcomes in patients with COPD during 1-year treatment with tiotropium. Eur Respir J 2002; 19:209–216.
10. ZuWallack R, Mahler D, Reilly D, et al. Salmeterol plus theophylline combination therapy in the treatment of COPD. Chest 2001; 119:1628–1630.
11. Burge PS, Calverley PM, Jones PW, Spencer S, Anderson JA, Maslen TK. Randomised, double blind, placebo controlled study of fluticasone propionate in patients with moderate to severe chronic obstructive pulmonary disease: the ISOLDE trial. Br Med J 2000; 320:1297–1303.
12. The Lung Health Study Research GroupEffect of inhaled triamcinolone on the decline in pulmonary function in chronic obstructive pulmonary disease. N Engl J Med 2000; 343:1902–1909.
13. Hay JG, Stone P, Carter J, Church S, Eyre-Brook A, Pearson MG, Woodcock AA, Calverley PM. Bronchodilator reversibility, exercise performance and breathlessness in stable chronic obstructive pulmonary disease. Eur Respir J 1992; 5:659–664.
14. Friedman M, Serby C, Menjoge S, Wilson J, Hilleman D, Witek T. Pharmacoeconomic evaluation of a combination of ipratropium plus albuterol compared with ipratropium alone and albuterol alone in COPD. Chest 1999; 115: 635–641.
15. O'Donnell D, Lam M, Webb K. Spirometric correlates of improvement in exercise performance after anticholinergic therapy in chronic obstructive pulmonary disease. Am J Respir Crit Care Med 1999; 160:542–549.
16. Mac Mahon S, Rodgers A. The effects of blood pressure reduction in older patients: an overview of five randomized controlled trials in elderly hypertensives. Clin Exp Hypertens 1993; 15:967–978.
17. Blood Pressure Lowering Treatment Trialists' CollaborationEffects of ACE inhibitors, calcium antagonists, and other blood-pressure-lowering drugs: results of prospectively designed overviews of randomized trials. Lancet 2000; 356: 1955–1964.
18. Rennard S, Carrera M, Agusti A. Management of chronic obstructive pulmonary disease: are we going anywhere? Eur Respir J 2000; 16:1030–1035.
19. Nocturnal Oxygen Therapy Trial Group. Continuous or nocturnal oxygen therapy in hypoxemic chronic obstructive lung disease. Ann Intern Med 1980; 93: 391–398.
20. Medical Research Council Working Party. Long-term domiciliary oxygen therapy in chronic hypoxic cor pulmonale complicating chronic bronchitis and emphysema. Lancet 1981; 1:681–686.
21. Dean NC, Brown JK, Himelman RB, Doherty JJ, Gold WM, Stulbarg MS. Oxygen may improve dyspnea and endurance in patients with chronic obstructive pulmonary disease and only mild hypoxemia. Am Rev Respir Dis 1992; 146:941–945.

22. Criner GJ, Celli BR. Ventilatory muscle recruitment in exercise with O_2 in obstructed patients with mild hypoxemia. J Appl Physiol 1987; 63:195–200.
23. Ries A, Carlin B, Carrieri-Kohlman V, Casaburi R, Celli B, Emery C, Hodgkin J, Mahler D, Make B, Skolnick J. Pulmonary rehabilitation: joint ACCP/AACVPR evidence-based guidelines. Chest 1997; 112:1363–1396.
24. Griffith T, Burr M, Campbell I, Lewis-Jenkins V, Mullins, Shiels K, Turner-Lawlor P, Payne N, Newcombe R, Lonescu A, Thomas J, Tunbridge J. Results at 1 year of outpatient multidisciplinary pulmonary rehabilitation: a randomised control trial. Lancet 2000; 355:362–367.
25. Brochard L, Mancebo J, Wysocki M, et al. Noninvasive ventilation for acute exacerbation of chronic obstructive pulmonary disease. N Engl J Med 1995; 333:817–822.
26. Bott J, Carroll MP, Conway JH, et al. Randomised controlled trial of nasal ventilation in acute ventilatory failure due to chronic obstructive airways disease. Lancet 1993; 341:1555–1557.
27. Kramer N, Meyer T, Meharg J, Cece R, Hill NS. Randomized prospective trial of non-invasive positive pressure ventilation in acute respiratory failure. Am J Respir Crit Care Med 1995; 151:1799–1806.
28. Geddes D, Davis M, Koyama H, et al. Effect of lung volume reduction surgery in patients with severe emphysema. N Engl J Med 2000; 343:239–245.
29. Decramer M, Gosselink R, Troosters T, Verschueren M, Evers G. Muscle weakness is related to utilization of health care resources in COPD patients. Eur Respir J 1997; 10:417–423.
30. France AJ, Prescott RJ, Biernacki W, Muir AL, MacNee W. Does right ventricular function predict survival in patients with chronic obstructive lung disease? Thorax 1988; 43:621–626.
31. Schols AM, Slangen J, Volovics L, Wouters EF. Weight loss is a reversible factor in the prognosis of chronic obstructive pulmonary disease. Am J Respir Crit Care Med 1998; 157:1791–1797.
32. Hodgkin JE. Prognosis in chronic obstructive pulmonary disease. Clin Chest Med 1990; 11:555–569.
33. Anthonisen NR, Wright E, Hodgkin JE, the IPPB trial group. Prognosis in chronic obstructive pulmonary disease. Am Rev Respir Dis 1986; 133:14–20.
34. Intermittent Positive Pressure Breathing Trial Group. Intermittent positive pressure breathing therapy of chronic obstructive pulmonary disease. Ann Intern Med 1983; 93:126–620.
35. Gerardi DA, Lovett L, Benoit-Connors ML, Reardon JZ, ZuWallack RL. Variables related to increased mortality following out-patient pulmonary rehabilitation. Eur Respir J 1996; 9:431–435.
36. Landbo C, Prescott E, Lange P, Vestbo J, Almdal TP. Prognostic value of nutritional status in chronic obstructive pulmonary disease. Am J Respir Crit Care Med 1999; 160:1856–1861.
37. Ferrer M, Alonso J, Morera J, Marrades R, Khalaf A, Aguar C, Plaza V, Prieto L, Anto J. Chronic obstructive pulmonary disease and health related quality of life. Ann Intern Med 1997; 127:1072–1079.

38. Dewan N, Rafique S, Kanwar B, Satpathy H, Ryschon K, Tillotson G, Niederman M. Acute exacerbation of COPD. Factors associated with poor treatment outcome. Chest 2000; 117:662–671.
39. Sweet L, Zwillich CW. Dyspnea in the patient with chronic obstructive pulmonary disease. Clin Chest Med 1990; 11:417–445.
40. Mahler D, Wells C. Evaluation of clinical methods for rating dyspnea. Chest 1988; 93:580–586.
41. Ries A, Kaplan R, Limberg T, Prewitt L. Effects of pulmonary rehabilitation on physiologic and psychosocial outcomes inpatients with COPD. Ann Intern Med 1995; 122:823–832.
42. Hajiro T, Nishimura K, Tsukino M, Ikeda A, Koyama H, Izumi T. Comparison of discriminative properties among disease-specific questionnaires for measuring health-related quality of life in patients with chronic obstructive pulmonary disease. Am J Respir Crit Care Med 1998; 157:785–790.
43. Szekely L, Oelberg D, Wright C, Johnson D, Wain J, Trotman-Dickenson B, Sheppard J, Kanarek D, Systrom D, Ginns L. Preoperative predictors of operative mortality in COPD patients undergoing bilateral lung volume reduction surgery. Chest 1997; 111:550–558.
44. Sha M, Hasselblad V, Gheorgiadis M, Adams S, Swedberg K, Califf R, O'Connor C. Prognostic usefulness of the 6 minute walk in patients with advanced congestive heart failure secondary to ischemic and non-ischemic cardiomyopathy. Am J Cardiol 2001; 88:987–993.
45. Miyamoto S, Nagaya N, Satoh T, Kyotani S, Sakamaki F, Fujita M, Na N, Miyatake K. Clinical correlates and prognostic significance of 6 minute walk in patients with pulmonary hypertension. Comparison with cardiopulmonary exercise testing. Am J Respir Crit Care Med 2000; 161:487–492.
46. Pinto-Plata V, Girish M, Taylor J, Celli B. Natural decline in 6 minutes walking distance in COPD. Am J Respir Crit Care Med 1998; 158:A20.
47. Cote CG, Celli B. In COPD patients the 6 minutes walking distance predicts health care resources utilization better than FEV1, MRC dyspnea scale and arterial blood gases. Eur Respir J 1998; 14:A383.
48. Jones PW. Interpreting thresholds for a clinically significant change in health status in asthma and COPD. Eur Respir J 2002; 19:398–404.
49. Whitney C, Farley M, Hadler J, Harrison L, Bennett N, Lynfield R, Reingold A, Cieslak P, Pilishvili T, Jackson D, Facklam R, Jorgensen J, Schuchat A. Decline in invasive pneumococcal disease after the introduction of protein-polysaccharide conjugate vaccine. N Engl J Med 2003; 348:1737–1746.
50. Kackson L, Neuzil K, Yu O, Benson P, Barlow W, Adams A, Hanson C, Mahoney L, Shay D, Thompson W. Effectiveness of pneumoccocal polysaccharide vaccine in older adults. N Engl J Med 2003; 348:1747–1755.
51. COMBIVENT Inhalation Aerosol Study Group. In chronic obstructive pulmonary disease, a combination of ipratropium and albuterol is more effective than either agent alone. An 85-day multicenter trial. Chest 1994; 105:1411–1419.
52. Dahl R, Greefhorst LA, Nowak D, Nonikov V, Byrne AM, Thomson MH, Till D, Della CG. Inhaled formoterol dry powder versus ipratropium bromide in

chronic obstructive pulmonary disease. Am J Respir Crit Care Med 2001; 164:778–784.
53. Khoukaz G, Gross NJ. Effects of salmeterol on arterial blood gases in patients with stable chronic obstructive pulmonary disease. Comparison with albuterol and ipratropium. Am J Respir Crit Care Med 1999; 160:1028–1030.
54. Van Noord JA, de Munck DR, Bantje TA, Hop WC, Akveld ML, Bommer AM. Long-term treatment of chronic obstructive pulmonary disease with salmeterol and the additive effect of ipratropium. Eur Respir J 2000; 15:878–885.
55. Celli B, ZuWallack R, Wang S, Kesten S. Improvement in inspiratory capacity with tiotropium in patients with COPD. Eur Respir J 2002; 20:491.
56. Martinez F, Montes de Oca M, Whyte R, Stetz J, Gay S, Celli B. Lung-volume reduction surgery improves dyspnea, dynamic hyperinflation and respiratory muscle function. Am J Respir Crit Care Med 1997; 155:2018–2023.
57. Chrystyn H, Mulley BA, Peake MD. Dose response relation to oral theophylline in severe chronic obstructive airways disease. Br Med J 1988; 297: 1506–1510.
58. Callahan C, Dittus R, Katz BP. Oral corticosteroids therapy for patients with stable chronic obstructive pulmonary disease: a meta-analysis. Ann Intern Med 1991; 114:216–223.
59. Dompeling E, van Schayck CP, van Grunsven PM, van Herwaarden CLA, Akkermans R, Molema J, Folgering H, van Weel C. Slowing the deterioration of asthma and chronic obstructive pulmonary disease observed during bronchodilator therapy by adding inhaled corticosteroids: a 4-year prospective study. Ann Intern Med 1993; 118:770–778.
60. Vestbo J, Sorensen T, Lange P, Brix A, Torre P, Viskum K. Long-term effect of inhaled budesonide in mild and moderate chronic obstructive pulmonary disease: a randomised controlled trial. Lancet 1999; 353:1819–1823.
61. Pauwels RA, Lofdahl CG, Laitinen LA, Schouten JP, Postma DS, Pride NB, Ohlsson SV. Long-term treatment with inhaled budesonide in persons with mild chronic obstructive pulmonary disease who continue smoking. N Engl J Med 1999; 340:1948–1953.
62. Albert R, Martin T, Lewis S. Controlled clinical trial of methylprednisolone in patients with chronic bronchitis and acute respiratory insufficiency. Ann Intern Med 1980; 92:753–775.
63. Sin DD, Tu JV. Inhaled corticosteroids and the risk for mortality and re-admission in elderly patients with chronic obstructive pulmonary disease. Am J Respir Crit Care Med 2001; 164:580–584.
64. Soriano JB, Vestbo J, Pride N, Kin V, Maden C, Maier WC. Survival in COPD patients after regular use of fluticasone propionate and salmeterol in general practice. Eur Respir J 2002; 20:819–824.
65. Petty TL. The National Mucolytic Study: results of a randomized, double-blind, placebo-controlled study of iodinated glycerol in chronic obstructive bronchitis. Chest 1990; 97:75–83.
66. Poole P, Black P. Oral mucolytic drugs for exacerbations of chronic obstructive pulmonary disease: systematic review. Br Med J 2001; 322:1271–1274.
67. Poole PJ, Black PN. Mucolytic agents for chronic bronchitis or chronic ob-

structive pulmonary disease. Cochrane Database of Systematic Reviews [computer file] CD001287, 2000.
68. Dirksen A, Dijkman JH, Madsen F, Stoel B, Hutchison DC, Ulrik CS, Skovgaard LT, Kok-Jensen A, Rudolphus A, Seersholm N, Vrooman HA, Reiber JH, Hansen NC, Heckscher T, Viskum K, Stolk J. A randomized clinical trial of alpha(1)-antitrypsin augmentation therapy. Am J Respir Crit Care Med 1999; 160:1468–1472.
69. Davies L, Angus RM, Calverley PM. Oral corticosteroids in patients admitted to hospital with exacerbations of chronic obstructive pulmonary disease: a prospective randomized controlled trial. Lancet 1999; 345:456–460.
70. Nieweohner DE, Erbland ML, Deupree RH, et al. Effect of glucocorticoids on exacerbations of chronic obstructive pulmonary disease. N Engl J Med 1999; 340:1941–1947.
71. Thompson WH, Nielson CP, Carvalho P, et al. Controlled trial of oral prednisone in outpatients with cute COPD exacerbation. Am J Respir Crit Care Med 1996; 154:407–412.
72. Nouira S, Marghli S, Belghith M, Besbes L, Elatrous S, Abroug F. Once daily oral ofloxacin in chronic obstructive pulmonary disease exacerbation requiring mechanical ventilation: a randomized placebo-controlled trial. Lancet 2001; 358:2020–2035.
73. Adams SG, Melo J, Luther M, Anzueto A. Antibiotics are associated with lower relapse rates in outpatients with acute exacerbations of COPD. Chest 2000; 117:1345–1352.
74. Anthonisen NR, Manfreda J, Warren CPW, Hershfield ES, Harding GKM, Nelson NA. Antibiotic therapy in exacerbations of chronic obstructive pulmonary disease. Ann Intern Med 1987; 106:196–204.
75. Miravitlles M. Epidemiology of chronic obstructive pulmonary disease exacerbations. Clin Pulm Med 2002; 9(4):191–197.

Index